Ethics at the Bedside
A Source Book for the Critical Care Nurse

American
Association of
Critical-Care
Nurses

J. B. Lippincott Company   Philadelphia

London   Mexico City   New York   St. Louis   São Paulo   Sidney

Ethics at the Bedside
A Source Book for the Critical Care Nurse

Marsha D. M. Fowler, PhD, MS(N), RN
Consulting Ethicist
Associate Professor, Department of Nursing
California State University at Los Angeles
Visiting Associate Professor, School of Nursing
Azusa Pacific University, Azusa, California

June Levine-Ariff, MSN, RN
Assistant Director of Nursing
Childrens Hospital of Los Angeles
Los Angeles, California

With 9 Contributors

Sponsoring Editor: Patricia L. Cleary
Manuscript Editor: Judith A. Ebbert
Indexer: Ann Cassar
Interior Design and Production: Nora Barry Leary
Cover Design: Tom Maciag
Production Manager: Carol A. Florence
Compositor: J. B. Lippincott Company
Printer/Binder: R. R. Donnelley & Sons

6   5   4   3   2   1

LIBRARY OF CONGRESS CATALOGING IN PUBLICATION DATA
Ethics at the Bedside.
    Bibliography: p.
    Includes Index.
    1. Intensive care nursing—Moral and ethical aspects.
2. Nursing ethics.   I. Fowler, Marsha Diane Mary.   II. Levine-Ariff, June.   III. American Association of Critical-Care Nurses.   [DNLM: 1. Critical Care.   2. Ethics, Nursing.   WY 85 E8514]
RT120.I5E84   1987   174'.2   87–4112
ISBN 0–397–54642–4

The cases in this book are true. All names and places, except those in the public record, have been fictionalized to protect the parties involved.

Preface

Nursing ethics has a long and honorable history. In 1893 Lystra Gretter composed the Florence Nightingale Pledge, the first acknowledged "code" of ethics for nurses in the United States. Three years later, the Trained School Delegates and Representatives from the American Society of Superintendents of Training Schools (the precursor to the National League for Nursing) met at the Manhattan Beach Hotel for the purpose of establishing an alumnae association for nurses in the United States and Canada (eventually to become the American Nurses' Association), and to establish the purposes of the group. The articles of incorporation set forth the objectives of the group as ". . . to establish and maintain a code of ethics." Thus, their first concern centered on the ethics of the profession.

Early organizational concern for nursing ethics is not the only evidence of a longstanding attention to ethics. The first formal literature of the profession probes and discusses a variety of aspects of ethical discourse. When, in the 1880s, the first official journal of nursing, the *Trained Nurse and Hospital Review*, inaugurated its publication, it featured a six-part series on nursing ethics. The *American Journal of Nursing*, which began in 1900, has published literally hundreds of articles principally concerned with nursing ethics. No fewer than 65 books are devoted to the topic of nursing ethics between 1900 and 1960, one of the first of which was Isabel Hampton Adams Robb's *Nursing Ethics: For Hospital and Private Use* (1900). Nursing ethics is neither new nor transient.

Neither is it identical to medical ethics. Nursing has an ethics and a moral tradition that are distinctive. That distinctive ethics, and that distinctive moral tradition, informs nursing practice and policy. Though contemporary works in nursing ethics are moving in the direction of an ethics that is uniquely nursing's, they reflect certain problems.

First, they do not always relate to nursing. Rather, they present a standard medical ethical treatment of an issue, then reflect on its application to nursing. It is not unusual to find that that application to nursing is strained. Nursing practice gives rise to a variety of ethical problems unique to the profession, or significantly modified by it. A second problem relates to the interpretation of the term *ethics*. It is not uncommon for works on ethics to deal predominantly with topics such as moral development or values clarification. Though those topics fall within the domain of descriptive ethics, and are certainly pertinent to ethics, ethicists generally regard descriptive ethics as within the realm of the social or psychological sciences such as anthropology, sociology, or psychology. A third difficulty with nursing ethical literature is that it tends to remain at a descriptive level, refraining from normative explorations. It is the normative analyses that need to be linked with nursing's moral tradition and would provide the most definitive source of guidance to the nurse in practice.

This work attempts to overcome these limitations by centering on discussions of ethical principles, virtues, and values that are grounded in nursing concerns and reflected in nursing policies. A serious attempt has been made to provide a book that will serve as an ethics resource, yet at the same time remain intelligible, applicable, and practical. This work is further intended to focus on issues and cases in critical care nursing.

The organizing framework has a twofold thrust: principles and values in bioethics as the basis, the tools, for decision making; and the policies, procedures, and mechanisms that are used to operationalize those principles and values. Chapter 1 presents a brief overview of the history of critical care nursing and the ethical questions such care raises. Chapter 2 sets forth an overview of the field of ethics and its divisions and the place of principles and values in normative ethics. The principles of autonomy, advocacy and accountability, nonmaleficence, beneficence, fidelity and veracity, justice, and duties to self will be discussed. A special section on values (Chapter 9), as the cornerstone of nursing's art, is designed to assist the reader in exploring both personal and professional values that interact with ethical decision making. The final chapters (11–12) discuss law, policies, and mechanisms essential to the implementation of nursing ethics at the bedside and at the societal levels. For, without the mechanisms to put ethics into action, we can only achieve a high level of moral frustration. The text also includes, as a postscript, though not an afterthought, a special section on exploring library resources to aid in ethical deliberation.

Amidst the chaos and confusion of contemporary health care, particularly in the light of both increasing fiscal constraints and the scientific and technologic revolution with its potential to change the quality and duration of human life, nurses are faced with ethical dilemmas that seem almost insurmountable. Yet, amidst that chaos, nurses are not set adrift; nursing itself can provide an anchor, a stable point in the storm, a source of moral values and a tradition that is rich in direction, understanding, and compassion for the human dilemma of illness and health.

Marsha D. M. Fowler, PhD, MS(N), RN
June Levine-Ariff, MSN, RN

About the Authors and Contributors

Mila Ann Aroskar, EdD, MS, RN, FAAN

Mila Ann Aroskar is Associate Professor and Chairperson, Public Health Nursing Major, School of Public Health, University of Minnesota. She has a BA in religion from the College of Wooster; a BS from the Department of Nursing, Columbia University; an MS from Teachers' College, Columbia University; and an EdD in curriculum development from the State University of New York at Buffalo. She was a Joseph P. Kennedy, Jr., Fellow in Medical Ethics at Harvard University (1976–77). She co-authored *Ethical Dilemmas in Nursing Practice*. Dr. Aroskar is a fellow and former vice president of the Hastings Center. She was a member of the national nursing panel for the President's Commission for the Study of Ethical Problems in Medicine and Biomedical and Behavioral Research. She is the Chairwoman of the American Nurses' Association Committee on Ethics, and the Nursing and Humanities Interest Groups of the Society for Health and Human Values. Dr. Aroskar lectures and consults nationally and internationally on issues in ethics in nursing and has published widely in the field. She has received numerous honors for her work.

Elizabeth A. Chaney, JD, MSN, RN

Dr. Chaney is an attorney at law, in private practice, in Monrovia, California. Her practice emphasizes health, labor, business, and licensing law related to nursing, and preventive elder law for persons with catastrophic and long-term illness. She holds a part-time clinical appointment as lecturer in community health nursing at California State College, Bakersfield, where she teaches courses in nursing law and community health nursing practice. She received her JD from Loyola University School of Law, Los Angeles; her MS in Nursing from Yale University; her BS from California State

University, Los Angeles; and her diploma in nursing from Queen of Angeles School of Nursing/Immaculate Heart College, Los Angeles. Dr. Chaney publishes and lectures frequently on topics related to law and nursing as well as the relationship between law and ethics in health care.

Joyce A. Crump, MLS

Joyce Crump is Head of Reference Services at the library of the Los Angeles County Medical Association. Previous experience includes developing and directing the medical library at Saint Agnes Medical Center in Fresno, California, serving as an information manager with Savage Information Services, and working as a reference librarian with the Palos Verdes Library District, California. Ms. Crump majored in physiology at Vassar College and received her MS in Library Science from the School of Library Science of the University of Southern California. She has been certified by the Medical Library Association since 1979 and is an active member of the Medical Library Group of Southern California and Arizona.

Anne J. Davis, PhD, RN, FAAN

Anne J. Davis, Professor of Nursing at the University of California was a Kennedy Post-Doctoral Fellow in bioethics at Harvard University, 1976–77. Since then she has written two books and numerous articles and has undertaken research in bioethics. She chaired the American Nurses' Association Committee on Ethics and established and chaired the California Nurses' Association Ethics Committee. She is on the boards of the American Society for Law and Medicine and of the American Hospital Association Ethics Committee. Dr. Davis has been a visiting professor at eleven universities in the United States, China, and Europe. She has received numerous honors including an honorary Doctor of Science degree from Emory University, Atlanta, and the ANA's first human rights award in 1986. At the University of California at San Francisco, she teaches a course in bioethics to master's degree and doctoral students and holds an appointment in Nursing Service where she conducts ethics rounds.

Patricia A. R. Flynn, MA, RN

Patricia Flynn is an adult health nurse practitioner and a clinical specialist in psychiatric mental health nursing. She was educated at Englewood Hospital School of Nursing, Emory University, and New York University. Ms. Flynn taught at the City University of New York and the State University of New York at Binghamton. She is currently on the faculty of St. Mary's College, where she teaches graduate and undergraduate health law and ethics, the United States' health care delivery system, and research and critical thinking. Ms. Flynn has written on holistic health and human behavior. She is currently a doctoral student in medical sociology at the University of California at San Francisco.

Marsha D. M. Fowler, PhD, MS(N), RN

Marsha Fowler is currently Associate Professor, Department of Nursing, California State University, and Adjunct Associate Professor, School of Nursing, Azusa Pacific University, Azusa, California. Dr. Fowler was a Joseph P. Kennedy, Jr., Fellow in Medical Ethics, Faculty of Medicine, Harvard University in 1978–79. She is currently a member of the American Nurses' Association Committee on Ethics, and Chairwoman of the California Nurses' Association Ethics Committee. She holds a PhD in religion and social ethics with a focus on bioethics, social criticism, and social change; an MS degree in biological dysfunctions and physiological nursing; a BS in nursing; and a diploma from Kaiser Foundation School of Nursing, Oakland, California. Dr. Fowler has been active in ethics consulting, teaching, and research since the early 1970s. She has published widely in ethics and nursing. Her current research is on the moral identity of nursing, the history of nursing ethics, and moral policy formulation in nursing.

Sara T. Fry, PhD, MS, RN

Dr. Fry is Assistant Professor at the University of Virginia School of Nursing, Charlottesville, Virginia, where she teaches the philosophy of nursing and nursing ethics. She received a PhD in philosophy, with a focus on biomedical ethics, from Georgetown University; an MS in public health nursing education from the University of North Carolina at Chapel Hill; and a BSN from the College of Nursing, University of South Carolina, at Columbia. Dr. Fry has published widely and presented numerous papers, nationally and internationally, on the topics of ethics and moral accountability in nursing practice.

Donna H. Groh, MSN, RN

Donna H. Groh is an Assistant Director of Nursing at Childrens Hospital of Los Angeles. She received her diploma in nursing at the Bryn Mawr Hospital School of Nursing and completed her baccalaureate and master's degree programs in nursing at the University of Pennsylvania. She was a recipient of the Louise Mellen Graduate Fellowship in Critical Care Nursing. Ms. Groh's practice focus is pediatric critical care and administration of nursing services. She has published and lectured frequently on topics related to pediatric critical care nursing and ethical decision making.

Andrew Jameton, PhD

Dr. Jameton is Assistant Professor in the Department of Medical Jurisprudence and Humanities, University of Nebraska Medical Center. He is author of the highly regarded book, *Nursing Practice: The Ethical Issues*. Dr. Jameton has a PhD in philosophy and has been teaching, consulting, and conducting research in ethics in health care centers since 1972. He is currently completing a project to study the responsibilities of residents of long-term-care facilities.

June Levine-Ariff, MSN, RN

June Levine-Ariff is Assistant Director of Nursing at Childrens Hospital of Los Angeles. Ms. Levine-Ariff received her baccalaureate and master's degrees in nursing from Ohio State University and received certification in nursing administration from the American Nurses' Association. She has had extensive experience as a clinical nurse specialist in neonatal and pediatric intensive care and as a nursing administrator in both maternal-child health and pediatrics. Ms. Levine-Ariff has lectured frequently in the areas of nursing administration and ethical decision making. She is a member of the California Nurses' Association Ethics Committee, chairs the Nursing Ethics Council at Childrens Hospital of Los Angeles, and is a member of that hospital's institutional ethics committee.

Diann B. Uustal, EdD, MS, RN

Diann B. Uustal is the founder and director of an independent educational and consulting network: Educational Resources in Nursing and Wholistic Health. Dr. Uustal received her BS in nursing from the University of Rhode Island, 1968, and her MS in nursing from the University of Massachusetts, 1974. She earned her doctorate in psychological education at the University of Massachusetts, 1983, concentrating in the areas of values and ethics in health care. Dr. Uustal was an assistant professor at Arizona State University, College of Nursing, master's degree program in adult health nursing, from 1982 to 1986. She was President of the Beta Upsilon chapter of Sigma Theta Tau, the National Honor Society of Nursing. She has authored numerous articles on values clarification in nursing and has published a workbook entitled *Values and Ethics: Considerations in Nursing Practice*, 1978. She has recently published a second workbook, entitled *Values and Ethics in Nursing: From Theory to Practice*, 1985. Dr. Uustal is a nationally recognized consultant and facilitator of values education and ethics workshops and seminars for colleges of nursing, hospitals, and various professional nursing organizations.

Acknowledgments

No book is ever written by its authors alone. The support of kith and kin has a great bearing on the realization of any publishing goal. Such is the case with this book.

Lest they fear that they are forgotten, we are grateful for the men, women, and children, related by blood, marriage, or affection, who have tolerated much for what must have seemed an eternity. It is a tribute to their fortitude that they never actually abandoned us. Honorable mention is due specifically to the children and spouses of the contributors and editors who endured real or imagined maternal or spousal deprivation. These include Benjamin, Michael, Tyler, Tak, Sara, Amy, and a host of others.

We are also indebted to numerous nursing colleagues whose persuasive influence, reassurance, and other input compelled us to both start and complete this book. In particular, we would like to thank Dr. Ingeborg G. Mauksch for her encouragement and support at the outset of the project, Dr. Phyllis Gallagher, Dr. Jeannette Hartshorn, Dr. Ruth Wu, Marilyn Chrisman, Bonnie E. Siegal, and our contributors.

We are grateful to the computer mavens who devoted hours to untangling myriad computer dilemmas in order to bring this book about. Specific thanks are due to Lee S. Blackburn, William Y. Martin, and Frank S. Waitkus. Production of the manuscript itself was greatly aided by the clerical and editorial contributions of Dorothy Waterhouse Smoker, Thea Kubota, and David Brashear.

Early on, the discovery and appropriation of obscure library resources were largely the work of Alice Reinhardt of the Medical and Nursing Libraries of the Los Angeles County Medical Center. It is true that a superlative librarian is the right arm of the researcher and writer.

And last, but never least, we are grateful to the American Association of Critical-Care Nurses, its members, and its board of directors for recognizing the need for additional work in ethics in critical care nursing. We especially acknowledge the excellent assistance of Jeannette Hartshorn, member of the board of directors and President-Elect of AACN; Ellen French, Director of Communications of AACN; and Patricia L. Cleary, nursing editor at J. B. Lippincott. Their efforts facilitated the abbreviated production time required by the book. We would like, further, to thank the numerous critical care nurses, for whom this book is intended, who have watched, and encouraged, and prodded us to bring this project to fruition.

Contents

Chapter 1

Treatment or Torture: Why Critical Care?

Donna H. Groh

The demands are very real, but the rewards are unforgettable. All the problems of the day are gone and forgotten when a mother breast feeds her infant for the first time. . . . An infant who was dependent on a ventilator two weeks ago finally goes home with his parents . . . and a child who was "the sickest baby in the unit" two years ago comes running in ahead of her parents for a visit. . . . We're brought closer together by the rewards and the responsibilities we share in the NICU.[1]

The need for nursing care is as old as mankind itself. Nurses are the glue that holds a modern hospital together, and nurses in an intensive care unit are the integral force that keeps the milieu of the technological environment, the multidisciplinary health care team of specialists, and the patient in proper balance. However, the history of intensive care nursing is very young, and to view it in perspective, one must appreciate events that preceded and led to its development.

Pre–Modern Era Nursing

Reports of nursing activity in primitive history are scattered and rare. What is recorded is interwoven with reports of magicians, priests, and medicine men. The first nurse to be recorded in history is Deborah, in the story of Rebekah in the Bible.[2] There are references to nurses and their knowledge regarding administration of drugs, as well as other attributes in early Indian writings hundreds of years before Christ.[3,4] However, a continuous history of nursing begins with the dawn of Christianity.[5,6] Several early religious orders such as the Poor Clares, the Third Order of St. Francis, and the Augustinian Nuns were devoted entirely to nursing the sick. The Reformation began a "period of darkness" for nursing, when hospitals were removed from church

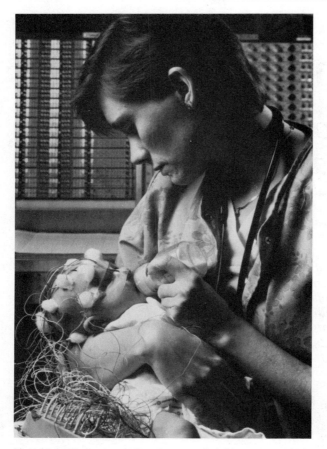

Figure 1-1. The neonatal ICU. Courtesy of Childrens Hospital of Los Angeles

control and the services of the religious orders were replaced with poorly paid workers, many assigned nursing duties in lieu of a jail sentence.

The three centuries between 1550 and 1850 saw numerous advances in the physical and biological sciences, including the birth of the contemporary scientific method of inquiry, the growth of anatomical knowledge, the discovery of the microscope, and the development of smallpox vaccine. By the late 19th century the stethoscope, the thermometer, and roentgenograms had become diagnostic aids to medicine, but there had been no concomitant advances in nursing care. No one who could earn a living by any other means would have become a nurse. Nurses were drawn from the lowest levels of society and were often illiterate and morally reprehensible.[7] "Hospitals were as a rule in a disgraceful state of degradation. They were dirty and ill-ventilated, they reeked with infection . . . the death rate was fearfully high, sometimes actually more than 50 percent."[8]

The first step toward establishing the modern profession of nursing is generally recognized to be the establishment of the Deaconess Institute at Kaiserswerth, Ger-

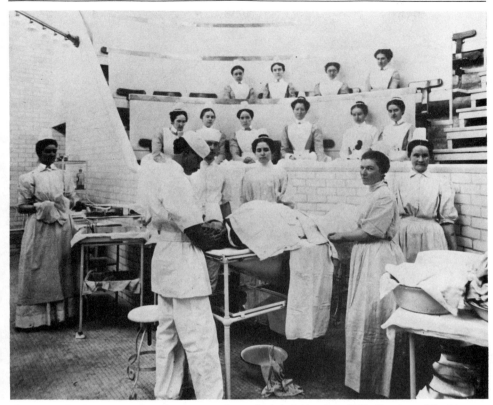

Figure 1-2. Student nurses observing an operation at St. Luke's Hospital, 1899. Courtesy of the Museum of the City of New York

many, in 1836 by Theodor Fliedner and his wife, Friederike. In 1849 four deaconesses trained there were sent to assume responsibility for the Pittsburgh Infirmary in Pittsburgh, Pennsylvania. Similar institutions were established in Alexandria, Beirut, Istanbul (then Constantinople), Jerusalem, and Smyrna.[9] This was the stage on which Florence Nightingale appeared, as a revolutionary in nursing care in the English-speaking world.

The Nightingale Era

It is beyond the scope of this chapter to provide a detailed account of the life of Florence Nightingale. Though it has been challenged in some contemporary revisionist histories, Nightingale is credited with altering the course of the nursing profession and the modern hospital. She was born to wealthy parents and was well educated, indeed better than many men of her time. She expressed a desire to enter nursing at an early age and, not surprisingly, her parents tried to dissuade her. She traveled ex-

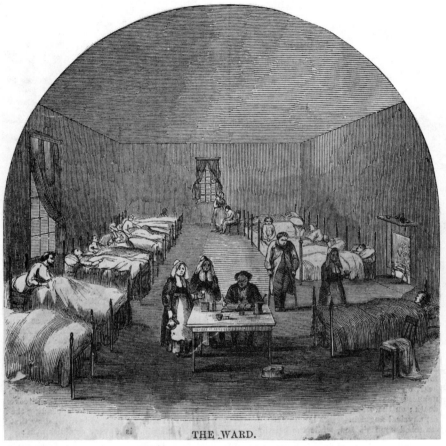

Figure 1-3. *The Ward*. New Orleans, 1859. Courtesy of the Bettmann Archive, New York

tensively, observed various hospitals, and eventually studied briefly at Kaiserswerth and with the Sisters of Charity in Paris. Afterward, she served as superintendent of the Establishment of Gentlewomen During Illness.

Because of her efforts at that institution, her social position, and her education, she was asked by Sir Sidney Herbert, Secretary of War for England, to lead a group of female nurses and to supervise the military hospitals in Turkey during the Crimean War. Despite rather rancorous beginnings, Nightingale arrived in the Crimea with a small band of nurses in tow. The conditions she found upon her arrival were appalling. An open sewer, infested with rats and vermin, ran under the building, which had no water, soap, linens, or dietary and laundry facilities. There were few medical supplies. The building encompassed miles of beds with 3000 to 4000 patients crammed into spaces designed for 1700. The death rate was 42.7%.[10]

Although hampered by military authorities, Nightingale managed to obtain supplies and establish diet kitchens, a laundry, recreation areas, and reading rooms. Al-

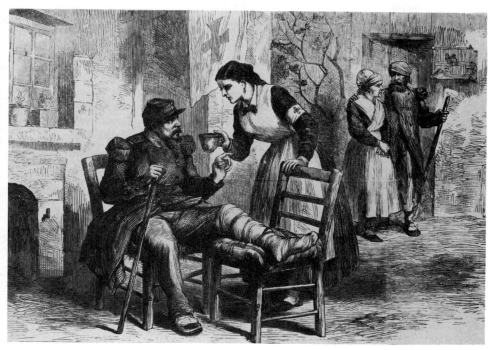

Figure 1-4. *Cared For.* Wood engraving published in *Harper's Weekly* (January 21, 1871) illustrating nursing work done by the Red Cross. Courtesy of the National Library of Medicine, Bethesda

though she consistently rejected the germ theory, despite supporting evidence in its favor, she had a penchant for cleanliness and fresh air and succeeded in reducing the mortality rate to 2.2% within six months.[11]

After the war she insisted on a comprehensive investigation of military health care and published her own views, complete with statistical studies, in an 800-page book. Her efforts were instrumental in establishing new sanitary codes and the formation of a military medical school, as well as other advancements. These new practices were carried over into civilian hospitals. In 1850 she published her study on hospital planning and administration, *Notes on Hospitals*.

In 1860 Florence Nightingale realized her goal of establishing the first organized school of nursing, The Nightingale Training School for Nurses, which was a financially independent educational institution affiliated with St. Thomas Hospital. *Notes on Nursing*, which Nightingale wrote in 1859, served as the primary textbook.

Nursing in the United States

Civil War

At the outbreak of the Civil War, there was no group of trained nurses available for service, nor was there any established group within the military to organize medical care for the wounded. Numerous religious groups volunteered, as well as other in-

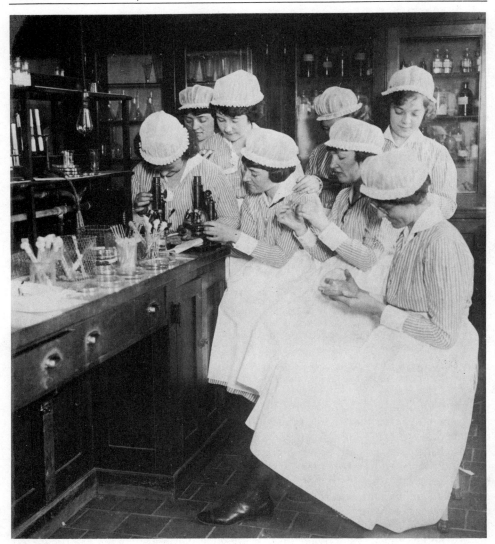

Figure 1-5. Nurses in training at Bellevue Hospital, c 1900, during instruction in a bacteriological lab. Courtesy of the Bettmann Archive, New York

dividuals, many of whom lacked training and experience. In 1861 Dorothea Lynde Dix was appointed superintendent of the Female Nurses of the Union Army.[12] Not trained as a nurse, Dix possessed administrative skills and was given the responsibility (without the accompanying authority) for organizing hospitals, supervising supply distribution, and appointing nurses.[13] Clara Barton, who later founded the American Red Cross, was another prominent lay nurse during the Civil War who functioned in large part outside the organized agencies.

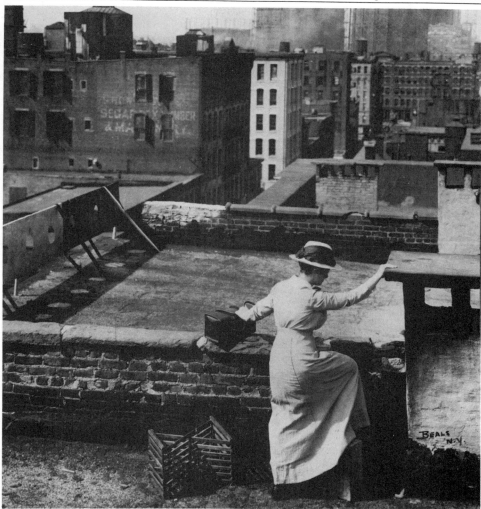

Figure 1-6. A visiting nurse, 1908, taking a shortcut across tenement roofs. Courtesy of the Museum of the City of New York

After the Civil War, because of heightened public awareness, there was significant interest in the establishment of organized educational programs for nurses. There were basically two suggested formats for the structure of these programs. One, which was based on the Nightingale model, recommended that the schools be created independently of hospitals and follow a well-planned curriculum that would generate "professional nurses." The other type of proposal (endorsed by the American Medical Association) recommended that "every large and well-organized hospital should have a school . . . the teaching to be furnished by its own medical staff."[14]

7

By 1873, three schools (Bellevue Training School, the Connecticut Training School, and the Boston Training School) had been established and were based partially on the Nightingale model. Unfortunately, they were soon absorbed by their affiliated hospitals because of a lack of independent funding. This development affected the direction of nursing in this country and delayed the development of nursing as a profession. This set the stage for an apprenticeship model of training that would persist through much of the 20th century, with hospitals using the schools to serve their own needs by supplying a steady source of virtually free labor.

Spanish-American War

The Spanish-American War was the first war for which trained nurses were available. Interestingly, the offer of the Nurses' Associated Alumnae of the United States and Canada (forerunner of the American Nurses' Association) to coordinate the soldiers' medical needs was rejected because the organization was too new to be recognized as an official voice for nursing. Instead, the Daughters of the American Revolution were given responsibility for organizing the Army Nursing Service; a female physician was appointed to head this effort.

Turn of the Century

The largest problem confronting nursing at the turn of the century was the establishment of standards for education and practice. Schools had proliferated as hospitals sought to profit from the cheap (free) labor provided by student nurses. There were no standards to protect the public from unsafe care.[15] During that era most graduate nurses went into private duty practice or into the newly developed arena of public health nursing. The settlement house movement was prominent during that period. The now famous Henry Street Settlement was founded by Lillian Wald, who besides being the founder of public health nursing is generally credited with laying the groundwork for modern social work. Nurses also began going into the home to supply health education and health screening of infants and mothers.

Despite these achievements, it is important to recognize that nursing was still subservient to a predominantly male world of physicians and hospital administrators. Early nursing practice acts, which were first passed as state statutes in the early 1900s, did not provide professional privileges, but restricted nurses' independent actions and gave them the right to practice only under the supervision of physicians.[16]

The early feminist movement, which fought to release women from some of the social restrictions they experienced, was fighting for the right to vote; with but a few noteworthy exceptions, professional women (including nurses) were on the side of the conservatives. Lavina Dock was one nursing leader who was an exception in this regard. She fought vigorously for suffrage and warned her colleagues of the threat of male dominance. She urged nurses to organize and work as a group toward establishing a strong professional identity. Dock also had definite views regarding the ethical responsibilities of nursing. She was outraged that "Nursing has not made itself a moral force; is not a public conscience; takes no position in large public questions; is not feared by those of low standards."[17]

World War I

The outbreak of World War I in 1914 created a large demand for nurses. Prior to the entry of the United States into the war in 1917, units of nurses were sent by the American Red Cross to assist the warring nations. Once America entered the war, the American Red Cross Nursing Service acted as the army and navy reserve. A plan was developed to recruit additional women into nursing by establishing a training camp for college graduates at Vassar College. The camp provided a preparatory nursing course whose graduates were then taken into selected nursing schools for their clinical training.[18]

Conditions of warfare had changed dramatically since the Spanish-American War, and military hospitals and nursing services had to be revised to meet the needs. During that period of revision, the concept of establishing several staging areas was first put into practice.

Advanced dressing stations were located at the front lines to treat emergencies and prepare the wounded for transportation to field hospitals and eventually to base hospitals. Female nurses never served at the front-line stations and only rarely at the field hospitals.[19]

Post–World War I

It was not until the 1930s that trained nurses began to shift their place of work from the public health and private duty arenas into the hospital setting. *Nurses, Patients, and Pocketbooks,* a study that focused on the supply and demand of nursing services, was released in 1928. Two major findings in that study were that salaries and working conditions were extremely poor and that an overproduction of graduate nurses had resulted in widespread unemployment.[20] Remember that graduate nurses did not staff hospitals; students did. Gradually, hospitals began to employ graduate nurses, sometimes with great reluctance. During that period nursing duties still included tasks such as delivering meal trays, scrubbing floors, and cleaning beds and equipment.

In the 1940s hospitals became safer and more efficient, with a resultant increase in the number of admissions for a greater variety of treatments and procedures. Prepaid hospitalization insurance was a new concept that became a significant factor in the development of an expanding health care system. Nurses were still primarily task oriented in a functional type of delivery system, taking on more procedures and integrating new technology.

> Nurses managed the apparatus for Wangensteen suction, tidal irrigation, and bladder decompression. They irrigated eyes, cecostomies, colostomies, and draining wounds. They did artificial respiration, and applied sterile compresses, and painted lesions. . . . They did catheterizations, sitz baths, and turpentine stupes. They gave insulin and taught the patient or his relatives to give the drug and examine urine. They administered . . . medications daily, by mouth or hypodermic. They assisted with lumbar punctures, thoracenteses . . . and phlebotomies.[21]

World War II

The nursing role in this war was dramatically different from previous wars throughout history. Members of the Army and Navy Nurse Corps during World War II numbered nearly 69,000 at its peak; these nurses were an integral part of the military health structure. Nurses served at the front lines, in evacuation hospitals, in base hospitals, on hospital ships, and in air ambulances. Flight nursing opened as a new field to military nurses. The use of sulfonamides, the introduction of penicillin, the ready availability of blood products, and the increased speed of rendering care were contributory factors in keeping the death rate lower than that of World War I.[22]

The Korean War

The Mobile Army Surgical Hospital (MASH), an experimental concept in World War II, was put into operation under combat conditions in Korea. This type of unit could be moved from place to place on a moment's notice and was typically located a few miles from the fighting front, with casualties being transported by helicopters. Efficient methods were instituted to sort patients by severity of injury for prioritization of treatment. These concepts of transporting seriously ill or injured patients by air and rapid triage for emergency care, along with innovative new surgical techniques and developing technology, would begin a revolutionary change in the way health care in hospitals was organized and delivered.

The Vietnam War

This war was the longest military conflict in the history of the United States. Between 1962 and 1973, more than 5000 nurses served in Vietnam.[23] At the end of the war, nurses assisted homeless people in refugee camps and provided nursing and medical education to Vietnamese nurses and doctors. Although the war caused extensive conflicts in this country, nursing's dedication to care was unequaled.

Early Development of Intensive Care

The modern intensive care unit (ICU) can trace its origins to the postanesthesia recovery room. Recovery rooms located in the operating suite were established in some hospitals in the early 1940s when it was realized that up to one third of postanesthetic deaths could be prevented by early detection and treatment of life-threatening complications such as airway obstruction and postoperative hemorrhage.[24] The need for nurses who were specially trained and able to function in an enlarged role was recognized by some of the early pioneers of these units.

During this period (early 1950s), nursing units were still generally organized on the large multibed ward concept. After World War II, many nurses had stopped practicing to rear their children, thus producing a shortage of nurses in civilian hospital care. The use of large wards enabled fewer nurses to observe large numbers of patients. Functional nursing, the delivery system of that era, organized nursing practice so that assignments were made according to the task to be performed. There were treatment nurses, medication nurses, and others who were assigned specific tasks, with a given task frequently taking precedence over a given patient. Team nursing was introduced to optimize patient care. Team nursing was designed, in theory, to make the best use of a scarce resource—the professional nurse. In team nursing, the registered nurse (RN) directs and supervises a team of personnel with differing levels of knowledge and training in providing care to the patient. The RN is responsible for making assignments, leading team conferences to plan care, and writing care plans to ensure continuity of care. In practice, patient care became efficient but fragmented. The RN responsible for the team usually ended up "nursing the desk" instead of patients. She checked doctors' orders, answered the telephone, made rounds with physicians, and was generally engaged in nonpatient-related activities.

Respiratory Care Units

It has been said that necessity is the mother of invention. The poliomyelitis epidemics of the late 1940s and early 1950s forced the establishment of respiratory care units, which resulted in a dramatic decrease in the polio mortality rate. In Scandinavia, the institution of manual ventilation via tracheostomy proved far superior to the cuirass respirator.

> At an early stage the following measures were adopted: Patients who were likely to develop respiratory complications were transferred to special wards for observation, and recording vital signs, etc. . . . Manual intermittent positive-pressure ventilation was used instead of or to supplement respirators. . . . At one time during the epidemic when 900 poliomyelitis patients had already been admitted, 75 patients were under manual artificial ventilation on the same day. For this it was necessary to employ 250 medical students to do the ventilation, 260 nurses from outside to sit at the bedside and attend to the patients' requirements and 27 hospital workers to change cylinders and control the machinery.[25]

In 1953, North Carolina Memorial Hospital established a multidisciplinary medical surgical intensive care unit. After a close call with a patient whose room was at the end of a hall the question was asked, "Why can't we put all of our critical patients in one room, have available everything we need for an emergency and give them the best care possible?"[26] Once the unit was established, it was calculated that the patients received 9.6 hours of direct patient care per day (combined registered nurse and practical nurse).[27] While this was undoubtedly an increase over the hours per patient day (HPPD) delivered on a general ward, many ICUs today deliver as many as 18 to 24 HPPD, provided solely by RNs.

Coronary Care Units

Advances in cardiac resuscitation were also taking place with the advent of cardiac pacing and AC defibrillation in the 1950s. In the early 1960s closed-chest cardiac massage and DC defibrillation were reported to be effective techniques. Coronary care units were first established in 1962 in three separate hospitals.[28] After disappointing results with monitoring patients on general medical floors and responding to emergencies with mobile crash carts, it became obvious that a specific area staffed by specially trained nurses was needed to meet the needs of patients with coronary disease.[29] An early coronary care unit at Presbyterian Hospital in Philadelphia has been described as follows: "Two small rooms were utilized with an aperture in the wall through which defibrillator paddles could be passed to either patient. At a small nursing station just outside, the coronary care nurse watched an oscilloscope and gave medical care to two patients."[30]

Neonatal Intensive Care Units (NICUs)

Premature infant nurseries had been established as early as 1896. The first hospital premature nursery in the United States was started in 1927.[31] However, it was not until the 1960s that improved resuscitation methods in the delivery room and mechanical ventilation techniques stimulated the growth of NICUs as they are known today. Regionalization of services and improved transport systems have also been major factors contributing to the development and success of NICUs.

Growth of ICUs

During the late 1960s and the 1970s, specialty ICUs proliferated. There are now burn, trauma, pediatric, spinal cord, neurological and neurosurgical, hypothermal, respiratory, and cardiovascular units, not to mention transplant units for heart and bone marrow. By 1983 there were at least 81,000 ICU beds distributed among 6900 ICUs in 6300 hospitals.[32] According to the American Hospital Association (AHA) surveys, ICU beds increased by 30% between 1979 and 1983.[33] It is estimated that 20% of total hospital charges relate to ICU care.[34]

Prior to the introduction of prospective reimbursement schemata, there were major financial factors that provided incentives to the development of ICUs. Under charge-based reimbursement plans, the cost of treating an ICU patient could be calculated retrospectively and charges established to more than cover the actual costs. The only constraint to the level of care provided was the limit of technological expertise.[35]

The Rise of Science and Technology

The explosion of scientific advances and the ability to translate that knowledge into technology that can be applied to health care in the 20th century has had a phenomenal impact on the development of ICUs.

The introduction of antibiotics, the capability to preserve and store blood products for transfusion, and improved skin-grafting techniques were major factors in improving mortality rates for the first time in World War II. While x-rays had been available since the latter part of the 19th century, there were marked improvements in diagnostic and therapeutic radiology during and following World War II, in part due to availability of fission products from uranium. The early 1970s saw the development of computed axial tomography (CAT), which radically enhanced diagnostic capabilities. The full significance of magnetic resonance (MR) imaging, introduced in the early 1980s, may not yet be completely realized. Other scientific advances within the past 30 years that have widespread applicability include renal dialysis, microsurgical techniques, plasmapheresis, and laser surgery.

Mechanical Ventilation

The introduction of ventilators along with their ongoing refinement has been one of the most significant technological achievements related to the evolution of intensive care units. Resuscitation equipment consisting of endotracheal tubes and a hand-operated bellows had been devised for victims of drowning in the early 19th century. Because of concerns about the danger of pneumothorax, these devices were declared unsafe.[36] In the early 20th century a patient-triggered, pressure-cycled ventilator had been invented, but it was not until the poliomyelitis epidemics of 1948–49 and 1952–53 that physiologic principles were understood well enough to be applied effectively to the development of mechanical ventilators.[37] It was soon after this that mechanical ventilation was used as supportive therapy following thoracic and general surgery and began to replace chest-wall traction as the preferred management of crushed-chest injuries.[38]

Cardiovascular Advances

Intracardiac catheterization, pioneered in 1929, was essential to later advances for medical and surgical treatment of cardiovascular disease.[39] This early innovation enabled investigators to conduct detailed physiologic studies and, of course, was a prerequisite technique for development of transvenous cardiac pacing and measurement of cardiac output via thermodilution methods, both of which are accepted routine practices in ICUs today.

Until the 1950s operative repairs of various congenital heart defects were performed entirely by feel without direct visualization, since the heart had to be kept pumping. It was not until 1953 that John Gibbon and his team constructed a cardiopulmonary bypass machine that paved the way for rapid advances in operative techniques for cardiac surgery.[40] Cardiac assist devices such as intra-aortic balloon pumps have become valuable adjuncts to medical and surgical treatment regimens.

Neurologic Advances

As early as 1866, techniques existed for direct measurement and graphic recording of intracranial pressure (ICP) using a trephine hole and the intact dura. However, it was not until 1951 that studies by Guillaume and Janny demonstrated that changing neurologic signs were unreliable indicators of increasing intracranial pressure, thus establishing the rationale for continuous intracranial pressure monitoring.[41]

Techniques and methods were refined, and by the mid-1970s ICP monitoring was a valuable technique being used to guide treatment decisions. If 1950–60 was the decade of respiratory resuscitation and 1960–70 the decade of cardiac resuscitation, then 1970–80 may be viewed as the decade of brain resuscitation.[42] Methods of ventilatory management and pharmacologic intervention were refined to prevent or minimize neurologic damage as the result of traumatic or hypoxic insults. In addition, CAT scanning and microsurgical techniques are technological advances that have been instrumental in increasing the treatment options for patients with a variety of neurologic insults, including tumors, arteriovenous malformations, and aneurysms.

Organ Transplant

The first successful organ transplant in a human was the 1954 renal transplant from an identical twin to his brother. The transplantation of a kidney from an unrelated individual was unsuccessful until the advent of immunosuppressant drugs. Since that time renal transplant has become a feasible alternative to chronic dialysis. In 1967 the first heart transplant was performed by Christiaan Barnard in South Africa; however, it was not until the late 1970s and early 1980s that increased understanding of immunology facilitated methods to manage the rejection response. Throughout these two decades research has continued with heart and other transplants, such as liver and pancreas. The use of an artificial heart has been receiving attention, but thus far is primarily used as an interim measure until a compatible human heart is available. By the early 1980s the use of a new immunosuppressant drug, cyclosporine, showed promise of vastly improving the success of organ transplants.

Increased Specialization

Specialization in Nursing

From the time the earliest ICUs were established, it was recognized that the personnel were the most important element in what was then a very innovative approach to caring for the sick. Cadmus has described choosing "the most capable and dedicated nursing personnel," and Osborn and Gerbode have related that "the patient's prognosis was correlated with her [the nurse's] skill and experience."[43,44] That perspective of recognizing the value of skilled and knowledgeable staff continues. "I am impressed more and more with the importance of the qualifications of the personnel . . . and their motivations, and less with the monitors, lines in the patients, and drugs. Cathode ray oscilloscopes do not make a great CCU, but people do."[45] With the exception of nurse midwives and nurse anesthetists, specialization in nursing is as young as ICUs. In hospitals, patients were not segregated according to diseases until the early 20th century. As late as World War II the majority of nurses still worked as general staff nurses. The advent of specialized units such as ICUs spawned a corresponding trend toward specialization in nursing practice.

American Association of Critical-Care Nurses (AACN)

Following a highly successful educational program for coronary care nurses, a dynamic group of approximately 140 nurses met in 1969 to form a national organization, the American Association of Cardiovascular Nurses. The goals of the founding group were "to set educational and practice standards, to communicate with other health care groups, to publish a periodical, to disseminate knowledge through educational programs and to establish a central source of information."[46] In 1972 the group reincorporated as the American Association of Critical-Care Nurses, a name that reflected the organization's intent to represent the expanding practice of its members.

By 1985, 15 years after its founding, the organization had grown to over 50,000 members. It publishes two periodicals, as well as membership newsletters, and sponsors numerous annual educational programs at local and regional levels; in addition, there is an annual National Teaching Institute. AACN has developed a credentialing process to grant certification status to nurses who "demonstrate the knowledge base and clinical expertise necessary for effective practice."[47] The organization has published standards of practice, has sponsored the publication of numerous books, and has developed several position papers pertinent to issues in the field of critical care nursing.

AACN has defined critical care nursing as follows: "In Nursing, a Social Policy Statement, the American Nurses' Association defines nursing as 'the diagnosis and treatment of human responses to actual or potential health problems.' Critical care nursing is that specialty within nursing that deals specifically with human responses to life-threatening problems."[48]

The trend toward specialization has not been isolated solely to nursing. There has been a proliferation of health care providers, each focusing on a particular area of specialization. Physicians have become specialized; there are cardiologists, endocrinologists, gastroenterologists, pulmonologists, and nephrologists. There are now subspecialists within specialties: pediatric cardiology, neuroradiology, and neonatology. The advent of ICUs has led to the emergence of medical intensivists.

The health care team for an individual patient in the ICU might now easily be comprised of several physician specialists consulting with the intensivist, the ICU nurse, a social worker, respiratory therapist, physical therapist, dietician, pharmacist, psychologist, and (in pediatrics) a child life therapist. Beyond this group of people, the patient and family may also be exposed to an array of technicians for x-rays, EKGs, EEGs, echocardiograms, pulmonary function, and laboratory testing. Some ICUs have monitor technicians and research technicians who collect data and massage computers. Teaching hospitals have interns, residents, fellows, nursing students, and graduate nursing students. Some hospitals have nurse practitioners and physician assistants.

The combination of the simultaneous explosions in technology and specialization has resulted in the creation of an environment in which virtually every vital life function can be monitored, recorded, analyzed, supported, or altered. It is an environment that is bewildering in its complexity, awesome in its magnitude of accumulated knowledge, and frightening in its potential. The modern ICU has engendered spectacular advances in the treatment of human illness and injury, but these advances have brought new problems, new challenges, new questions, new costs, and new dilemmas.

What effect has the increased technology, specialization, and growth of the ICU had on the patient, the nurse, and even the public's expectations? As technological advances are reported, people expect that these innovations will be available to them. ICUs are depicted (at times unrealistically) by the media as places where miracles are wrought and technology is seen as being synonymous with "quality care."

Fragmentation of Care

One potential effect of increased specialization is fragmentation of care. Prior to the development of ICUs, nurses practiced in a model of team nursing. One of the primary advantages of the ICU is that of discarding the team-nursing model and having one nurse responsible for the total care of the patient during a given shift. That nurse renders basic care, administers medication, monitors the patient closely for changes and response to treatment, and performs necessary procedures. With increasing technology, the role of the nurse has expanded to encompass more activities that formerly had been within the realm of medicine. The increasing array of high-tech machines takes more and more of the nurse's time. Technical personnel have been introduced into some units, frequently with undefined roles and unclear competencies.[49] Increased specialization has led to increased numbers of personnel involved with each patient. The high stress load and changing social trends have created demands for flexible work schedules such as 12-hour shifts. The result of all these factors can be fragmentation of care and distancing of the nurse from the patient.

The nurse is the individual central to any patient's care. Nursing is the only discipline that is with the patient 24 hours a day. AACN's Scope of Critical Care Nursing Practice states that "the critical care nurse is . . . committed to ensuring that all critically ill patients receive optimal care."[50] Further, the Principles of Critical Care Nursing Practice state that "the critical care nurse . . . *coordinates* care delivered to patients and supports families within the critical care environment" [emphasis added].[51]

While total care was the method of nursing care delivery from the outset in most ICUs, the concept of primary nursing, introduced during the 1970s, has now been adopted by many ICUs. Primary nursing has as its central concept the notion that one professional nurse is designated as the individual responsible and accountable for coordinating and planning the patient's care on a 24-hour basis, from the time of admission to the time of discharge. The primary nurse cares for the patient when she is there and leaves instructions for others to follow when she is not. Primary nursing can be very effective in preventing fragmentation of care.

Hazards of Technology

Technological advances have sometimes been applied before all potential effects have been fully understood. One example is the indiscriminate use of increased levels of oxygen with premature infants in the 1940s, and the subsequent discovery of its role in the development of retrolental fibroplasia. The indiscriminate use of x-rays soon after their discovery resulted in an increased rate of cancer years later among those patients. Female children of women who were given diethylstilbestrol (DES) during pregnancy have also shown, as adults, an increased incidence of cancer years afterward.

New diseases have resulted from the application of some technological innovations. Bronchopulmonary dysplasia (BPD) develops in some infants following prolonged ventilator use for respiratory distress syndrome. BPD has a mortality rate of 30% to 40%, and significant morbidity may persist in survivors for months or years.[52] Necrotizing enterocolitis (NEC) is suspected to be related to certain feeding practices for immature infants.[53]

Thus, while many of the new technologies advanced in ICUs over the past 30 years have saved lives that otherwise would have been lost, huge risks are associated with some of those innovations. Some complications become apparent almost immediately, but others may not be understood until much later, after many patients are affected.

New Dilemmas

What will be the effects of some of the technologies now being used? Will the use of laser surgery result in an increased rate of some form of cancer 20 years from now? Will those patients who undergo MR imaging develop a syndrome, as yet unidentified, in the next decade? Will intra-aortic balloon pumping cause weakening of the aortic wall resulting in formation of aneurysms 15 years later? Will cyclosporine cause genetic defects that will affect the children of recipients of the drug? We must ask whether new technologies have been thoroughly tested—and their effects carefully evaluated—before being used. Are new methods applied correctly to the entity/population for which they have been evaluated? Are the known risks and effects carefully explained, and is adequate informed consent obtained before a treatment is administered? Is society prepared to accept, deal with, and pay for the burdens that may result from new technological achievements? These are some of the new questions that health care professionals, particularly in ICUs but also in society at large, must confront.

Efficacy of ICUs Questioned.   Subjectively, there has been the sense, on the part of many physicians, nurses, and the public, that ICUs are effective and beneficial. However, there has only recently been any objective evaluation of the efficacy of intensive care therapy. There has been an increasing trend to evaluate the effectiveness of care provided by examining outcome statistics correlated with severity of illness measurements. The stimulus for this trend comes from the national awareness of and interest in health care economics, and the emergence of biomedical ethical issues as a matter of public concern.

Patients are generally admitted to ICUs for one of two reasons. They are either critically ill and require life support for organ-system failure, or they are in stable condition and their physician believes that close monitoring may prevent sudden complications or rapid deterioration.[54] These stable, monitored patients may account for up to half of the admissions in some units.[55]

Several studies since 1976 have described a category of ICU admissions consisting of the elderly, those in chronically poor health, and those with poor short-term survival prognosis as a group in which ICU therapy can do little except prolong death.[56,57,58] A Consensus Development Conference on Critical Care Medicine held at the National Institutes of Health (NIH) in 1983 concluded that:

> The highly favorable outcomes derived from these [early ICUs] served as the stimulus for establishing large numbers of such units. Over the past two decades, the availability of physical resources, nursing staff, and related specialized procedures, as well as patients' expectations, have resulted in an expansion of the original indications for admission to categories for whom the achievable benefits are less clear.[59]

Knaus and associates have posed three questions that must be answered to improve the utilization of ICUs.

1. Can we improve our ability to select patients for intensive care?
2. Is it appropriate ethically and possible legally to be more selective?
3. Can we design policies to provide incentives for physicians and hospitals to use intensive care more selectively?[60]

Regardless of the eventual answers to those questions, nurses must be actively involved in the attempt to address them. Intensive care units were originally established, in large part, because of the need for a higher level of nursing care and supervision. If patients are excluded from ICUs on the basis of being medically stable, regardless of nursing care needs, how will these needs be met? Selection criteria and patient placement guidelines must be established in a way to ensure that the total range of patient care needs is considered.

Dilemmas—New and Old

Surely there were ethical dilemmas in the Nightingale era, although it is unclear how they were acknowledged or addressed. The issue of risk to the nurse versus her duty or obligation to the patient is clearly present throughout history. Is the risk of caring for patients with acquired immune deficiency syndrome (AIDS) any greater than was the risk of caring for victims of the plague, or serving in the Spanish-American War when yellow fever was epidemic? One could argue, indeed, that the risk with AIDS is less because there is a greater body of knowledge and understanding of the mechanisms of transmission as well as the precautions for safety. In addition, there are clearly defined standards (as defined in the ANA Code for Nurses) relating to how the nurse can ethically discharge responsibilities to the patient if the risk outweighs the duties.[61]

There have also surely been issues related to allocation of scarce resources throughout nursing history. When Nightingale had few or no medical supplies for thousands of patients, how did she decide who got what little was available? The issue that nurses must not lose sight of in the technologically oriented ICU is that they themselves are the most precious resource. Bed space in the ICU is of little value if there is not a competent nurse to attend the patient in that bed. Recent studies (cited earlier in this chapter) indicate that for some units a significant percentage of patients may be inappropriate admissions. It is incumbent upon nurses to be actively involved in formulating policies regarding admission and discharge criteria.

It is certain, too, that nurses have always been concerned about doing good for patients and avoiding the infliction of harm. The difference in the ICU of today is that it has become much more difficult to draw the line between what constitutes doing good and what constitutes doing harm.

Dilemmas Arising From Science and Technology

Numerous ethical dilemmas currently confront health care providers and are receiving considerable attention in both the professional literature and the public media. Almost without fail these dilemmas have arisen from the scientific and technological advances of the past 30 years. Withdrawal of life support was certainly not an issue before cardiorespiratory function could be supported technologically almost indefinitely. The allocation of resources such as heart and liver transplants, extracorporeal membrane oxygenation (ECMO) for neonates, and ICU beds has become even more puzzling in an era of prospective reimbursement. Where is the nurse in some of these issues? What is the distinction between the dilemma for the nurse and that of the physician?

Withdrawal of Life Support.   Like the physician, a nurse may be concerned about determining that life support is a burden for the patient that outweighs its benefit. There are, however, additional issues for the nurse. The nurse is the individual who must continue rendering physical care while medical treatment decisions are being deliberated. The nurse may be in the position of feeling that she is inflicting continued suffering, pain, or indignity. The nurse is concerned with helping the family cope with its anguish and assisting with the grieving process. The nurse must know if the family wants to be present at the withdrawal of life support—if they want to say good-bye before or after support is withdrawn. In some units, a nurse who has not participated in the decision to withdraw life support may be the individual who receives the order to disconnect the ventilator. It is the nurse, finally alone after all is done and everyone else has gone, who wonders if enough was done, or if too much was done.

Guidelines for ''Do Not Resuscitate'' (DNR) Orders.   Physicians have been socialized into a philosophy aimed at the mastery of disease. There has been long-standing resistance to ''admitting defeat'' by writing orders not to resuscitate, even when the inevitable is obvious. Nurses have often been caught in the middle, between the patient and the physician. They have been told to ''walk slowly,'' to ''do everything but . . . ,'' and even not to resuscitate, in the absence of written orders. Some units have policies that *every* patient is *always* resuscitated. Nurses have been begged by their competent patients to allow them to die and have been compelled by such orders and policies to ignore those pleas and proceed with resuscitation. These are truly examples of how treatment can become torture. Situations such as these have been the reason some nurses have left the ICU or nursing entirely. How do we decide when enough is too much?

Nursing Art Versus Nursing Science

Nursing is both an art and a science. Throughout nursing history there have been periods when one was emphasized over the other. In modern nursing's struggle to achieve recognition as a profession, the emphasis has frequently been placed on the science. Demonstrating adherence to scientific principles, documenting a defined body of knowledge, and conducting research to guide practice and validate the effectiveness of interventions are elements that stress the science of nursing. Aspects that comprise the art of nursing have sometimes been confused with roles that are considered less than professional, perhaps mundane or even menial. Nursing is linked with maternal types of behavior such as nurturing, caring, laying on of hands, and comforting, which have not always been highly valued by society.[62] As nursing has evolved in ICUs, there has been an exceedingly high value placed on science. The integration of new knowledge, application of rapidly expanding technology, strong focus on numbers, and correlation of data are essential for the critical care nurse. One must monitor and record the vital signs, measure the output, calculate the drug infusions, perform the cardiac output measurements and compute the index, set the timing for the intra-aortic balloon pump, and much more. However, it is the art of nursing that remains the aspect that initially drew many into the profession—and ultimately what keeps them there.

> Nursing is not merely a technique, but a process that incorporates the elements of soul, mind and imagination. Its very essence lies in the creative imagination, the sensitive spirit, and the intelligent understanding that provide the very foundation for effective nursing care.[63]

If the ICU nurse practices science in her attention to numbers, data, procedures, and machines, she also practices art in her attention to form, context, and meaning. Her assessments must be attuned to the smallest change in color, rate, rhythm, odor, size, and movement. She must be sensitive to nuances in speech, tone, and expression. She must listen to what patients do and do not say. She must plan for what has and has not happened. She must anticipate the responses of others and move the members of the team in a never-ending dance to the music that is unique to each patient. She must see each patient as a person, with unique hopes and dreams, fears and pains, needs and values. The way the nurse goes about meeting those needs, calming those fears, recognizing those hopes, and abiding by those values forms the essence of the art of nursing.

Nurses in the ICU who practice the science, but exclude the art of nursing, focus on the technological aspects of care and disregard the importance of involvement with the human element. The phrase "high tech/high touch" has been coined to emphasize the importance of maintaining a high degree of human interaction in high-tech environments such as the modern ICU.[64] Many ICUs, however, have become "low touch" environments not only because of the extent of technological advances, but also because of administrative, sociocultural, and educational factors.[65] Physicians and nurses have distanced themselves emotionally from each other, from other providers, and ultimately from the patient and family. We have paid so much attention to the numbers, the machines, and the technical skills that we have overlooked the people. We have lost the *care* from the critical care unit and we have turned treatment into torture. This kind of environment—these attitudes, the drive to use technology to its fullest application—questions the very purpose of an intensive care unit. The ethical dilemmas faced daily in every ICU are what have forced these questions to surface.

The ethical issues that confront nurses are sometimes quite different from those that confront physicians. Both the nurse and the physician may be concerned with questions of whether a given technology should be used if there is little hope for success. Should we resuscitate? Does the patient understand the risks of surgery? Beyond those issues, however, are others particularly of concern to nursing. Are there enough nurses to provide safe care? Should the patient continue to be suctioned with "Do Not Resuscitate" orders? Are the patient's wishes being respected? The list of questions is almost endless.

Subsequent chapters in this book will explore these dilemmas. A foundation in ethical theory will be provided, ethical principles will be defined and presented as tools for decision making. The intent of this book is to improve the nurse's knowledge about and ability to address ethical dilemmas in the practice setting.

Notes

1. Whitworth H: The World of Childrens Hospital, p 1. Los Angeles, Childrens Hospital, 1985
2. Donahue MP: Nursing—the Finest Art, an Illustrated History, p 56. St Louis, CV Mosby, 1985
3. Ibid, p 61
4. Lyons AS, Petrucelli RT: Medicine—an Illustrated History, p 143. New York, Abrams, 1978
5. Donahue, op cit, p 163
6. Lyons, Petrucelli, op cit, p 543
7. Donahue, op cit, p 193
8. Ibid, p 271
9. Ibid, pp 236–238
10. Ibid, p 243
11. Ibid, p 244
12. Ibid, p 293
13. Ibid

14. American Medical Association: Proceedings, New Orleans, May 1869. Medical News 20:339–351, 1969

15. Donahue, op cit, p 358

16. Ashley JA: Nurses in American history, nurses and early feminism. Am J Nurs 75:1465, 1975

17. Dock LL: The duty of this society in public work. In Proceedings of the Tenth Annual Convention of the American Society of Superintendents of Training Schools, Pittsburgh, Oct 7–9, 1903, pp 78–79. Baltimore, JH Furst, 1904

18. Dreves KD: Nurses in American history—Vassar training camp for nurses. Am J Nurs 75:2000, 1975

19. Donahue, op cit, p 404

20. Ibid, p 385

21. Dennison C: Nursing service in the emergency room. Am J Nurs 42:777, 1975

22. Donahue, op cit, p 415

23. Shields EA (ed): Highlights in the History of the Army Nurse Corps. Washington, DC, US Army Center of Military History, 1981

24. Hilberman M: The evolution of intensive care units. Crit Care Med 3:159, 1975

25. Lassen HCA: Preliminary report in the 1952 epidemic of poliomyelitis in Copenhagen. Lancet 1:37, 1953

26. Cadmus RR: Intensive care reaches silver anniversary. Hospitals 54(2):98, 1980

27. Cadmus RR: Special care for the critical case. Hospitals 28(9):65, 1954

28. Hilberman, op cit, p 162

29. Day HW: History of coronary care units. Am J Cardiol 30:405, 1972

30. Ibid, p 406

31. Hilberman, op cit, p 163

32. Richards G: Critical care under PPS. Hospitals 59:66, 1985

33. Ibid

34. Knaus WA, Draper EA, Wagner DP: The use of intensive care: New research initiatives and their implications for national health policy. Milbank Mem Fund Q 61:561, 1983

35. Lave JR, Knaus WA: The economics of intensive care units. In Bensch K et al (eds): Medicolegal Aspects of Critical Care. Rockville, Aspen Systems, 1986

36. Hilberman, op cit, p 160

37. Ibid

38. Ibid

39. Lyons, Petrucelli, op cit, p 594

40. Ibid

41. Bruce DA: The Pathophysiology of Increased Intracranial Pressure. Upjohn, Current Concepts, 1978

42. Safer P, Grenvik A: Organization and physician education in critical care medicine. Anesthesiology 47:82, 1977

43. Cadmus 1980, op cit, p 98

44. Hilberman, op cit, p 162

45. Burch GE: Changing concepts in cardiovascular therapy—a quarter century perspective. Am Heart J 93:413, 1977

46. AACN: Historical Archives. Disk 100: AACN HIST, 1985

47. Ibid

48. AACN: Position Statement. Definition of Critical Care Nursing, 1984

49. AACN: Position Statement. Use of Technical Personnel in Critical Care Settings, 1983

50. AACN: Position Statement. Scope of Critical Care Nursing Practice, 1980

51. AACN: Position Statement. Principles of Critical Care Nursing Practice, 1981

52. Cone TE: History of the Care and Feeding of the Premature Infant, p 130. Boston, Little, Brown & Co, 1985

53. Ibid, pp 14–142

54. Knaus, Draper, Wagner, op cit

55. Knaus WA et al: The range of intensive care services today. JAMA 246:2711, 1981

56. Chassin MR: Costs and outcomes of medical intensive care. Med Care 20:165, 1982

57. Cullen DJ et al: Survival, hospitalization charges and follow-up results in critically ill patients. N Engl J Med 294:982, 1976

58. Thibault GE et al: Medical intensive care: Indications, interventions, and outcomes. N Engl J Med 302:938, 1980

59. National Institutes of Health Consensus Development Conference. JAMA 250:798, 1983

60. Knaus, Draper, Wagner, op cit

61. ANA: Code for Nurses with Interpretive Statements. Kansas City, MO, ANA, 1985

62. Fagin C, Diers D: Nursing as a metaphor. N Engl J Med 309:116, 1983

63. Donahue, op cit, p ix

64. Naesbitt J: Megatrends: Ten New Directions Transforming Our Lives. New York, Warner Books, 1982

65. Birnbaum ML: High tech/low touch. Crit Care Med 12:1006, 1984

Chapter 2

Introduction to Ethics and Ethical Theory: A Road Map to the Discipline

Marsha D. M. Fowler

> *You, reader, whoever you are, are not a complete beginner in this subject. You already have some idea of what "good" and "bad," "right" and "wrong," mean, and you know some acts to be right, others wrong, some things to be good and some bad. Now these are precisely the topics with which Ethics as a subject of systematic study deals.*[1]

Most persons do, indeed, have some sense of what is right and wrong, virtuous and evil, good and bad, apart from any formal study of ethics. This knowledge arises at least partially from the common social morality, accessible even to the very young, through social rules, expectations, and prohibitions. Morality tells us not to harm others, not to kill, to be good persons, to keep promises, and to tell the truth.

Ethics, however, goes beyond morality and is a very specialized field of endeavor, usually seen as one of several different divisions of either philosophy or theology. Ethics, particularly as applied to clinical practice, is concerned about more specific issues, such as when doing good (providing critical care) becomes harmful (as in prolongation of suffering). Critical care nursing, too, is a very specialized area of concern and is part of the larger discipline of nursing in general. The combination, then, of ethics and critical care nursing goes considerably beyond the interests of everyday morality and becomes an intricate and complex area of concern to a relatively small segment of society, comprised of critical care nurses and the recipients of critical care nursing.

To understand nursing ethics in critical care, one must understand both critical care nursing and nursing in general, their philosophy and tradition, and ethics. The task of this book is to merge the two fields so that the critical care nurse can evaluate and choose in the moral realm, with the tools necessary to do so. The purpose of this chapter is to clarify what ethics is and is not, to give an overview of the field of ethics and its divisions, and to define some basic ethical concepts and terms.

Morality and Ethics

Ethics deals with what "ought" to be, and the ways in which we discuss or think about that ought. Morality arises, in part, from the social nature of the community, though in some respects it stands apart from it, and is necessary for the realization of values such as human dignity, freedom, and faithfulness to one another.

Though it is common to use the terms *ethics* and *morality* interchangeably, and for the most part that will be the case here, there is a distinction between the two. Morality exists more at the level of social convention, codes of behavior, and community expectation. Morality provides us with general rules of conduct and standards of evaluation. It tells us that certain kinds of actions (like lying), or certain specific actions (like pocketing patient narcotics), are either right or wrong. It also tells us whether the consequences of an action, or the motives or character traits of an individual, are good or bad. Morality provides the conventional or customary rules of conduct or standards of evaluation for a given social group. Morality also refers to the additional personal rules or standards, within conventional morality, that guide the individual.

Ethics is the broader, over-arching, more reflective endeavor. In a sense, it takes up where morality leaves off. When a person goes beyond the acceptance and internalization of traditional rules of the social group and moves into the realm of reflecting upon those rules, ethical thinking has begun. The ultimate end of ethical thinking is to shape a critical and reflective morality to embrace as one's own personal ethics. Ethical thinking permits one to give a reasoned accounting of an ethical position, to move beyond a viscerohormonal, seat-of-the-pants response or an undefended assertion that something is right or wrong, virtuous or evil, good or bad, simply because we know that to be the case. Though that sort of response may ultimately give the correct answer, ethics looks for responses that are both right and reasoned.

The terms *ethical* and *moral* need some clarification. They are frequently used to mean ethically right or morally good. The terms *unethical* or *immoral*, then, are used to mean wrong, bad, or evil. In the field of ethics, *ethical* and *moral* refer to a *category* or *class* of actions, values, judgments, or thinking, and not to their rightness or goodness. In this respect, to claim that an action or value is ethical is simply to assert that it *pertains to morality*, not that it is either right or good. The terms used in this book are used as they would be used in the field of ethics.

The focus of this text is ethical, which necessitates setting forth a distinction between law and ethics, as there is generally a commingling and confusion about their distinctiveness. Although Chapter 10 explores that distinction and examines areas of convergence, congruence, and divergence, a few preliminary comments are in order here.

Law and Ethics

Both law and ethics have social sanctions and functions, and both serve as so-called action guides. Law is created or promulgated for the purposes of maintaining order and continuity in society; it generally sets a minimum standard for social behavior.

25

The force behind the law is that of imprisonment or fine or some other enforceable form of punishment. The police powers of the state assure that members of a society will conform to its laws. Though law itself—and specific laws themselves—predates the individual's birth, it is constantly renewed, revised, or created as new social conditions or situations arise.

Ethics is a bit different. It, too, exists before the individual and arises from the social context, but it is not created in the same sense that law is. Ethics makes demands on the individual, some of which may exceed or even conflict with the demands of the law. It is often regarded as being higher than the law, and a source of judgment of the law itself. However, at the level of everyday decision making, disobedience of the law can bring punishment if an issue is pressed. Disobedience to ethical norms does not carry the same force.

Violation of a moral rule may elicit moral disapproval from others—even anger, hostility, ostracism, or mistrust. The violator may even be condemned to eternal punishment, the wrath of God, or the avenging sword of St. Michael, but not to imprisonment or fine. The force of morality is the force of *moral suasion* (influence, persuasion, or urging), much of which has lost its ability to elicit obedience in a society that is not particularly threatened by heavenly vengeance.

Moral suasion, when connected to professional codes or specific bodies such as Congress, does have censure or expulsion from the group as an instrument of punishment. In its document *Guidelines for Implementing the Code for Nurses,* the American Nurses' Association (ANA) provides for either censure or expulsion from the association for violation of either the code or the association's bylaws.[2]

In some cases, impeachment and conviction on moral grounds could lead to a loss of reputation or standing in the community. Usually, though, the offense has to be of such enormous magnitude that proceedings are rarely invoked.

Ethics does set standards, but the standards it sets are more than minimum expectations. Ethics also identifies ideals (as maximal standards toward which we strive—such as confidentiality in a teaching hospital) and actions that, while not morally obligatory, are morally praiseworthy. Nonobligatory, morally praiseworthy actions are termed *supererogatory* and include things like risking one's own well-being to care for a patient under disaster conditions. Consistent conformity to an ideal, going beyond one's duty, and meeting one's duty under conditions in which others would fail or flee are actions that differentiate persons who meet their moral duties from those who are nursing's saints or heroes.[3]

Where ethics deals with the sorts of persons we are to be—whether good persons or saints or heroes—and where it deals with the ends we ought to seek—and the duties and obligations we ought to meet—its specific concerns fall within the area of normative ethics. Ethics has several divisions that require some explanation in order to proceed with a discussion of ethical issues in critical care nursing.

The Discipline of Ethics

Its Divisions

It is easy to get lost in ethics and not unusual to wonder if you are "maze-bright" or "maze-dull." However, it is hoped that if we look at the maze from above and have something of a roadmap, navigation will be a bit easier. Here we must provide an overview of the discipline to give a picture of the sorts of categories into which that discipline is divided, and the concerns that those categories generate.

Because any classification (whether it be nursing diagnoses, nursing theories, or divisions of the field of ethics) is a reflection of the assumptions and presumptions that undergird it, there are inevitably several ways to formulate these categories. Contemporary American ethics is often divided into two major subcategories: metaethics and normative ethics. Another area of ethical concern, *descriptive ethics,* while morally relevant, is not actually a formal division of ethics.

Metaethics is the division of ethics that largely remains the domain of professional ethicists. It is non-normative and is primarily concerned with theoretical issues of meaning and justification, or logical, epistemological (how we know), and semantic questions in ethics. Metaethics addresses questions such as "Is the good good because the gods have ordained it, or do the gods ordain the good because it is good?"[4]

Metaethics also asks questions such as "What do we mean when we say that *X* [a particular value or action] is good or right or just [or any moral term]?" Or, "Why be good?" These sorts of ethereal or speculative questions are what people often think of as "ethics." It is also not unusual for these sorts of questions to be viewed wrongly as impractical theorizing. Debate about these questions is useful and important, though not immediately practical to the nonethicist.

A second area of ethical concern is not actually regarded by ethicists as a true division of ethics itself. *Descriptive ethics,* though linked to ethics, represents the work of sociologists, anthropologists, psychologists, historians, and others who describe or attempt to explain moral behavior or ends.[5,6]

The scientific study of moral behavior is relevant to, but not part of, the philosophical study of moral behavior. The former seeks to answer questions such as "What does *X* group of people believe is right and good?" or "Why do these people behave, morally, as they do?" Nurses who have contact with the scientific study of moral behavior most frequently encounter it in the form of either "values clarification" or theories of "moral development." The purpose of values clarification is to help the individual identify those values—personal or professional—that influence behavior, including moral decision making. In this sense, values "provide a frame of reference, a basic comprehension of reality through which we integrate, explain, and appraise new ideas, events, and personal relationships."[7] As some values are "central motivating values" and others are "supporting values," it is essential that the critical care nurse examine and understand those values, especially in terms of how they influence personal moral decision making.[8] Yet, values clarification is descriptive and not normative, is a part of descriptive ethics, and most often addresses psychological, sociological, or anthropological questions.

Likewise, moral development, as seen in the theories of Kohlberg and others, though pertinent to ethics falls within the realm of psychology and is part of descriptive ethics. The theories do claim to be value neutral—an assertion that has been strongly challenged.[9] Developmental theories, including moral developmental studies, focus on what the developmental theorists hold to be universal stages that follow laws of development in their structure, and vary in content according to the individ-

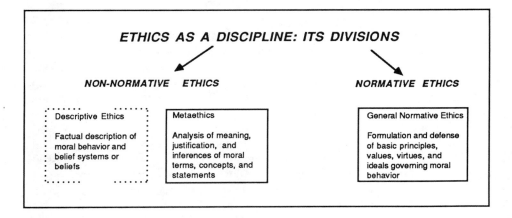

Figure 2-1. The divisions of ethics. Copyright © 1984, Marsha D. Fowler, adapted with permission

ual's cultural and life experiences. Moral developmental theories target stages of moral reasoning as their concern. Work in moral development is principally conducted in the fields of psychology or education, and is directed toward both analysis of moral development and application to moral education in the schools.

Normative ethics, the second major division of ethics, is about norms or standards of behavior and value and their ultimate application to daily life. The focus is on evaluative judgments, and the goal is to identify moral obligations, duties, and values that ought to guide individual or group moral action. Normative ethics asks questions like "What is a just allocation of social resources?" or "What characteristics does a 'good' person possess?" Normative ethics, which leads to applied ethics, is thus the division of ethics that most health professionals are concerned about. (See Fig. 2-1.)

There are two major divisions within normative ethics. The first division focuses on decisions about what is *right* or *wrong to do.* These judgments are called *norms of obligation* because they tell us what our moral obligations and duties are. (All duties are obligations, but not all obligations [e.g., charity] are duties.)

Normative ethics also tells us what is *good* and *bad* in persons, groups, motives, or things. Judgments of what is good or evil in persons are called *norms of moral value,* and would pose questions such as "What is a 'good' critical care nurse?" Examples of moral values, sometimes called virtues, include honesty, courage, and trustworthiness.

Judgments of what is good or bad in things or ends we seek or desire are called *norms of nonmoral value.* Norms of nonmoral value answer questions that often seem of peripheral interest to ethics, for example, "What is a 'good' cough?" There are literally hundreds of categories of nonmoral values. Some are things that "are good in themselves," or intrinsic goods (such as human dignity). Some are instrumental values, goods that allow us to reach other ends. Health can be considered an instrumental value because it allows us to reach other, more important values. Though judgments of nonmoral value are in fact normative judgments, they really belong to

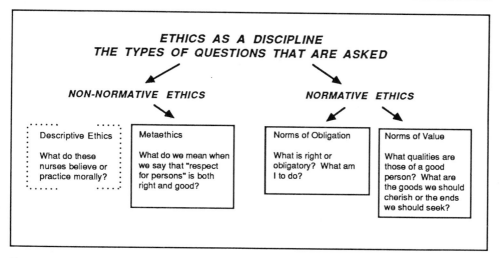

Figure 2-2. Types of questions that ethics addresses. Copyright © 1984, Marsha D. Fowler, adapted with permission

the field of *axiology* and are not always regarded as a part of ethics proper. This is not to say, however, that they are not important: they are, and they pertain to ethics because they influence our ethical decisions and designate the goods or ends we seek, such as health, well-being, or dignity. (see Fig. 2-2).[10]

Norms of Obligation

There are various ways by which to specify what is right or wrong. These various methods distinguish one ethical theory from another. Most persons, irrespective of their formal background in ethics, have heard the terms *hedonistic* and *stoic*. Hedonism and stoicism are two different ethical theories and determine what is right or wrong in two different ways. In hedonism (and there are multiple forms), an action is right or wrong in proportion to the amount of pleasure it produces, or the proportion of pleasure over pain. It should be mentioned that in hedonism pleasure is not necessarily defined as one usually thinks of pleasure. In stoicism (again, there are variant types), an action is right or wrong in proportion to its conformity to sound reason and nature, which includes freedom from passion and indifference to joy or grief.[11] There are other theories in ethics that specify what is right and wrong in yet other ways.

Within normative ethics, under norms of obligation, there are two major subdivisions, teleological and deontological systems of ethics. It is customary in bioethics books to discuss both systems, a brief introduction to which is given here. The importance of the teleological-deontological discussion differs here from that of other books. In the end, most theories (though not all) in either category focus on ethical principles and rules as action guides. This book focuses on the principles and rules themselves, rather than on any involved discussion of the theories that generate those rules.

Teleological theories (from *telos,* Greek for "end") determine an action to be right or wrong based on the consequences the action produces. Teleological ethics is sometimes called consequentialist ethics. Because hedonism and stoicism determine the rightness or wrongness of an action based on the consequences produced, they both fall within the category of consequentialist ethics. In teleological theories, however, more than just consequences must be examined. An action is right or wrong based on the consequences produced, *as measured over against a specific end that is sought, a nonmoral value,* such as pleasure or utility or dispassion. This is precisely the point at which norms of nonmoral value become important to ethics. For it is nonmoral values, such as pleasure, that are the *telos,* the ends of teleological theories. Or, stated another way, that which is right (to do) is a function of that which is good (to seek or cherish) in teleological theories.

The most important teleological theory for contemporary health care is *utilitarian* ethics. John Gay developed the philosophy of utilitarianism, from a theological base, in the 1700s in England. Subsequent prominent exponents of utilitarianism, all British, were Jeremy Bentham, John Stuart Mill, Henry Sigwick, Hastings Rashdall, and G. E. Moore.

Utilitarianism asserts that a right act is one that produces the greatest amount of pleasure or happiness over pain. However, if you wish to gauge whether pleasure is produced in the greatest amount or whether pleasure exceeds pain, there must be a way to measure the pleasure that is produced. Bentham, one of the most influential of the utilitarians, formulated a "calculus" by which pleasure could be measured. Given his sensitivity to social issues (what he called "public ethics"), pleasure was to be understood in terms of utility, and especially social utility. The calculus included an assessment of the intensity, duration, certainty/uncertainty, propinquity (remoteness), fecundity, and purity of the pleasure. Actually, this calculus is not too dissimilar to assessing the dimensions of symptomatology in which the patient is asked the intensity, duration, location, and other aspect of his or her pain.

Many of us remember important, though obscure, bits of information through jingles or acrostics: "Every good boy does fine" for the treble clef, HOMES for the Great Lakes, "King Philip sailed . . ." for kingdom, phylum, species. In a wonderful recognition of the frailties of the human mind, Bentham composed the following (not easily remembered or understood) verse to assist in remembering the qualities of his calculus:

> *Intense, long, certain, speedy, fruitful, pure—*
> Such marks in *pleasures* and in *pains* endure.
> Such pleasures seek, if *private* be thy end:
> If it be *public,* wide let them *extend.*
> Such *pains* avoid, whichever be thy view:
> If pains must come, let them extend to few.[12]

J. S. Mill, Bentham's disciple, modified Bentham's utilitarianism. It is Mill who is credited with the principle of the "greatest good for the greatest number." This is a popular understanding of Mill, but does a disservice to his work by oversimplifying it. His utilitarianism is better understood as seeking "the greatest possible balance of value over disvalue for all persons who would be affected."[13]

Utilitarian theories can judge the rightness or wrongness of an action on a situation-by-situation basis. Mill and subsequent utilitarians, however, have leaned toward the form of utilitarianism that is based on the premise that *adherence to certain moral rules* will generally produce the greatest value over disvalue in their consequences. That is, rather than judging the utility of single acts situationally (referred to as *act utilitarianism*), Mill and others have preferred to judge utility through the use of rules (called *rule utilitarianism*).

There are other ethical theories that depend on something other than consequences to determine the rightness or wrongness of an action. These theories do not maintain that consequences are unimportant, only that they do not determine what is right or wrong. These theories are usually termed *deontological* (from *deon*, Greek for "duty") or *formalist* theories.In deontological ethics, the intrinsic quality of the action itself or its conformity to a rule determines the rightness or wrongness of the action. For instance, breaking a promise could be considered to be intrinsically wrong. Most situations, however, have extenuating circumstances; in some instances it would be better to break than to keep a promise, particularly if the promise were minor and breaking it would save a life.

Immanuel Kant, a brilliant German philosopher, is the chief representative of formalism. Ethical formalism generally results in the use of principles or their derivative rules to guide decision making. Thus the issue of promise keeping produces the rule that promise keeping is right. Given that rules can produce untoward results when viewed as absolute, perhaps it is better stated that promise keeping is "right making," if not always right. In ethical formalism rules are regarded as *contentless forms* (hence the term *formalism*). Forms are rules without specification, without content. For example, "thou shalt not kill," is a contentless form. It neither defines killing nor specifies conditions under which killing might be socially permissible. Yet it is clear that killing is done in civilized societies (war, capital punishment). It is also clear that killing must be justified, as unjustified killing is severely punished. "Thou shalt not kill" is a general contentless rule that society upholds but which must be given content when applied to specific situations. One contentful reformulation of the rule is, "It is always wrong directly to take innocent human life." This restatement adds content, sufficient to permit limited types of killing while prohibiting others and upholding the general rule.

Rules can be valid only when they meet certain conditions. Kant formulated one condition, in three restatements, that must be satisfied for a moral rule to be considered valid. He called this condition the "categorical imperative." That the restatements are identical, despite Kant's claim, is not clear. Paul Taylor has provided a lucid "translation" of the categorical imperative in its reformulations:[14]

1. For a rule to be a rule, it must be consistently universalizable.
2. For a rule to be a moral rule, it must be such that, if all men follow it, they would treat each other as ends in themselves, and never as means only.
3. For a rule to be a moral rule, it must be capable of being self-imposed by the will of each person when he is universally legislating.

What these reformulations say, in part, is that valid moral rules should be applicable to all persons, without exception. Second, rules must lead to treating the persons involved as persons of absolute worth—as ends, not merely as means to another's ends. Third, persons who choose to embrace a rule as self-chosen, and are not coerced to accept it, acknowledge the universally valid nature of that rule. These conditions give rise to the principles and rules that are often discussed in the bioethical literature: principles of justice, autonomy, nonmaleficence, beneficence, fidelity, veracity, confidentiality, and so forth.

The distinction between principles and rules is generally that principles are basic and rules are derived from principles. Different authors identify principles differently, but this does not reflect a difference in views of the importance of the different principles. Rather, it reflects differences in opinion as to which are basic principles and which are derived rules.

A detailed discussion of deontology and teleology, specifically Kantianism and utilitarianism, has been deliberately avoided here for good reason. Even if space would allow, both utilitarianism and Kantianism result in the use of *principles* and *rules* in ethical decision making, though their justification of the use of rules does differ. Utilitarians use rules because their use will generally produce consequences that most closely approximate the ends they seek. Deontologists use rules because the rules are intrinsically "right making," irrespective of the consequences they may produce in a particular situation. Because both systems employ rules, it is presumably more beneficial to focus on the principles and rules themselves rather than on the nuances of the underlying theories. These principles and rules are discussed individually in Chapters 3 to 8 and include autonomy, nonmaleficence, beneficence, fidelity, veracity, justice, and duties to self.

Norms of Moral Value

Norms of obligation specify our duties and obligations. Norms of value specify what we are to be or to seek as goods or ends. Those norms of value that identify what is good or bad, or virtuous and evil, in *persons* are called *norms of moral value*. Norms of moral value are also called *virtues*. Virtues are habits of character that predispose a person to meet his or her duty, to do what is right.[15] They are learned and practiced, not inherited or associated with personality.

A subset of virtues, *excellences,* is of more interest to us here. Excellences are those habits of character that predispose a person to do a specific skill or task well.[16] They are the traits of character that one would see in a "good critical care nurse." Too little attention is given these days to identifying and fostering the excellences neces-sary to critical care nursing. This is not to say that nursing should return to the days of scrutinizing the moral purity of its members. Rather, the profession must give greater thought to identifying the virtues and excellences it considers essential for its practi-tioners, both in general and specialty practice.

In addition, nursing must attend to the proper construction of a moral milieu that will cultivate and support the desired excellences. For example, work loads should not be so heavy that they prohibit nurses from being compassionate, patient, wise, or knowledgeable. The moral environment should be such that knowledge, skill, professional growth, and competence are both expected and rewarded. In terms of excellences, the practice, research, or education environment that is created must be commensurate with the virtues and excellences that are demanded of the nurse.

Norms of Nonmoral Value

Norms of nonmoral value specify what we are to cherish or seek as ends; they specify what are intrinsic goods or values to be sought for their own sake. Nonmoral values form the ends that teleological theories seek. They are also inherent in every human endeavor, nursing included. Nursing itself cherishes intrinsic values such as human dignity, well-being, and human worth. Other less global goods are also part of nurs-ing: comfort, care, respect, and meaningful life. Certainly, critical care nursing, as a member of the broader nursing community, also holds these generic nursing values dear. Perhaps, however, there are values, specific to critical care nursing, which go beyond the goods or ends general nursing seeks? This question will be explored fur-ther in Chapter 9.

Professional Ethics and Policy Formulation

Normative ethics gives rise to several subdivisions of relevance to nursing practice (see Fig. 2-3). Norms of obligation and norms of value combine to produce two areas. The first is the field of applied ethics and the various subcategories of applied ethics. Every discipline or profession has its particular ethical concerns. Medicine has its own, law its own, divinity its own, business its own, and nursing its own. Profes-sional ethics is one type of applied ethics. Bioethics, ethics applied to the life sci-ences, is also a form of applied ethics. Both nursing and medical ethics can be viewed as subtypes of bioethics.

In addition to applied ethics, a second area arises from both norms of obligation and norms of value: the area of moral policy formulation. Moral policy formulation involves the process of giving voice, through policies and position statements, to professional obligations and values in terms of their contact with specific societal is-sues. Policies and position statements can be formulated to represent the moral ac-tion guides of a group of virtually any size. In some instances, groups that are power brokers within society may not actually prepare policies, but may instead present documents that function as either the ground for policy development or as quasi-policies themselves.

The President's Commission for the Study of Ethical Problems in Medicine and Biomedical and Behavioral Research is an example of one such body. Authorized by Congress in 1978, the Commission was convened in 1980. Its 21 members represented the disciplines of law, theology, ethics, medicine, sociology, economics, and biomedical sciences. Nursing was not initially represented, but a nurse was subsequently appointed to the Commission upon the resignation of an attorney.

The Commission's task was to "[study] problems whose value components are at least as important as their technical aspects."[17] As a result of its work, the Commission produced nine reports, one of which is *Deciding to Forego Life-Sustaining Treatment*,[18] the largest and most controversial of the Commission's documents. Though this and the other reports are not themselves statements of policy, they are consensus reports that lay the groundwork for policy statements. The Los Angeles County Bar and Medical Associations and the Hospital Council of Southern California's "Principles and Guidelines Concerning the Foregoing of Life-Sustaining Treatment for Adult Patients," which cites the President's Commission report, is an example of a policy document that draws upon the Commission's report.[19]

In addition to consensus reports, the federal government produces actual policies enacted through regulation or legislation. As part of the Department of Health, Education, and Welfare (DHEW), the National Commission for the Protection of Human Subjects of Biomedical and Behavioral Research made recommendations to DHEW and Congress for regulation of research using human subjects. The recommendations were published in the *Federal Register* and deal with special categories of human subjects, such as research involving children, prisoners, and the institutionalized mentally infirm. What the recommendations (later adopted as regulations) set forth are the conditions that must be met for any research grant to be considered for support or sponsorship by DHEW or other divisions of the government. The control of research that does not satisfy the regulations is indirect; the recommendations serve as the basis for refusal of funding (which itself may prevent the research from going forward).

Policy formulation gives ethics both bark and bite through actual policy statements, as well as through position statements, guidelines, and similar documents of varying degree of enforceability. As noted above, enforcement is sometimes indirect, and depends on granting or withholding funding or endorsement of a project. Policy and position statements are also developed by professional organizations and professional specialty groups. In late 1983 the American Nurses' Association (ANA) published a position statement on the nurse's participation in capital punishment by lethal injection.[20] (Statements like this are generally understood to represent the position of the profession as a whole on an issue.) The Massachusetts Nurses' Association, a state nurses' association (SNA) of the ANA, has a policy statement on "whistleblowing," formally entitled "Ethics for Patient Protection: Guidelines for Nurses."[21]

Specialty organizations, such as the American Association of Critical-Care Nurses (AACN), also formulate policy and develop position statements on specific issues of social import. AACN recently published a statement entitled Statement on Ethics in Critical-Care Research.[22] (The statement is reproduced in Appendix I.) As with the federal guidelines, this statement cannot prohibit research that does not meet AACN's guidelines. It does mean that, by way of sanctions, research projects that do not conform to the statement will not receive organizational support or endorsement, and findings of such projects would not likely be published in any of the organization's publications. The usefulness of specialty organizational work on policy statements is that they may develop statements that address concerns of the nurse-specialist that are not encountered by the nurse-generalist. There is, though, a need for greater collaboration among the various nursing organizations in preparing policy and position statements on generic issues common to all nurses (such as reporting irregular medical practice).

Individual hospitals, agencies, and nursing schools also develop policies. With increasing frequency, hospitals are preparing guidelines on a variety of issues, such as writing "do not resuscitate" (DNR) orders. Health care organizations are also preparing policies on admission or treatment of indigent persons, and others who cannot pay for services. Nursing schools, which have lagged behind in some areas, have finally begun to formulate human subjects guidelines, particular to the values and norms of nursing and to the individual schools represented. It is generally unwise for nursing to rely on the policies established by medicine or institutions, such as a university, to reflect the particular concerns of this profession. Nursing must give voice to its own values and obligations through the formulation of its own policies and positions. Policy issues and policy formulation are crucial to ethics from at least two perspectives. First, it is through policy statements and guidelines that the norms of a group are given public voice and force. Second, there are few policy issues that do not have a moral aspect.

Sound policy formulation and enactment are critical to the practitioner. It is policy that allows the professional to act on the norms of the profession within society. Policies set forth official professional expectations and allow for the development of mechanisms and processes for relevant action. These expectations, then, become the standards of the profession by which individual professional actions are judged. Policies also serve as standards for professional groups themselves in terms of their long-range goals, the allocation of organizational resources, or the establishment of professional priorities.

Moral policy formulation is also important to a profession in that it is one aspect of broader policy formulation processes. There are few issues in society or within a profession that are solely moral issues and of no interest to the law or other regulation. However, there are few significant policies that do not contain a moral element. It is ludicrous to think that a policy on the allocation of health care resources for the elderly could be free of any consideration of justice, a specifically moral concern. Likewise, "Baby Doe" and "Grandpa Doe" policies or regulations cannot be written without some regard for treatment and the moral discussion surrounding the quality of life–sanctity of life debate. Thus, when moral policy does not stand alone, it can be incorporated into broader policy concerns that address large social issues.

35

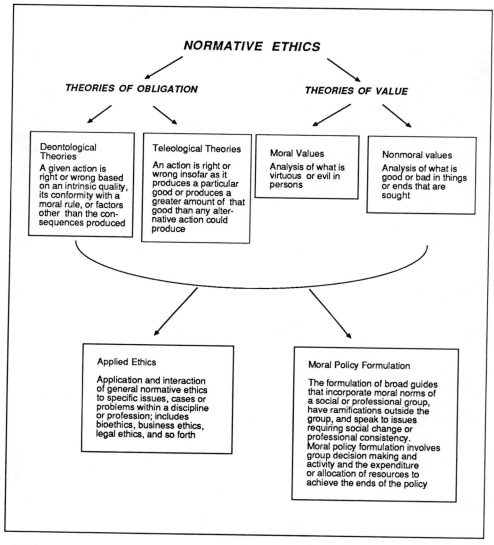

Figure 2-3. Divisions of normative ethics. Copyright © 1984, Marsha D. Fowler, adapted with permission

Conclusion

This book emphasizes normative ethics and its application to the moral concerns of the critical care nurse. Succeeding chapters focus on an overview of norms of obligation, and nursing's interpretation of those norms, as well as norms of moral and nonmoral value. It is critical that the reader never lose sight of the importance of character to obligation and obligation to character. The nurse who knows his or her moral obligations must have the character to meet them. If, however, the nurse has the character to do what is right but does not know her or his obligations, that nurse drifts without direction. Norms of obligation must always be joined to norms of moral value.

Care must be taken to understand, in each moral discussion, that terms can be used in different ways. Nursing discussions of autonomy often collapse when a speaker fails to make clear to another whether autonomy is being discussed as a principle (as in respect for autonomy), a virtue (the autonomous nurse), or an end that is sought (patient autonomy). In some cases, the term remains the same whether the discussion is focused on a norm of obligation or a norm of value. This book discusses both obligations and values.

Often, the place where obligations and values come together is in the nurse-patient relationship. Chapter 9 will discuss the nurse-patient relationship in terms of duties, virtues, and nonmoral values. Chapter 11 will move one step further and explore the processes and mechanisms whereby the nurse can act, within an institution or the profession, to live out those duties and values.

Nursing is an inherently moral endeavor, with a long, rich, and heroic moral tradition that suffuses its practice. At every point in the book, an effort has been made to deal with nursing-specific concerns within the critical care environment and to pose questions and responses that reflect nursing's distinguished ethical tradition and moral perspectives. We agree with Jameton, who has written:

> Nursing is the morally central health profession. Philosophies of nursing, not medicine, should determine the image of health care and its future directions. In its anxieties to control the institutions and technology of health care, medicine has allowed the central values of health care—health and compassion—to fall to the hands of nursing. Nurses thus supply the real inspiration and hope for progress in health care, and among health professionals, represent the least equivocal commitment to their clientele.[23]

We would go further and assert that those values have always been and remain a large part of nursing's moral tradition. Nursing is, indeed, the hope and inspiration for progress in health care.

Notes

1. Ewing AC: Ethics, p 1. London, English Universities Press, 1953
2. ANA: Guidelines for Implementing the Code for Nurses. Kansas City, MO, ANA, 1980
3. Beauchamp TL, Childress JF: Principles of Biomedical Ethics, pp 228–229. New York, Oxford University Press, 1979
4. Plato: Euthyphro, Apology, Crito, and Symposium, Hadas, M (trans), p 13. South Bend, IN, Gateway Editions Ltd, 1953
5. Frankena W: Ethics, 2nd ed, p 4. Englewood Cliffs, Prentice-Hall, 1973
6. Taylor P: Principles of Ethics: An Introduction, p 5. Belmont, CA, Dickinson, 1975
7. Uustal D: Values Education in Baccalaureate Nursing Curricula in the United States. PhD diss (unpublished), University of Massachusetts, Amherst, 1982

8. Ibid
9. Gilligan C: In a Different Voice. Cambridge, Harvard University Press, 1982
10. Frankena, op cit, p 10
11. Jones WT: The Classical Mind: A History of Western Philosophy, 2nd ed. New York, Harcourt Brace Jovanovich, 1969
12. Bentham J: The principles and morals of legislation. In Melden AI: Ethical Theories: A Book of Readings, 2nd ed, p 385. Englewood Cliffs, Prentice-Hall, 1967
13. Mill JS: Utilitarianism (1861). Priest O (ed): Indianapolis, Bobbs-Merrill, 1957
14. Taylor, op cit, p 88
15. Frankena, op cit, pp 62–63
16. Aristotle: Nichomachean Ethics, p 33. Ostwald M (trans): Indianapolis, Bobbs-Merrill, 1962
17. President's Commission for the Study of Ethical Problems in Medicine and Biomedical and Behavioral Research: Summing Up, p 3. Washington, DC, Government Printing Office, 1983
18. President's Commission for the Study of Ethical Problems in Medicine and Biomedical and Behavioral Research: Deciding to Forego Life-Sustaining Treatment. Washington, DC, Government Printing Office, 1983
19. Los Angeles County Bar Association: Deciding to Forego Life-Sustaining Treatment. Los Angeles, LA County Bar Association, 1985
20. ANA: Statement on Nurses' Participation in Capital Punishment. Kansas City, MO, ANA, 1983
21. Massachusetts Nurses' Association: Ethics for Patient Protection: Guidelines for Nurses. Boston, MNA, 1986
22. AACN: Ethics in Critical Care Nursing Research. Newport Beach, CA, AACN, 1986
23. Jameton A: Nursing Practice: The Ethical Issues, p xvi. Englewood Cliffs, Prentice-Hall, 1984

Chapter 3
Autonomy, Advocacy, and Accountability: Ethics at the Bedside

Sara T. Fry

During the past few years, the need for technical competence in the care of the critically ill patient has increased partly as a result of the growing number of complex technical functions assumed by the nurse in critical care units. To meet this need, educational programs in nursing are emphasizing the use of new technologies in health care and are developing specialized programs of study in critical care nursing. Nurses who have undertaken these programs of study are considered to be skilled practitioners capable of utilizing highly sophisticated technologies in carrying out the nursing process in critical care areas. They epitomize the "very best" in terms of nursing competence and skill.

Yet these same nurses are often criticized for participating in or even compounding the impersonal and dehumanizing methods of providing needed critical care services. Despite the severity of illness or the need for critical care services, patients have basic human needs to have their choices respected and to be protected from harm. Patients especially need protection from manipulation by others or to be protected from outright harm from the use of new technologies and treatment plans during times of diminished autonomy due to illness states or lack of information. Thus, some of the traditional values of nursing have gained new importance in the face of new technologies and advances in critical care nursing and medicine. These values—respect for patient self-determination (or autonomy), patient advocacy, and nurse accountability—and their dimensions in critical care nursing are the subject of this chapter.

Autonomy

The term *autonomy* is used to refer to different characteristics of the concept of autonomy. The term can refer to self-determined choice, or freedom of action, or individual liberty, or self-governance according to a principle that the individual would will for everyone. These different uses of the term reflect two origins of the concept of autonomy in modern thought.[1]

The value of autonomy expressed as respect for the unconditional worth of a person is based on the view of autonomy expounded by the 18th-century philosopher Immanuel Kant.[2] Kant argued that persons are rational individuals capable of making choices according to moral principles that could be willed universally valid for everyone. Because of this capacity, persons *ought* to be treated as ends in themselves and never as a means to the ends or means of others. To be an autonomous agent is to be self legislating in terms of valid moral principles that the individual would will for everyone. To respect autonomy is to respect this capacity in other persons and to allow them to make choices according to the principles that they would will or legislate for themselves. To respect persons in this manner is to treat them as an end in themselves and not as a means to one's own ends or the ends of others.

The value of autonomy expressed as respect for individual thought and action is based on the view of the 19th-century philosopher John Stuart Mill.[3,4] Mill was a utilitarian and believed that autonomous thought and action are beneficial to the welfare of individuals and the welfare of the state. He argued that persons have the right to make autonomous choices of any type according to their personal convictions. Other persons cannot interfere with this right as long as the choices made do not limit the freedom of choice of others and do not harm others. According to Mill, it is in the public interest to allow persons to have the opportunity to make individual choices in this manner in order that they might develop their full potential and contribute to the state. In fact, Mill would even argue that one role of government is to foster social conditions that would allow the development of a person's character to choose according to self-determined plans developed by the individual. The development of this right is fundamentally important to the moral order of the state and the concept of government.

Components of Autonomy

Respect for Unconditional Worth of the Individual—Respect for Individual Thought and Action

Both views on the value of autonomy are contained in the definition of autonomy usually discussed in the bioethical literature. According to Beauchamp and Childress, "the autonomous person determines his or her course of action in accordance with a plan chosen by himself or herself."[5] Such a person is able to legislate principles of conduct (Kant) and is able to follow a plan of action in accordance with the principles chosen (Mill). Persons who have diminished autonomy are not capable of acting according to a plan of action that they have chosen. They are incapable of either willing their principles of conduct, choosing a plan of action, or of acting on the plan.

To respect autonomy is to respect the individual right of self-governance according to a plan that is chosen and followed by the individual. Following the distinctions of autonomy raised by both Kant and Mill, to respect autonomy is to treat a person as an end in himself or as someone who has legislated his own principles of conduct that he would also will as valid moral principles for everyone. It also means to respect the plan of action that has been chosen or implemented by that individual. To reject an individual's plan of action or to restrict the freedom of an individual to act on the plan of action that they have chosen is to disrespect autonomy.

To say that nurses ought to respect autonomy is to assert a principle of autonomy as a guideline for action on the part of the nurse. It is a broad principle in that it is binding on all nurses. For example, to say that the nurse respects the autonomous choices of patients is to follow procedures for gaining the informed consent of the patient before initiating procedures or treatment involving the patient. Nurses believe that it is important to gain the permission (or consent) of the patient before beginning nursing or medical treatment. The treatment offered must be one that the patient would choose or that would be congruent with the course of action that he would want implemented on his behalf. Therefore, soliciting the informed consent of the patient or making sure that the patient receives all the information that he needs to make an informed consent are ways that nurses respect the autonomy of the patient. The statement that nurses ought to respect autonomy also presents autonomy as a prima facie principle, meaning that it is to be followed unless it is overridden by another moral principle of greater weight or standing. For example, it may not always be possible to allow patients to make their own choices or to follow the course of action that they have chosen. The choice of action might be perceived harmful to the person or harmful to other parties. Furthermore, the capacity of the individual to make autonomous choices might be in question. In these situations, the obligation to prevent harm to others or to benefit the patient is perceived as having greater weight than the obligation to respect autonomy.

Autonomy and Respect for Persons

This principle is also different from the principle of respect for persons in that it entails respect for self-determined choice of action. To respect persons *simpliciter* is to respect another individual as someone who shares the same human destiny as oneself. To respect self-determined choice is to respect choice as one way that an individual may autonomously realize his or her destiny, even though a person may realize his or her destiny through other means as well. Thus, respect for persons is a more abstract principle, whereas respect for autonomy is a specific principle regarding principles of conduct that can be willed by the individual that result in a *principled* plan of action chosen and followed by the individual.

As a principle guiding nursing actions, respect for autonomy does not apply to patients who are not capable of acting autonomously. In other words, the obligation to follow the principle of autonomy does not apply if the patient is a young child or is comatose, severely mentally retarded, or mentally ill. Obviously, it may be a difficult principle to follow in critical care settings where autonomy is often compromised by the use of technologies that reduce autonomous action on the part of the patient, by the administration of potent life-saving medications that affect judgment, and by the severity of illness that affects the patient's ability to make choices, however temporarily. Although it is a moral principle that is highly valued by the nursing profession, it is often compromised due to illness or the inability of the patient to articulate his or her choices. In these situations, another value of the nursing profession helps assure that the basis of autonomy—respect for persons—is protected when patients are substantially nonautonomous.

Advocacy

The term *advocacy* is one that primarily means active support of an important cause. It is often used in a legal context to refer to the defence of basic human rights on behalf of those who cannot speak for themselves. For example, many hospitals employ patient advocates who are expected to defend and speak for patients who cannot, by virtue of hospitalization or diminished autonomy as a result of illness, voice their own choices or assert their own rights. The role of the advocate is, therefore, to assert the patient's choices or desires on his behalf, similar to the way a lawyer presents the case of his client, pleads for an interpretation of the case, and defends his client's right in the case.

Models of Advocacy

Rights Protection Model

In the nursing literature, at least three views of advocacy can be found. The first view is the legal metaphor or *rights-protection model*. The nurse is viewed as the defender of patient rights against an impersonal health care system that violates patient rights. The nurse has the responsibility to inform the patient about his or her rights in the hospital (for example, discussing the American Hospital Association's Patient's Bill of Rights), making sure the patient understands these rights and knows how to exercise them within the health care system. It is presumed that the nurse also serves as the one to whom the patient reports infringements of his rights and is the appropriate member of the system to ameliorate infringements and prevent further violations.

This view of advocacy has been extensively discussed by Winslow as a basic model of ideal nursing practice.[6] According to Winslow, the metaphor of advocacy in nursing involves the defense of the patient against infringements of his or her rights and has been "adopted" by nursing to protect and enhance the personal autonomy of patients. Advocacy is, in fact, "nursing's new ethic" as evidenced by nurse advocate stories in the literature,[7,8] the requirement of "advocacy projects" in basic nursing education,[9] and the language of advocacy in the interpretive statements of the American Nurses' Association's Code for Nurses.[10] Even though Winslow recognizes that the advocacy metaphor in nursing needs further clarification, is not widely accepted by patients, is not protected by state nurse practice acts, is controversial, and engenders conflicting loyalties and interests for the majority of nurses, he still views

crucial to the well-being of the nation."[28] Other authors have discussed the value of accountability in primary care nursing,[29] in research,[30] or have focused on legal accountability and its relationship to other concepts such as autonomy and authority.[31]

Throughout all these discussions of accountability, the value of accountability is consistently noted. It is a value related to the social responsibilities of nursing, and to the moral and legal requirements of nursing practice. Yet no specific model of accountability is supported in the nursing literature. Accountability is valued by the nursing profession, but it remains without substantive description and material evaluation in various areas of nursing practice. Clearly, the need for accountability in nursing has increased partly as a result of the growing use of new technologies in caring for the critically ill individual and partly as a result of growing recognition that answerability for what is done in the nursing role has economic and political, as well as moral and legal, dimensions. Accountability is related to power in the health care arena and is a value that needs to be cultivated and developed within the individual nurse practitioner. Accountability is also a value that seems consistently intertwined with the values of autonomy and advocacy. How are these values related? What are their implications for critical care nursing?

Value Relationships

The relationships of autonomy, advocacy, and accountability are demonstrated by the following case situation in critical care nursing:

When the Wishes of the Patient Are Uncertain

Cecily Thornton is a nurse in a critical care unit in a large midwestern medical center well known for the excellence of its critical care facilities. One day, J. Clive Smythe, a 62-year-old man was admitted to the intensive care unit (ICU) from the recovery room following cardiac arrest post–surgical repair of an inguinal hernia. He had received CPR in the recovery room, was intubated, and his blood pressure was being maintained by vasopressors. While in the recovery room, a physician who had treated Mr. Smythe several months ago for myocardial infarction, recognized the patient and informed the resident in charge of the code that Mr. Smythe had been a DNR on his last admission because he had a living will and did not want to receive extraordinary support measures. The attending physician made a note on the chart that Mr. Smythe might have a living will and transferred the patient to the ICU.

When admitted to the ICU, Mr. Smythe's systolic BP was in the 70s while on vasopressors. He responded to commands, opened his eyes, gripped Ms. Thornton's hands, and responded to pain in the upper extremities (his lower extremities were still under the effects of the spinal anesthesia from his surgery). Cardiac monitoring showed that the patient was still having sinus tachycardia; $CO = 6.8$, $SUR = 800$; $PCWP = 28$; temp 35.5 core; resp ABG improving with 730/42/60 on 100%; $IMV = 12$, $Peep = 5$.

After some consultation, the ICU resident and fellow approached Ms. Thornton and told her that they thought the continued treatment of Mr. Smythe was inappropriate considering his previous DNR orders on his last admission and the fact that he apparently had a living will. Although no relatives had, as yet, produced the living will, they felt that maintaining his blood pressure with vasopressors should be slowly discontinued. They asked Ms. Thornton to slowly turn off the IV drip of dopamine and dobutamine over the next hour. It was assumed that Mr. Smythe would not be resuscitated if he arrested again.

Obviously, this case raises several important issues about living wills and the appropriate mechanisms to communicate patient wishes contained in a living will. Its main value, however, concerns the meaning of significant human values and the relationships of the values of autonomy, advocacy, and accountability in nursing practice.

To respect autonomy is to respect self-determined choices according to a plan chosen by the self. If Mr. Smythe has previously requested no resuscitation if cardiac or respiratory arrest occurs, does he still want to maintain this request? Has anyone asked him what he wants? Is the nurse expected to follow through on presumed wishes of the patient or does the nurse have an obligation to make sure that the patient's requests are congruent with his current physical and mental condition? Respecting the value of autonomy seems to require that treatment be continued unless the patient has validly requested otherwise. Since Mr. Smythe seems to be responsive to his surroundings and able to communicate his wishes to some degree, it is surprising that no one has thought to *ask* the patient whether he has a living will, what his wishes for this situation are, if he understands what has happened to him, and how he is currently being treated. Even if it is established that Mr. Smythe does have a living will, it may still be uncertain that the will is even applicable to this illness and his treatment, and even if it is, there is no guarantee that it will be recognized by his attending physician in this situation. Does the patient know this? For Mr. Smythe to make informed choices about his treatment, he first needs information. Here, the value of advocacy interfaces dramatically with the value of autonomy in critical care nursing.

Ms. Thornton will need to consider whether there is an important cause surrounding Mr. Smythe's care that will need her active support. If Mr. Smythe needs information to make informed choices about his treatment, is this sufficient reason for her to assume an advocacy role on behalf of this patient? In this situation, there is a life-and-death issue, but does there need to be for there to be sufficient cause for the nurse to assume the advocacy role? Or is the fact that the patient needs information sufficient for the advocacy role? These are all questions that are best discussed *prior* to a situation similar to the case of Mr. Smythe. Realistically, they are rarely discussed until the acute moral discomfort created by a situation forces the nurse to assess the competing values of this type of situation and the importance of these values to the patient, the nurse, and other members of the health care team. Ms. Thornton might also consider the model of advocacy that is applicable to this patient and to her value system. If Mr. Smythe is capable of discussing his wishes and values, then she might follow the values-based decision model of advocacy. After providing information to Mr. Smythe, then she would assist him to make decisions concerning his care that are consistent with his wishes, beliefs, and desires. If Mr. Smythe is not capable of making his own decisions, even temporarily, she might need to consider the respect-for-persons model of advocacy. In this model, the nurse might have to act according to the welfare of the patient as perceived by herself or significant others to preserve Mr. Smythe's dignity, privacy, and previously made self-determined choices. Regardless of the model of advocacy that is chosen, Ms. Thornton will eventually need to provide some justification for the actions she has performed in the role of advocate. She will need to assume accountability for her actions or be answerable for how she has respected the basic human dignity of the patient unrestricted by other considerations. This means that she will be answerable for the quality of the services that she has rendered in response to the moral dimensions of the values of accountability, advocacy, and autonomy. All these values are anchored in the implicit trust relationship between client and nurse and are balanced by the nursing profession's obligation "to provide services with respect for human dignity and the uniqueness of the client, unrestricted by . . . the nature of health problems."[32]

Accountability: The Foundational Value

It has been suggested by some theorists that a superior moral standard in health care might entail that the health professional should act on the basis of a duty-based ethic to protect or respect self-determination in conjunction with the duty to keep promises.[33,34] Acting on this basis would be acting in accordance with what is right by the client rather than what is judged to be in his best interests. Once the health professional acts in accordance with the rightness of acts, in response to duties, then a foundation is made for a contractual relationship between the professional and client in matters of health care. This contract relationship is considered ethically superior to other types of relationships in health care because it is created by doing what is right by the client according to what duty requires, instead of on the basis of consequentialistic outcomes.

The profession of nursing has already taken a strong stand on the duty to respect autonomy and keep promises by the Code for Nurses' recognition that the nurse provides services with respect for human dignity unrestricted by other considerations. Because clients have rights to self-determination in health care, the nurse acts to preserve and safeguard this right through appropriate actions. Acting to preserve self-determination is thus couched in terms of a duty toward the preservation of the human dignity of the client. This duty is derived from the ethical principle of respect for persons, the foundational principle of the Code. This interplay between the principle of respect for persons and the duty to respect autonomy and the human dignity of the patient suggests that there is a partial foundation in nursing for the kind of contract relationship based on superior moral standards rather than on consequentialistic outcomes.

In nursing, the substance of this tentative contract relationship is articulated by the value of accountability. As the Code for Nurses acknowledges, the nurse meets the requirements of legal accountability through licensing procedures. Because society expects certain safe, minimum standards of competence from nurses, nurses are held legally accountable through their license to practice. However, the Code also claims that the nurse is ethically accountable, meaning that the nurse is morally answerable to someone for what one has done in the nursing role. To be answerable in this sense is to be able to provide moral justification, in terms of standards or norms recognized by the profession, for one's actions in the role of nurse.

Accountability, therefore, involves a relationship between at least two parties. It is a contract relationship in that the nurse is an agent who has entered into a contractual agreement to perform services and to be held answerable for performing them according to agreed-upon terms. Being answerable in this regard is a moral obligation and is derived from the nature of the implicit trust relationship between client and nurse. It is an obligation correlative to the patient's right to self-determination and competent nursing care.

Hence, accountability is the foundational value on which the values of autonomy and advocacy find sustenance in nursing. Accountability is the value that helps define the relationships of patient, nurse, and the public at large and is broadly articulated by the professional ethic. It sustains the moral dimensions of the nurse-patient relationship and also sustains the tradition of nursing, providing both the practice of nursing and the social role of nursing with its necessary historical content.

Conclusion

In critical care nursing, the complex and highly technical nature of nursing functions requires an astute knowledge of values important to the practice of nursing. The values of autonomy, advocacy, and accountability are traditional values of the nursing profession. However, in critical care settings, these values have interesting moral dimensions that are not well articulated in the nursing literature. This chapter has discussed these values in terms of their meanings, origins, and moral dimensions. All three values are demonstrated, through the use of a case situation, to have interrelationships that shape the performance of nursing functions in critical care settings. The foundational role of accountability in nursing practice is discussed in terms of its answerability requirements or the moral justifications provided by the nurse for protecting autonomy and assuming an advocacy role with the critically ill patient. It is argued that fulfilling moral requirements of nursing practice in critical care settings involves a contract relationship based on a duty-based ethic that respects autonomy and keeps promises. The value of accountability is viewed as the superior moral standard in nursing that provides the foundation for the contract relationship required in critical care nursing.

Notes

1. Beauchamp TL, Childress JF: Principles of Biomedical Ethics, 2nd ed. New York, Oxford University Press, 1983
2. Kant I: Groundwork of the Metaphysic of Morals (1785). Patton HJ (trans): New York, Harper & Row, 1964

3. Mill JS: On Liberty (1859). New York, Liberal Arts Press, 1956

4. Mill JS: Utilitarianism (1861). Priest O (ed): Indianapolis, Bobbs-Merrill, 1957

5. Beauchamp, Childress, op cit, p 59

6. Winslow GR: From loyalty to advocacy: A new metaphor for nursing. Hastings Cent Rep 14:32–40,1984

7. Smith CS: Outrageous or outraged: A nurse advocate story. Nurs Outlook 28:624–625, 1980

8. Tuma J: Letter: Professional conduct. Nurs Outlook 25:546, 1977

9. Namerow MJ: Integrating advocacy into the gerontological nursing major. Journal of Gerontological Nursing 8:149–151, 1982

10. ANA: Code for Nurses with Interpretive Statements. Kansas City, MO, ANA, 1985

11. Winslow, op cit, pp 32–40

12. Kohnke ME: The nurse as advocate. Am J Nurs 80:2038–2040, 1980

13. Fry ST: Ethics in community health nursing practice. In Lancaster J, Stanhope M (eds): Community Health Nursing: Process and Practice, pp 77–96. St Louis, CV Mosby, 1984

14. Gadow S: Existential advocacy: Philosophical foundation of nursing. In Spicker SF, Gadow S (eds): Nursing: Images and Ideals, pp 79–101. New York, Springer-Verlag, 1980

15. Abrams N: A contrary view of the nurse as patient advocate. Nurs Forum 17:258–267, 1978

16. Kohnke, op cit, p 2038

17. Gadow, op cit, pp 79–101

18. Ibid, p 85

19. Murphy CP: The moral situation in nursing. In Bandman EL, Bandman B (eds): Bioethics and Human Rights: A Reader for Health Professionals, pp 313–320. Boston, Little, Brown & Co, 1978

20. Murphy CP: Models of the nurse-patient relationship. In Murphy CP, Hunter H (eds): Ethical Problems in the Nurse-Patient Relationship, pp 9–24. Boston, Allyn & Bacon, 1983

21. Greenfield HT: Accountability in Health Facilities. New York, Praeger, 1975

22. Geekie DA: Professional accountability and evaluation. Can Med Assoc J 20:346, 1973

23. Churchill L: The professionalization of ethics: Some implications for accountability in medicine. Soundings 60:40–53, 1977

24. Downie RS: Roles and Values: An Introduction to Social Ethics. London, Methuen London Ltd, 1971

25. Bowie N: Role as a moral concept in health care. J Med Philos 7:57–63, 1982

26. McIntyre A: After Virtue. Notre Dame, University of Notre Dame Press, 1981

27. Fromer MJ: Professional accountability. In Ethical Issues in Health Care. St Louis, CV Mosby, 1981

28. Schlotfeldt RM: Accountability: A critical dimension in health care. Health Care Dimensions 3:137–148, 1976

29. Ciske KL: Accountability: The essence of primary nursing. Am J Nurs 79:891–894, 1979

30. Fry ST: Accountability in research: The relationship of scientific and humanistic values. Advances in Nursing Science 4:1–13, 1981

31. Murchison I, Nichols TS, Hanson R: Legal Accountability in the Nursing Process. St Louis, CV Mosby, 1978

32. ANA, op cit

33. Veatch RM: A Theory of Medical Ethics. New York, Basic Books, 1981

34. Veatch RM, Fry ST: Case Studies in Nursing Ethics. Philadelphia, JB Lippincott, 1987

Chapter 4

The Boundaries of Intervention: Issues in the Noninfliction of Harm

Anne J. Davis

Roger Kingston is a 58-year-old married man who was admitted to intensive care immediately following a truck-to-auto accident in which a truck driver fell asleep at the wheel, jumped the median, and collided head-on with the Kingston car. He has multiorgan system failure, multiple fractures, disfiguring burns of the left arm, and a traumatic amputation of the left foot. He is in excruciating pain, but awake and aware of what has happened. He can communicate with staff. There is some question as to whether or not he can be made to survive, even with intensive efforts. In that accident, he saw his wife, his childhood sweetheart, killed instantly. His two adult children, who were in the back seat of the car, escaped with minor injuries and were released from the emergency room within hours. He has now been in an intensive care unit for 10 weeks. He sees no reason to struggle to live and knows that you, the nurse, have the means to actively end his suffering. He asks you again, as his primary nurse and the person with whom he has the closest relationship, to overmedicate him, or to discontinue the ventilator. He knows that you are very uneasy about helping in this way. If you cannot, he wants you to stay with him and hold his hand while he pulls out his tracheostomy tube; it is understood that you would not call for help. He has also asked that you not tell others of his discussions with you. He pleads extreme pain, no reason to live, poor chances of survival, and pointless suffering. His situation is heartrending, and you fundamentally agree with his wish to end what seems to be extraordinary pain and intense suffering. The quality of his life seems to make it truly not worth living, both from the patient's perception and your own. How is a nurse to think about a situation such as this? What are the moral principles pertinent to this sort of dilemma? What are the nurse's options?

In the Western philosophical tradition, several ethical principles remain central to our notion of what constitutes the right thing to do. One of these principles, autonomy (discussed in Chapter 3), indicates the importance that we attach to the idea that competent adults should make their own decisions about health, life, and death. Another principle or duty central to our thinking, nonmaleficence, will be discussed in this chapter. Nonmaleficence is the duty to do no harm.

While both of these principles play central roles in our ethical decisions, nonmaleficence has long been a tradition in medicine and in nursing. Autonomy, on the other hand, has developed in the health sciences in a central way only relatively recently. If we were to summarize the present situation in health care ethics today, one description would identify uneven movement from more nonmaleficent ethics to ethics in which patient autonomy has become a more significant force in the decision-making process.

The way these two ethical principles have been presented here pits them, at least to some extent, against one another. Historically, in the name of nonmaleficence, health care professionals did not inquire about patients' values, hopes, wishes, or other personal perspectives. Nor did those professionals inform patients about their diagnosis and prognosis. The norm that functioned said that health professionals knew what was best for patients. Patients were neither to know too much about their condition or treatment nor to interfere in any way with that treatment. These behaviors were paternalistic on the part of the professionals and were often justified on the basis of "doing no harm."

This concept of doing no harm can be found in the earliest documents that serve to guide physicians and nurses in their practice. Documents such as the Hippocratic Oath and the much more recent Nightingale Pledge are two examples. In the Nightingale Pledge the nurse swears that she[1] " . . . will abstain from whatever is deleterious and mischievous, and will not take or knowingly administer any harmful drug."[2]

In the past we had fewer ways of doing good; we also had fewer methods of inflicting harm to the extent now possible. Formerly, infliction of harm was principally the result of nontreatment or inappropriate treatment. However, with the vast developments in scientific knowledge and the attendant technology necessary to implement it, a new category of harm has arisen. In today's technology, harm can result from carrying treatment too far because the use of technology generates additional physical problems (physical harm), the patient has been forced to receive treatment that was refused (personal harm), or the patient's life has been prolonged beyond all reasonable measure (harm to dignity and the sanctity of life). Obviously, few persons would wish to return to previous centuries when people died or were grossly debilitated by diseases or conditions that are no longer seen. But, as in much of our progress, technology creates situations in which trade-offs must be made. Essentially, patients benefit from health science technology, but they can be victimized by it as well.

Because the principle of nonmaleficence has been so central for so long in medicine, and nursing has accepted that value, nurses have a stringent duty not to harm others. With that in mind, we must examine the issues and problems that confront nurses so that we can clarify the boundaries of intervention and how nonmaleficence may conflict with other ethical principles, such as autonomy or beneficence (doing good).

The Principle of Nonmaleficence

Nonmaleficence means that we must not inflict harm on another person. There are many kinds of harm that lead us to employ specific subrules of nonmaleficence such as: do not kill; do not cause pain; do not disable; do not deprive another of her or his freedom or opportunity. It is important to understand that both the principle of nonmaleficence and these derivative rules are not absolute. That is, under certain circumstances it is ethically justifiable to inflict harm. Amputation, as a form of bodily mutilation, is a prime example of the justifiable infliction of harm. The use of invasive monitors, which yield information necessary to care for or heal patients, is another example. In instances in which we will do harm, that harm must ultimately be justifiable, usually to achieve some greater good or to prevent a greater harm.

Along with the duty to prevent intentional harm, nonmaleficence dictates that we minimize the probability of harm. Many activities and events in life have a risk of harm. For example, patients are asked to serve as research subjects when there is some risk of harm. Questions that arise in such situations are: (1) what is the level of risk? (2) what is the balance of potential harm over benefit? (3) what is the nature of the risk that is involved (physical, psychological, social), and (4) who benefits—this patient, future patients, science, society? Levels of risk vary according to (1) the procedure itself (e.g., research questionnaire versus an experimental drug protocol), (2) the nature of the harm that might occur (social, physical, financial, psychological, or other), and (3) the patient's value system (which ranks various harms).

Not all harm or even risk of harm is intentionally produced. The duty of nonmaleficence requires that we act carefully and thoughtfully toward others, so as not to knowingly inflict harm. Negligence is that conduct below a standard established by the law. While there is no moral rule against negligence per se, there is a moral rule to guard against risk of harm to others. Health professionals have a duty to practice within the standard of due care, which means they are knowledgeable, skilled, and diligent in their work. As part of due care, the Code for Nurses of the American Nurses' Association (ANA) requires that nurses keep abreast of new knowledge and skills to avoid doing harm.[3]

What constitutes due care will vary from place to place and from time to time. The policies and practices of a given health care profession in part define the applicable standard of care. For example, the ANA Code for Nurses requires that nurses act in ways that take into account selected ethical principles such as autonomy, beneficence, and nonmaleficence while practicing within the standards of due care. All such standards must acknowledge the inherent fallibility of clinical judgment, since due care cannot totally eliminate mistakes or prevent all harms.

Not only does nonmaleficence focus on issues of risk-benefit analysis, but also it takes into account the notion of detriment-benefit analysis. Risk-benefit analysis focuses on the harms that occur at the time of a given procedure; detriment-benefit analysis focuses on the consequences of the benefits. Amputation of an extremity is an example that can be viewed from a risk-benefit analysis (risk of sepsis, death, etc.) and from a detriment-benefit calculation, since the loss of a limb is, itself, a harm or detriment.[4] This is an important distinction, especially in cases in which death is caused or permitted and is ethically justifiable.

Balancing Good and Evil: The Principle of Double Effect

In any discussion of nonmaleficence the rule of double effect must be considered. This principle or rule, developed within a Roman Catholic ethical tradition, has been used to support claims that an act having harmful effects is not always morally prohibited. In these cases the harmful effect is viewed as an indirect, unintended, or merely unforeseen effect and not as the direct and intended effect of the action.[5]

Four conditions must be present for the principle of double effect to be used to support claims that an act that causes harm is not morally prohibited. These four conditions are: (1) the action itself must be good or at least morally indifferent, (2) the individual must intend only the good effect and not the evil effect, that is, the evil effect may be foreseen but not intended, (3) the evil effect cannot be a means to the good effect, and (4) there is a proportionately grave reason for permitting the evil effect, that is, there must be a proportionality or favorable balance between the good and the evil effects of the action.[6]

We often appeal to the principle of double effect in situations of moral ambiguity in which a good action will have undesirable or harmful effects. In those instances, it is not possible to help the patient by that action and at the same time avoid harming him. In the classic example, we have a duty of nonmaleficence toward a terminally ill pulmonary patient who is in great pain with a respiratory rate of ten. Suppose, however, that to alleviate pain the nurse must administer morphine sulfate, which has been known to cause respiratory depression in this patient. It is possible that the dose of morphine, sufficient to quell the pain, will also quell the patient's respirations. The nurse has a duty not to harm the patient and, as will be discussed in the next chapter, to benefit him positively. Is it permissible to give the morphine? Does it meet all four of the criteria of the principle of double effect?

Yes. The action, giving an injection of morphine, is itself a morally indifferent act. The relief of pain, not respiratory depression, is the intended effect. Respiratory suppression is not the means by which pain relief is achieved. The fourth criterion, the most important one in contemporary Catholic ethics, looks at the proportionality of the good and the evil. Relief of pain—and the consequent reduction of suffering—is seen as a sufficiently grave reason, or a proportionately greater good than the harm that is incurred—in this case respiratory suppression and likely death. The Code supports this position when it declares that "the nurse may provide interventions to relieve symptoms in the dying client even when the interventions entail substantial risks of hastening death."[7]

Letting Die and Killing

While the distinction between letting die and killing has recently come under some attack, and the distinction has been called morally insignificant, it remains useful for health professionals to understand this distinction and the argument that simultaneously supports letting die and not killing in some ranges of cases. Killing is only ethically and legally supported in cases of self-defense, military combat, and other socially sanctioned defenses of individuals and society.

Critics attack the letting die/killing distinction from various perspectives. For example, some believe that in reality it is impossible to make this distinction now that we have biomedical technology. Disconnecting the respirator has become a standard example of this problem. Other critics say that the distinction that is attempted has no moral punch or bite to it. And yet others say that it would be absurd to affirm the moral significance of this distinction and then accept *all* cases of letting die as morally fitting. (This last criticism points to the fact that in those instances of letting die that can be ethically justified, other criteria, such as detriment-benefit analysis, must be taken into account.)

It is important to know that while some critics attack the distinction between killing and letting die, others favor it for both moral and practical reasons. They say that the distinction enables us to express and to maintain ethical principles such as nonmaleficence and to avoid certain harmful consequences. They argue that we must ground this distinction in the difference between acts and practice.[8] They make the point that it is one thing to ethically justify an act and say it is the right thing to do; it is quite another thing to justify a general practice. This means that while particular acts of letting die may not violate the duty of nonmaleficence and probably would be compassionate and humane, a policy authorizing killing would probably violate the duty of nonmaleficence by causing a grave risk of harm in most, if not all, cases.[9]

On the other side of the letting die coin lies the problem of vitalism. Health professionals place great stock in the value and worth of the patient as a human being. The sanctity of life position, while most important and well grounded in our religious and secular beliefs, can also lead us to treat patients beyond the limits of their wishes or beyond the point of benefit. Going beyond these limits is referred to as *vitalism*. Vitalism is morally unacceptable in nursing because it violates the dignity of the individual and, therefore, is defined as doing harm.

Wedge Argument

While the distinction between acts and practices is useful to help us sort out aspects of an ethical problem, we also need to know about the *wedge argument* because it is useful in determining the adequacy of moral arguments for or against an action such as killing the suffering patient. The wedge argument can take one of two forms. The first, the *slippery slope* form of the argument, hinges on "logical distinctions" between acts, distinctions that are not necessarily as sharp as they would seem. For example, if society prohibits killing innocent persons, and permits taking of noninnocent lives (war, self-defense), and we actively take the lives of some patients (actively end suffering/life), there is no *logical* ground for *not* extending that form of killing to other innocent persons. As another example, some who argue for abortion fail to make a logical distinction between abortion and infanticide. The same reasons used to justify abortion (e.g., a fetus is not a person; personhood requires a sense of personal history, ability to communicate, cognitive schemata, etc.) can also be used to justify infanticide. Thus, the first version of the wedge argument claims that a justification that we use for an act that seems right to us may have logical implications for the justification of another act that strikes us as wrong. The ethical principle behind this logical implication is that of universalizability, which says that we should treat similar cases in a similar way. In short, if we judge action A to be right and we can point to no relevant dissimilarities between actions A and B, then we cannot judge action B to be wrong. Essentially, in this and other questions focused on the logical implications of decisions, we need to ask if there are morally relevant dissimilarities. The wedge argument is used to argue against the claim that killing and letting die are one and the same. It says: if letting die and killing are morally the same, then if it is rational and morally defensible to allow patients to die under A, B, and C conditions, then it is rational and morally defensible to kill them under those same circumstances. Clearly, nursing does not claim that letting die and killing are the same.

The second version of the wedge argument concerns itself with the probable impact that changing rules or making exceptions in situations will have. The argument in general goes as follows: if we remove specific restraints against killing, killing will increase, a moral decline in our society will occur, and those who are socially "undesirable" will be allowed to be killed. The second type of wedge argument, sometimes called a "social consequences argument," relies on social concerns while the first form relies on logical concerns; the two forms of argument provide fairly powerful defenses against actively taking the life of a suffering patient.[10]

The preceding discussion draws on the principle of nonmaleficence and examines in a general way some of the problems and issues in the letting-die question. But we need to develop these ethical considerations by placing them in specific clinical situations. In doing so, we shall see how the duty of nonmaleficence can conflict with other ethical principles. This means that we then have the situation in which if we act according to one principle we will violate another.

Clinical Cases and Nonmaleficence

To reason through an ethical dilemma, one must raise several specific questions. The first question is whether or not there is an ethical problem. For a situation to be an ethical problem it must have conflicting moral claims. That is, (1) the situation has something that you both ought and ought not to do, or (2) it makes competing demands—it has two oughts. The earlier example of keeping a terminally ill patient comfortable—but by using medications that can suppress respirations and hasten death—is a very good example of an ethical problem. Another example is a situation in which a competent patient wants to be allowed to die in peace, and the health care professional wants to treat him or her perhaps by using an experimental procedure. This is a case of two conflicting ethical principles: autonomy and beneficence. Although in general there are some limits to autonomy, patients have the right to make their own decisions about themselves. But health care professionals have the obligation to do good for patients. Where nonmaleficence enters this picture is in the question: is it doing harm even in the name of doing good to violate a patient's autonomous decision? One problem with individuals having the right to make their own decisions is that they may make a decision that goes against the values of the health professional. For example, a patient's refusal of treatment can produce the ethical problem whereupon autonomy and beneficence must be examined in terms of nonmaleficence.

But what about those clinical situations in which patients cannot make their own decisions because of their young age, their psychological status, their physical status, or their level of cognitive development? There is a duty of nonmaleficence on the part of those who speak for patients who cannot speak in their own interest. But what constitutes doing no harm in these situations? If the family or other second party person knows what the patient values and what he or she would most likely want in this situation, then not to take this information into account in the decision-making process is doing harm. The ANA Code for Nurses makes just such a claim: "The measures that nurses take to care for the dying client and the client's family emphasize human contact. They enable the client to live with as much physical, emotional, and spiritual comfort as possible, and they *maximize the values the client has treasured in life* [italics added]."[11] In addition, if the family were not sure what the patient would choose in a given situation, but were aware that treatment at a particular stage in the illness would only cause or increase suffering, with little possibility of benefit, then this most likely would be a case of doing harm.

The most difficult cases are those in which patients cannot speak for themselves, in which there is a fair amount of clinical uncertainty, but in which clinical judgment tends to lean in the direction of treating. Interestingly enough, in cases that have less or little ambiguity about diagnosis and prognosis—even if the patient cannot speak in his or her best interest—the ethical issues do not seem as difficult. If the clinical situation is judged to be terminal or if it is judged to be more than just hopeful, with some probability of getting better if not recovering entirely, then professionals are inclined to feel that the decisions tend to be more easily reached and ethically justified. The certainty in either direction helps us make ethical decisions about a given situation. In cases in which there is much clinical uncertainty or both clinical and moral uncertainty, decisions are more difficult. In situations of clinical and moral uncertainty, the ethical argument usually errs on the conservative side, of treating based on the principle of nonmaleficence.

In all these types of clinical cases, we need to ask what constitutes doing harm. When we raise this question, we need to think of harm not only as something physical, but also as those actions that violate the patient's autonomy or the family's stance, which, we must assume without evidence to the contrary, speaks in the best interests of the patient when the patient cannot speak on his or her own behalf.

When Help Becomes Harm

From the preceding comments, it becomes obvious that in some instances what we think of as help can be harmful by other definitions. Because we have a fundamental duty to do no harm, these situations of harm in the name of doing good are serious not only clinically but also legally and ethically. The following clinical case makes this point dramatically.

> By everyone's clinical judgment, the 73-year-old man in the cardiac critical care unit was terminally ill. His two children (both physicians) had met with the staff and the decision was made to have a no code order written, to discontinue the antibiotic, and to discontinue tube feedings. The participants in the discussion spent much time detailing what the patient would want if he could speak for himself. While these decisions were difficult for both the family and the staff, there was an overriding sense that this was the best thing to do and that withdrawing treatment would not harm the patient. The attending physician, a well-known cardiologist, was not present when the medical and nursing staff and the family members met. In fact, he had been out of town for some days. When he returned, he canceled all the orders written by the chief resident and in their place wrote: "Code, continue antibiotic and tube feedings." No communication with the family had taken place, so the nursing clinical specialist was not sure of the basis for this reversal of orders. She wondered if the new orders were doing harm not only to the patient but also to the patient's two children.

Now the questions arise: What, if anything, should the clinical specialist do? Does she have an obligation in those situations in which she thinks harm is being done? In this actual case, the clinical specialist called the family members and told them what had occurred and suggested that they contact the cardiologist for further discussion and some resolution of the situation. Meanwhile, however, the staff nurse is usually faced with the decision of withholding what is ordered and questioning the order, as opposed to proceeding as ordered while questioning the order.

The case presents a dramatic example, and in some ways this may be a typical ethical problem. Indeed, one could argue that this case seems sufficiently clear-cut as an ethical problem, so that figuring out what the clinical specialist should do is easy. But other situations may be less dramatic. What about when nurses proceed with treatments without patient consent? Does that constitute harm? And consider those cases in which staff members withhold information such as diagnosis or prognosis from the patient. The reason given for such an action usually is a combination of viewing the patient as unable psychologically to handle bad news and of our obligation to do good. But is that doing good, or is it doing harm? We know that we have the greater duty to do no harm. There are no easy answers to this ethical problem, other than to say that some patients cannot handle information while many others can. Situations in which patients would be truly unable to cope with or handle information are extremely rare. (They occur with greater frequency when it is the professional who has difficulty coping with the information.) This means that we need to know our patients, their values, and their psychological state, all of which we must take into account before we make any decision—cautiously and with sufficient deliberation and rational justification—to withhold information. Here, we can often turn to the family for assistance. When, in rare cases, information is to be withheld from the patient, it is not necessarily withheld from the family, and certainly not withheld from others. That is, the decision to withhold information is not to be a secret one. At the baseline, withholding information is considered harmful because doing so makes it impossible for people to make decisions and to act autonomously. There are some exceptions to always informing the patient, but we must be honest with ourselves and ask whether we withhold information because it is best for the patient—even though it is doing harm from one perspective—or whether we withhold information because it is best for us in that we don't have to deal directly with the ensuing problem of the patient knowing.

These are but a few of the ethical problems that arise and the questions we need to think about. In our thinking we always need to raise the ethical principle of non-maleficence or do no harm.

The Ethical Use and Non-Use of Technology

We are all both beneficiaries and victims of modern technology. While none of us would want to live in the 14th century, the time of the Black Death that wiped out large segments of the population, we must realize that we live in a time when the major way of thinking about technology, as good and as progress, has begun to be questioned.

A discussion of the ethical and nonethical use of technology can be very broad and can include social and health problems such as air pollution, nuclear weapons testing, or artificial hearts. But this discussion will be limited to those aspects of technology that are central to critical care units in hospitals.

Not many years ago, hospitals had no critical care units. The very existence of these units resulted from the development of knowledge and technology. While lives have been saved in them, the use of technology in these units has raised some of our most difficult ethical questions. These questions include those surrounding dying and death, the allocation of scarce resources, and the use and non-use of technology. Another issue that often arises is the dilemma of the suffering of the patient in the name of treatment. If the patient will benefit from the treatment, then the issue of doing harm is removed, provided the patient has given informed consent. But if the patient will not benefit from the treatment using technology, then to avoid harm, alleviation of suffering must take precedence.

The general rule is that if the patient will not benefit from the use of technology, then to use it will constitute doing harm. While it is often difficult to withhold treatment, there may and often does come a time when the non-use of technology is the best course and the most likely way to avoid doing harm. It is harmful not only to the patient, but also as a misuse of scarce resources.[12]

Some argue that the driving force in critical care units is the technological imperative. This argument says that when we have technology we are compelled to use it and the ethical question in this argument becomes: should we use technology simply because we have it?

In this and other discussions of technology, one problem becomes the very definition of what can be called "technology." In short, what are the boundaries of the concept of technology? Obviously, respirators and such machinery are considered to be technology. Pacemakers are also technology, though no longer "high" technology because they have become more commonplace. But are feeding tubes technology? While they are very different from respirators, feeding tubes are technology too. A recent court case involving the now deceased Mary Conroy said that feeding (here by NG tube) was treatment and not just the basic substance that sustains biological life. So we now have definitions that say technology includes everything that is an extension of the person, such as blood pressure apparatus and feeding tubes, and that feeding and even fluids are treatment.

Not to use technology when it would be beneficial is another potential situation of doing harm. However, as has been maintained by various writers, the use of technology for the benefit of the individual is greatly dependent on certain factors besides medical benefit. Where someone lives and whether certain technology is available are basic factors. More recently, economic issues have become another concern. If we decided not to use technology, should factors other than medical benefit come into our deliberations? Should factors such as age, ability to pay, or gender be considered? If we do use these as major criteria in the decision not to use technology, could we justify this ethically? While this type of situation may be a problem, it is most likely that overuse of technology is more of a problem at the present time.

Overuse of technology has become a problem due to several interrelated factors. Factors include the traditional lack of patient autonomy, the traditional physician ethics to do good (which meant to treat), and the physician's fear of legal action on the part of patients or their families. Another factor is the professional socialization process of medicine, which teaches that physicians must do everything they can, coupled with the need to do clinical research, not only to do good but also to do better, if not for this patient then for future patients. Though contemporary nursing is focused principally on the individual patient rather than "the unknown patient" of the future, medicine's focus, nursing's increasing concern for conducting research, and the pressure of tightening health care economics are additional factors that put nurses in the middle of the dilemmas of the overuse of technology.

Examples of overuse of technology can be found in many situations, not all of which are dramatic. What about the nurse who prefers to give a sleeping pill rather than a back rub, a quiet chat, a glass of hot milk, or all three rather old-fashioned nontechnological remedies? If medications or hot milk and conversation would accomplish the same end, should the milk or the pill be the first response? Or could we think of this approach to a nursing problem as doing harm? Many other similar clinical nursing problems can arise. Before we take the easiest way out, we need to ask ourselves whether we are doing harm.

Values

Our values, much like our breathing, are part of our taken-for-granted world. Before we can thoroughly examine clinical cases in critical care, we need to have as much awareness as possible of our values as people and nurses. (This will be discussed in Chapter 9.) What seems natural and proper and doing good may not be viewed that way by everyone at all times. We, as health professionals, value technology and what it can do for our patients. But we need to remember that people do not always share the same perceptions or values to the extent that we might think. In order to do no harm, we must be aware not only of our own values, but also of those that patients have. We also value actively doing something for the patient, and this grows out of our basic obligation to care and treat. Obviously, health professionals share many of the same root values. Therefore, one could argue that patients in the critical care unit are potentially vulnerable not only because of their physical and psychological status, but also because the shared values of the nursing (and probably medical) staff might not be those of the patients. This is a major reason why the principles of autonomy and of nonmaleficence must so often be taken together in tandem.[13]

Conclusion

One aspect of nonmaleficence that has not been addressed is the responsibility of the nurse, who may be party to doing harm while not necessarily having the central decision-making responsibility for the action. Some people have dealt with this type of situation by saying that they were "only following orders." They seem to think that this reply protects them ethically (and legally), which absolutely is not the case. It can be difficult to refuse to carry out a physician's order, particularly if the physician is a person of power within the institution and if nursing administration or nursing peers do not support such nursing actions. However, "just following orders" goes beyond being simply an inadequate defense; it is unconscionable in today's nursing climate. (See Chapter 3 for a fuller discussion of autonomy, advocacy, and accountability.)

It is important for each nurse to examine and evaluate a situation to determine if harm is being done or if the risk of harm is too great. In the process of this analysis, it is necessary for the nurse to gather as much morally relevant information as possible from patient, peers, family, and physician. The nurse must not stop at analysis; he or she must actively decide, and act on the basis of the evaluation. Ethical obligations are not discharged by default; a more proactive position is called for. In the final analysis, the nurse must weigh values and principles, evaluate options for action, and act with full knowledge of the ethical import of her or his decision. Wherever possible, the nurse should use the mechanisms and processes available within the institution as a vehicle for minimizing harm to the patient. As part of the moral analysis, the nurse must also be aware of any personal consequences that may derive from moral action within the setting, and act with the courage or perseverance that the situation demands. In doing so, the nurse builds on a tradition rich with examples of nurses who, in devotion to the patient, have met the duty of the noninfliction of harm.

Notes

1. Early nursing codes, pledges, and literature invariably referred to the nurse using the female gender. That custom will be employed here, to remain faithful to the intent or substance of the original documents; nonsexist language will be used for that period of time when nursing documents became gender indifferent (after the 1960s).
2. Gretter L: The Florence Nightingale Pledge, 1893
3. ANA: Code for Nurses with Interpretive Statements. Kansas City, MO, ANA, 1985
4. Beauchamp T, Childress J: Principles of Biomedical Ethics, 2nd ed, pp 111–112. New York, Oxford University Press, 1983
5. Mangan JT: An historical analysis of the principle of double effect. Theological Studies 10:41–61, 1949
6. Ramsey P, McCormick R (eds): Doing Evil to Achieve Good: Moral Choice in Conflict Situations. Chicago, Loyola University Press, 1978
7. ANA, op cit, p 4
8. Rachels J: Active and passive euthanasia. N Engl J Med 292: 1, 1975
9. Steinbock B (ed): Killing and Letting Die. Englewood Cliffs, Prentice-Hall, 1980
10. Beauchamp, Childress, op cit, pp 122–124
11. ANA, op cit, p 4
12. Davis A: Ethical and legal issues in a technological age. In Hockey L: Recent Advances in Nursing: Current Issues in Nursing. Edinburgh, Churchill Livingstone (in press)
13. Davis A, Aroskar M: Ethical Dilemmas and Nursing Practice, 2nd ed. Norwalk, CT, Appleton-Century-Crofts, 1983

Chapter 5

Questions of Risk, Duty, and Paternalism: Problems in Beneficence

Patricia A. R. Flynn

The inscription at the entrance to a medieval hospital in Paris—*Guérir quelquefois, soulager souvent, consoler toujours*—states the essential nature of beneficence as applied to the health care field: "to cure sometimes, to help often, to comfort and console always." The early writing of Hippocrates about benefits and harms, while addressed to physicians, was reaffirmed by Florence Nightingale and is still found in contemporary nursing codes. In Hippocrates' writings, the primary moral injunction is: to benefit, or at least do no harm.[1] In referring to hospital care, Nightingale put it somewhat differently when she said, "It may seem a strange principle to enunciate as the very first requirement in a Hospital that it should do the sick no harm."[2] The general principle of beneficence states that we must do good and, on the other hand, must act to prevent harm. We have the duty to assist those in need. Although all people have a moral duty to do good, the principle of beneficence imposes greater duties on those who have chosen for their work caring for the welfare of others. Beneficence is traditionally seen as residing at the foundation of health care and refers specifically to the principle that the goal of actions in relation to patients ought to be to promote health, to relieve from unnecessary pain and suffering, and to prolong life.[3]

Beneficence "asserts the duty to help others further their important and legitimate interests."[4] In the nursing context beneficence may be treated as a duty. Nurses have a *duty* to benefit others, and to prevent and remove harmful conditions. The term *nonmaleficence* is reserved for the noninfliction of harm.[5] Equally important is the duty to balance possible goods against the possible harms of an action. Under the principle of beneficence two ideas may be considered. The first, requiring that we provide benefits, including the prevention and removal of harm, and the second, that we balance benefits and harms.[6]

The principle of beneficence in health care places a duty on us to behave in such a way that the important and legitimate *goods* and *ends* of the patient are pursued while at the same time avoiding harms. The *goods* of the patient include health; the prevention, elimination, or treatment of disease; relief from pain and suffering; and the prolongation of life. The good may be determined primarily by the values and beliefs of the health care providers, in which case they may be acting paternalistically. Or, they may be determined primarily by the patient and considered to be autonomous.

The principle of beneficence itself can be interpreted as having four separate meanings: (1) one ought not to inflict evil or harm, (2) one ought to prevent evil or harm, (3) one ought to remove evil or harm, and (4) one ought to do or promote good.[7] Anne J. Davis has dealt with the first three of these in the previous chapter on nonmaleficence. In this chapter, the focus will be on the fourth element: one ought to do or promote good.

A number of questions arise in contemplation of the injunction "one ought to do or promote good." When is "good" a duty and when is it beyond duty? What is "good"? Must we always "do good"? Whose "good" is it that we must consider? Can there be too much good? What does promoting good entail, and what risks must we accept in doing good? In other words, who decides what is good, for whom, when, to be done by whom, at what risk, under what circumstances, and what, after all, is good?

That a nurse tries at all times to do good seems so obvious that at first glance one may wonder what there is to say about it. The place of beneficence in nursing is so central that one might think it should pose no serious issues for philosophical reflection. However, there may be disagreements about what is meant by the *good*, about how to go about *doing good*, and how to interpret the clinical situation. For example, is one doing good when one continues to treat a critically ill patient who wishes no treatment? Is one doing good when one feeds a patient who is in irreversible coma? Is one doing good when one continues to turn every two hours a patient in whom the ventilator has been discontinued? We will look at the issues that arise in making clinical decisions, peering behind the thin veneer of good actions.

Beneficence: Doing Right by Doing Good

Doing good is linked to both duties and ends. Beneficence, as preventing harm, removing harmful conditions, and positively benefiting another, is a duty. It is, however, linked to nonmoral ends (discussed in Chapter 2), in that in attempting to benefit others we seek certain things or conditions that can be considered good. That is, beneficence moves toward achieving specific nonmoral goods and ends, such as human dignity and the alleviation of suffering.

For some, preservation of life at all costs is the overriding value or good that is sought. This makes decisions much simpler; all lives must be saved, whatever the quality of that life, whatever the costs. Others, believing also that life is indeed precious, feel that the principle of the preservation of life may at times have to be restrained if it is not to cause excessive suffering or distress.[8] The quality of life must be balanced against the sanctity of life. While recognizing that life is of great value one can also acknowledge that "the uncontrolled application of medical technology may be detrimental to individuals and families."[9]

Is the only good to prevent death, or is perhaps an equal good to prevent suffering? Is it perhaps possible that the greater good is to decrease suffering, not to prevent death? Is it not possible that the greater good is a meaningful life that deserves a meaningful death, not an agonized one? Is it really true that any life is better than any death? What life should be prolonged; what death should be?

The codes for nurses of both the American Nurses' Association (ANA) and the International Council of Nurses (ICN) stress the alleviation of suffering as a nursing function, over saving life. The ANA Code for Nurses states: "Nursing encompasses the promotion and restoration of health, the prevention of illness, and the alleviation of suffering."[10] The ICN Code declares that "the fundamental responsibility of the nurse is fourfold: to promote health, to prevent illness, to restore health, and to alleviate suffering."[11]

Those who argue against the position of life at any or all costs would urge us to keep in mind, while making deliberations, the great importance of the quality of the life we are so aggressively maintaining. Two key issues in any consideration of quality of life decisions include attending to the patient's capacity to experience or relate to others and a consideration of control of the patient's pain and suffering.[12]

To Whom Is Beneficence Owed?

In considering the scope and limits of beneficence in health care, we need to ask who will appropriately receive our efforts to do good? With whom will we have a special relationship—those who are part of our society, all of humanity, the most needy? Should the recipients of our beneficence extend to future generations who will need some of the earth's limited resources that are now at our disposal?

Nurses agree that beneficence is owed within the individual nurse-patient relationship. We owe beneficence to our patients as we fashion a web of commitments and understandings, explicit and implicit, that sustain a fabric of mutual understanding.[13] The more that individuals share a moral community and a single moral sense, as in the case of the nurse and the patient, the more clearly defined are the moral obligations of beneficence.

Beneficence and Autonomy: "For Their Own Good"

What are some of the ethical dilemmas that arise when applying the principle of beneficence? There may be a conflict with the principle of autonomy. The principles of beneficence and autonomy address two central moral points of view: one considers what it means to do good and avoid evil, and the other considers what it means to act with independent choice and self-determination.

The first moral point of view is that of beneficence: the good one ought to achieve for others within constraints of respect for others.[14] However, our mandate to act for the interests, or good, of the patient must not ignore the second moral point of view, that person's right to self-determination. Our overriding need to do good generally must not express paternalism in the provider-patient relationship.

Unfortunately, as so often in life, one aim will conflict with another. There will be times when beneficence and autonomy will conflict. This can be seen in the case of Elizabeth Bouvia, a quadriplegic cerebral palsy patient with extremely painful arthritis, who petitioned the court to have her forcible feedings stopped. The principles do not easily lead to a solution that is acceptable to all. Where one might hope to be guided by one noble principle one finds that such principles are liable to conflict.

Sometimes, prioritizing the goods and possible harms is based on different values. A young woman with breast cancer refuses surgery because she cannot tolerate the thought of living with a disfigured body. For her, beauty and the integrity of her body are higher goods than life. Is not life a higher good than beauty? Perhaps to some, but not to this patient. At issue here is for nursing to focus on what good the nurse can now provide for the patient. It is obvious that medicine's efforts to do good were not accepted by the patient. Nursing must look beyond medical interventions.

We want to do good and we also need to respect the autonomy of those whom we intend to help. In the case of conflict, the duty of beneficence must be balanced by the duty of respect for autonomy. As John Stuart Mill wrote in 1859:

> The only purpose for which power can be rightfully exercised over any member of a civilized community, against his will, is to prevent harm to others. His own good, either physical or moral, is not a sufficient warrant . . . In that part [of anyone's conduct] which merely concerns himself, his independence is, of right, absolute.[15]

Beneficence and Justice

Our duty to do what is best for one patient may conflict with the same duty to others. This involves the principle of justice where we must consider the wants, needs, and rights of others. The duty of beneficence must be balanced with the duty for justice. In the event of scarce health care resources, the fair allocation of scarce resources may mean that there is a conflict between our duty to two patients. If the intensive care unit is full, and a patient has a very good chance of recovery if a critical care unit is available, do we admit that patient to the ICU and transfer a patient with a poor prognosis to the medical service?

Beneficence and Nonmaleficence

Our efforts to help cannot be bought at too high a price. We must weigh the duty of beneficence with the duty of nonmaleficence. If the treatment is not appropriate to the cure, then it is not in the patient's best interest. We are treating a whole person, not a series of symptoms or discrete diseases. We must ask whether the treatment is proportionate or disproportionate to the benefits expected.

We must ask these difficult questions, and on the basis of our answers we may be led to difficult actions or nonactions. Shall we act to treat or not, shall we feed, or discontinue feeding, shall we withhold or withdraw a ventilator? Can we passively *not* do something and refrain from active intervention? The principle of beneficence can be used to justify action as well as to justify inaction. We need to discern the relevance of beneficence to action and nonaction as well as to other moral principles that might justify certain conduct or nonconduct.

How can we seek the greatest balance of good over harm for another as the beneficence principle would mandate? In the stark reality of the clinical situation, ethical principles must be considered in a delicate balance. One does not decide on the basis of autonomy, veracity, fairness, fidelity, or beneficence alone. Rather, one weighs the balancing demands of each duty in attempting to arrive at an appropriate moral decision.

Duty and Beneficence

In discussing beneficence we need to consider the legal and moral rights and duties that emanate from the principle. As will become clear, "the principles in a moral system both impose duties and confer rights."[16]

When do we have a duty to do good? We owe a duty when there is a duty of reciprocity.[17] As philosopher David Hume stated: "All our obligations to do good in society seem to imply something reciprocal. I receive the benefits of society, and therefore ought to promote its interest."[18] That is, we have already received benefits and this incurs a reciprocal duty of beneficence. In society, we have each accepted benefits and have each been voluntarily helped by others. This obligates us to help others. If we had never incurred any obligations, then we might have no duty to help others, but because we have all benefited, we all have obligations to help others, in a moral sense at least. This has specific application when we consider the duty of the nurse in a society that has sustained most of the costs of our professional education. We then have some obligations incurred from that social advantage.

Perhaps more than any other ethical principle, beneficence has special relevance in the health care context both as the philosophical basis for caring for patients as well as in the special circumstances arising in critical care situations. In a situation in which the participants in the transactions are in a relationship of relative strength and weakness, advantage and disadvantage in the pursuit of their goals, that is, of one person helping the other, the duty of doing good is vital.[19]

At least some aspects of beneficence are part of one's duty. What are the boundaries of the duty of beneficence in health care? What is the scope of how beneficent we must be? Should beneficence be considered a duty of health care professionals, but not a supererogatory one?[20]

What is the distinction between beneficent acts that are required by duty and beneficent acts that go beyond what is required. Are we obligated to pull patients from a burning bed in an intensive care unit? Are we obligated to care for patients with fulminant hepatitis, or with communicable or infectious diseases? Do our obligations change if we are well, if pregnant, or if our own immune systems are compromised? There are situations in which there is not a clear duty. In a legal sense, we have no obligation to stop at the scene of an accident. However, does the *need* for help impose a moral obligation on the health care professional who would be able to help as long as there is only minimal risk?

We have a duty to act beneficently if we can do so without excessive personal risk. Are we, however, in our role as nurse, obligated to act beneficently even in the face of significant personal risk? In other words, do we have a duty to be a good Samaritan or only "a minimally decent Samaritan?"[21]

Since beneficence potentially demands extensive positive acts, such as generosity, some moral philosophers have argued that it is virtuous and morally ideal to act beneficently, but not a moral duty to do so. We are not always morally obligated to benefit others even if we are in a position to do so. The line, however, between what is our duty and what is the moral ideal is difficult to determine.

There are some who feel there is a definite obligation to provide assistance, to act beneficently: ". . . if it is in our power to prevent something bad from happening, without thereby sacrificing anything of comparable moral importance, we ought, morally, to do it."[22]

Earlier we spoke of the moral obligation of beneficence as being a more stringent duty. The less individuals participate in a particular moral community, the more individuals are moral strangers to each other, and the more acts of beneficence become supererogatory rather than obligatory. Some ethicists maintain that if one stops at the scene of an accident to offer aid, one is not obligated to do so but is acting in a supererogatory way, above and beyond the call of duty. Others feel that if one has the knowledge to help, one has an ethical duty to do so—if it does not put oneself or one's family at great risk. This position holds that society has prepared professionals with special knowledge; professionals therefore have an obligation to act generously toward society. Health care providers have a duty of beneficence emanating from patients' needs. Professionals have "the duty to help others further their important and legitimate interests when we can do so with minimal risk to ourselves.[23]

The duty related to the principle of beneficence cannot be strictly specified: it is a contentless form. That is, the principle itself does not tell us how much help we are to give, what form that help is to take, or even whom we are to help, since there is a finiteness of time and resources that means choices must be made.[24]

Kant's categorical imperative directs one to act only on principle, which one can at the same time will to become a universal law. To will the universalization of a principle is to be willing for everyone to act on that principle under similar conditions. Kant used the categorical imperative to provide a justification for the principle of general beneficence. The general duty of beneficence is ultimately based, according to Kant, not on concern for the well-being of others, but on respect for autonomy.[25]

John Rawls is another philosopher with concerns related to beneficence and justice. His theory assigns a prominent role in the promotion of the good of others as a matter of justice.[26]

Beneficence and Risk to the Nurse

To what extent does the principle of beneficence require the nurse to assume personal risk or to suffer harm? We have discussed the risks that exist for the patient in terms of determining the degree of benefit that will accrue to the patient in withdrawing or withholding life-sustaining measures balanced with any harm that we might anticipate. We also need to balance the amount of risk or harm to the nurse who is placed in a situation with potential for harm.

A model describing criteria for the acceptance of risk for practitioners has been developed by Smith and Davis and may be helpful in sorting out issues in which doing good involves risk to the nurse. Risk can be loosely divided into low, moderate, and high.[27]

Health care entails some risk by virtue of the fact that nurses always work with patients who may have known or unknown illnesses, infectious or not. As part of the nurse's duty, the risk is accepted; nurses have a duty to accept some health risks in meeting the needs of patients.[28]

Moderate risks have traditionally been considered to be voluntary. That is, a nurse could volunteer to work on an infectious or communicable disease unit, in prisons, on locked wards in state mental hospitals, or under siege. While the nurse voluntarily works in this moderate risk environment, all measures to prevent infection or harm must be taken by the hospital. Hospital administration has a duty toward the nurse, to provide equipment or procedures that prevent harm and minimize risk for the nurse.

In the 1970s in one dialysis unit, virtually 95% of the staff contracted hepatitis. At the time, there were no risk management strategies in operation. The nurses were thus placed at inordinately high risk, by an administration that did not take the responsibility to establish precautions necessary to protect the well-being of the staff.

High-risk situations are those in which there is no duty to do good, for it would be at too high a cost to the nurse. The patient room in which a nurse is trapped represents too high a risk for another to be obligated to assume, although some would do so voluntarily.

When Doing Good Is Too Much: Court Decisions

Several major court decisions provide case law that addresses the issue of when doing good becomes a burden to the patient. When can we stop doing good? When can we stop treating because the patient does not want treatment? Do we have a duty to treat when the treatment is futile? When can we decide to stop treating because the burdens to the person clearly outweigh the benefits. These cases involve the competent adult who refuses treatment, the patient who expresses the wish not to be treated and then loses the ability to participate in treatment decisions, and the legally incompetent patient whose own wishes are never expressed but for whom treatment is futile. These involve both ethical and legal issues of beneficence: doing good for a person and that person's right to self-determination and to privacy, that is, the right to autonomy and freedom from unwanted assault.

In the critical care situation, proposed treatments are often viewed as constituting artificial means to the prolongation of life. If there is no hope for recovery, such as a terminally ill person who is sustained by a ventilator, can we stop "doing good" by treating when (1) the patient wants us to stop, (2) the patient wants but cannot say, and (3) staff wants to discontinue treatment because treatment is futile.

What is the difference between withdrawing or withholding treatment? The President's Commission report concludes that the distinction between stopping treatment and never starting treatment to begin with is morally meaningless; reasons sufficient to justify not initiating treatment are also sufficient to justify withdrawing it once begun.[29]

However, some jurisdictions still recognize a distinction and require court approval to *withdraw* treatment but not to *withhold* it.

The older distinction between what was once considered to be "extraordinary" treatment, such as a ventilator, and what was thought to be "ordinary" treatment, such as nutrition and medication, has also become blurred. In the landmark *Conroy* decision, which is discussed subsequently, the court approved the removal and withholding of artificial feeding from a patient using the more definitive distinction of what is proportionate versus disproportionate treatment in light of that person's life.[30]

When can we stop doing good? Whose good is served if we do *everything* possible to keep a permanently unconscious patient alive?

The Quinlan Case

Perhaps the best known case to illustrate this is that of Karen Ann Quinlan, a New Jersey resident who was in a persistent vegetative state as a result of ventilatory arrest in April 1975.[31] Her father, Joseph Quinlan, petitioned the court to be appointed her guardian. He requested the express power to authorize discontinuing all extraordinary procedures that were sustaining his daughter's vital life processes.

In balancing the state interest in preserving life, the court spoke of Quinlan's poor prognosis as overcoming any interest the state might have: "We think that the State's interest contra weakens and the individual's right to privacy grows as the degree of bodily invasion increases and the prognosis dims. Ultimately there comes a point at which the individual's rights overcome the State's interest [in maintaining life]."[32] The court concluded that she was alive and also a person with interests and rights, including the right of privacy and the right to refuse treatment. The court made it clear that this was a decision to be made by the patients and physicians, and that no court order was necessary. Further, the court ruled that "Karen's right of privacy may be asserted on her behalf by her guardian under the peculiar circumstances here present. . . ."[33]

This landmark case represents the first judicial decision to base the withholding or withdrawing of life-sustaining treatment from a patient on the constitutional right to privacy. In effect the court said: "[when the prognosis was such that] there is no reasonable possibility of Karen ever emerging from her present comatose condition to a cognitive, sapient state and that life support apparatus . . . should be discontinued, they shall consult with the hospital ethics committee." If the hospital ethics committee agrees with the prognosis, life-support may be withdrawn "without any criminal liability . . . on the part of any participant."[34]

An autonomous and constitutional right to privacy, including the right to refuse futile treatment, in this case superceded the duty to do good, to continue to treat. The *Quinlan* case decided that, for patients like Karen Ann Quinlan, staff did not have a legal duty to do everything possible to sustain life: ventilators could be turned off. What of the other aspects of care of a patient in persistent coma: food, water, antibiotics, and so forth?

The Barber Case

In 1983, eight years after the Quinlan decision, a case was heard that attempted to answer the questions of exactly what one must do, or could forgo doing, to keep a permanently unconscious patient alive. It addressed the issue of whether or not food, fluids, and antibiotics are logically different from ventilators or are a separate category of life-sustaining treatment. This is the California case of Clarence Herbert, whose two doctors, Nejdl and Barber, were charged with his murder. Herbert had entered the hospital for elective surgery but had become comatose in the recovery room. Three days later the doctors and family, judging that he was in an irreversible coma, agreed to turn the ventilator off. Like Karen Ann Quinlan, he breathed on his own without the ventilator. Unlike the *Quinlan* case, the family and physicians decided to remove the nasogastric tube feedings and the fluids and medications given by intravenous lines. Herbert died, and the case was taken to court. A charge of murder was upheld by the Superior Court but was reversed by the court of appeals. The court of appeals held that the physicians' decision to remove the life support and feeding lines "though intentional and with knowledge the patient would die" was not an unlawful failure to perform a legal duty since "a physician has no duty to continue treatment once it has been proved to be ineffective."[35]

The *Barber* court specifically rejected the distinction between ordinary and extraordinary care and cited the report of the President's Commission.[36] In this case the court ruled that life-sustaining treatment may be withdrawn from an incompetent patient provided that it is what the patient preferred. Furthermore, life-sustaining treatment may be withdrawn if it is in the patient's best interest. The court ruled that the pain and suffering of continued existence outweigh the benefits of prolonging life, that is, the treatment was disproportionate.

The 1983 California *Barber* court agreed that there is no distinction between medical procedures that provide nutrition and other forms of life support. The courts moved away from the specific treatment, the issue of feeding through a nasogastric tube, to the more general issue of treatment to support life.

An important point in all of the court cases thus far has been a search for what the patient would choose if he or she were able to choose. This is something that needs to be anticipated by the professional staff. Nurses need to discover ways to help patients talk about their wishes with someone while they can. They can invite patients to discuss their preferences about life-sustaining treatment and to consider whom they want to make health care decisions for them when they cannot. In an attempt to deal with the ambiguities about patient wishes, over 21 states have enacted natural death statutes and/or durable power of attorney for health care laws. Natural death statutes permit competent adults to direct that in the event the patient has a terminal illness they do not wish life-sustaining treatment. A durable power of attorney for health care (DPAHC) law permits a competent patient to appoint an attorney-in-fact who is authorized to make medical decisions on his or her behalf even after the patient becomes incapable or mentally incompetent.

With no directive from the patient, in the form of a living will, an advance directive to physicians, a DPAHC, or a record of discussions with the hospital staff or family, we are left in the difficult position of "guessing" what the person might want. It is a measure of "doing good" as well as of patient autonomy to consider these issues, and it is good nursing care to offer opportunities to discuss these matters. Critical care staff might discuss how best to handle this with each patient, understanding that sometimes it will, of course, be impossible.

One must always consider what the person will gain by instituting or continuing treatment. Will the patient, in fact, gain by it? What function will it serve? Will it affect the disease? Will it cause pain and suffering? All these things must be weighed.

There is no legal duty to provide useless or futile treatment. Prolonging dying is generally regarded as futile. Life-sustaining treatment can be withheld if the pain and suffering of the anticipated treatment would: "markedly outweigh any physical pleasure, emotional enjoyment, or intellectual satisfaction that a patient may still be able to derive from life."

> [It can also be withheld if] the net burdens of the patient's life with treatment clearly and markedly outweigh the benefits that the patient derives from life. Furthermore, the recurring, unavoidable and severe pain of the patient's life with the treatment should be such that the effect of administering life-sustaining treatment would be inhumane."[37]

Treatment must not be inappropriately withheld, but neither should patients be subjected to inappropriate life-sustaining treatment.

As the law is currently understood the staff will be acting within the law when they decide to withhold or withdraw life-supporting interventions if the following conditions are met:[38]

1. Further medical intervention will not attain any of the goals of medicine other than sustaining organic life.
2. The preferences of the patient are not known and cannot be expressed.
3. Quality of life clearly falls below the threshold considered minimal.
4. Family and members of the staff are in accord.

In cases where there is nonconcordance, it is valuable to have a review committee. Many hospitals have instituted ethics committees and have written policies that can be helpful in coming to difficult decisions.

Several other cases that were heard between 1975 and 1983 show the gradual evolution of decisions relating to doing good, which moved away from the interests of the state to keep *everyone,* even the dying person, alive by any means, to a focus on the self-determination of the individual and his or her constitutional right to privacy.

The Dinnerstein Case

The case of Shirley Dinnerstein involved a 67-year-old widow with advanced Alzheimer's disease, a coronary condition, and a recent stroke. Her daughter, son, and physician asked the court for a determination that would allow the physician to lawfully enter a "no-code" order directing hospital staff to refrain from resuscitation measures should Dinnerstein have cardiac or ventilatory arrest.

This ruling answers the question, "when can we cease to benefit another, refrain from treating?" The court said that the painful resuscitation procedures would only prolong death, not relieve or cure illness. This decision upholds the validity of no-code orders directing that resuscitative measures be withheld from irreversibly and terminally ill incompetent patients in the event of cardiac or ventilatory failure.[39]

The Fox Case

Brother Fox, an 83-year-old monk, had, prior to becoming ill, consistently expressed a wish that his life not be prolonged by medical means if there was not hope of recovery. He became comatose in 1979 during an operation. Neurologists concurred that he was in a "permanent vegetative state." A request to remove a ventilator was denied by hospital officials and physicians. His superior, Father Eichner, initiated court proceedings to obtain approval for removal of the ventilator.

The court approved the request, based on Brother Fox's "hopeless" condition and his common law right to refuse treatment. The court upheld the patient's right to decline treatment as guaranteed by common law, but also drew upon the constitutional right of privacy protection of that right stating that "as a matter of constitutional law, a competent adult who is incurable and terminally ill has the right . . . not to resist death and to die with dignity.[40]

That right, the court affirmed, is not lost when a person becomes incompetent; even if the patient has not made his or her wishes known when competent, that right can be exercised on his or her behalf. Treatment refusal is made easier, the court noted, when a patient has unequivocally expressed his or her desires before becoming incompetent.

Three decisions deal with the refusal of treatment by competent patients.

The Bartling Case

Bartling, in 1984, was a competent patient with emphysema, arteriosclerosis, an abdominal aneurysm, and a malignant lung tumor. During a biopsy the lung collapsed, and it did not reinflate. A tracheotomy was performed, and he was put on a ventilator. Bartling had stated in a living will, a DPAHC, and verbally that he understood that he might die if the ventilator were removed, that he did not want to die, but that he did not want to continue to live on the ventilator. The court found that he was seriously but not terminally ill; because he was not comatose, he was considered legally competent. The court ruled that life support could not be removed. Bartling died six months later; a day after his death, the court of appeals heard the case. They reversed the trial court decision and ruled that the right to disconnect life support was not limited to comatose or terminally ill patients or to their representative. The court said that "a clearly recognized legal right to control one's own medical treatment predated the [California] Natural Death Act . . . [and] that a competent adult patient has the legal right to refuse medical treatment."[41] The right to refuse medical treatment, the court said, is based on the constitutional right of privacy that "guarantees to the individual the freedom to choose or reject, or refuse to consent to, intrusions of his bodily integrity."[42] Further, the court considered the significance of the state's interest in preserving life:

> If the right of the patient to self-determination is to have any meaning at all it must be paramount to the interests of the patient's hospital and doctors. The right of a competent adult patient to refuse medical treatment is a constitutionally granted right which must not be abridged.[43]

Most of the decisions in these cases were based on the constitutional right to privacy. They uphold the right of a competent terminally ill person, or his or her guardian, to refuse further medical treatment. Courts have given much force to the patient's right to privacy but do not suggest that the expressed wishes of competent adults alone may determine medical treatment. For example, a patient should not be able to dictate a course of treatment that requires staff to ignore their own conscience or to commit malpractice.[44]

The Conroy Case

The case of Claire C. Conroy, an 84-year-old resident in a nursing home, deals with the issue of withholding and withdrawing life-sustaining treatment. Her case and others illustrate how the courts have become involved in clarifying the principle of beneficence. The principle of withholding food—an issue in this case—is germane to the critical care unit. The decisions relative to feeding and nonfeeding that were made in this case are important legal and ethical landmarks.

In 1984 a decision concerning appropriate nutrition and hydration had to be made regarding Claire Conroy. She had severe dementia and was being fed through a nasogastric tube because she was unable to get adequate nutrition by mouth. She had been hospitalized for an elevated temperature and dehydration and was confused and disoriented. She was confined to her bed, was incontinent, was unable to speak, and slept in a fetal position. She had necrotic ulcers of the foot as well as gangrene of her left leg. She was apparently not in a vegetative state, could follow people with her eyes, and smiled when her hair was combed and when her back was rubbed. She sometimes moaned when fed or moved, or when her bandages were removed. Two doctors testified about her ability to feel pain, but their testimony was inconclusive. It was estimated that she would live but a few months, even with a feeding tube.

In the 84 years before she became incompetent, she had avoided physicians, even when ill. On one occasion she had been taken to an emergency room, probably with pneumonia, but refused to sign in. Her nephew, her only relative, visited regularly, and all agreed that he would act in her best interests. He believed that her feeding tube should be removed and that that is what his aunt would want. When the physicians refused, he, as her legal guardian, petitioned the court to permit removal of the feeding tube. Members of the staff felt they had a duty to do good: to feed. The nephew felt that it was time to stop doing good and that his aunt would agree.

How would you decide on this case? What principles and values would you weigh? The New Jersey Supreme Court ruled that tube feedings, like other life-sustaining treatments, may be withheld if they are against the patient's wishes or best interests. This is consistent with the ethical and medical recommendations of the President's Commission for the Study of Ethical Problems in Medicine and Biomedical and Behavioral Research (1983).

The New Jersey Supreme Court held that life-sustaining treatment, including nasogastric feeding, may be withheld or withdrawn from incompetent patients in three circumstances:

1. When it is clear that the patient would have refused the treatment under the circumstances: the subjective test.
2. When there is some indication of the patient's wishes and the treatment would only prolong suffering: the limited objective test.
3. When there is no evidence of the patient's wishes but the treatment clearly and markedly outweighs the benefits that the patient derives from life: the pure objective test.

The Limits of Beneficence: Withholding and Withdrawing Treatment

The issue of how to proceed if a patient has suffered brain death has been clearly answered. If a person is brain dead, he or she is legally dead, and no treatment can or need be given to dead people legally or ethically. The difficult issues arise with patients who are terminally ill with irreversible conditions, whether competent or not. Before deciding on instituting life-sustaining treatment for a competent patient, it is important to discuss the treatment alternatives, including nontreatment. It is generally agreed that competent patients have the right to make treatment decisions for themselves, and this includes the right to refuse even life-sustaining treatment.

In the event of an incompetent patient, consult with the family to ascertain whether the patient, while competent, had expressed a preference regarding future medical treatment in case of incompetency. If the patient has a living will or DPAHC, these should be placed on the patient's chart. Other comments made by the patient about preferences should be considered. The critical care nurses treating the patient will often be the most knowledgeable about this because they have the greatest opportunity to find out the patient's wishes. Document all of this in the patient's record.

Before making a decision to discontinue life-sustaining measures, the patient, family, and staff must be consulted. The decision to discontinue life support includes all treatments used to maintain life, including ventilators, antibiotics, transfusions, intravenous therapy, vasopressors, and the like. Some feel that the decision to remove a feeding tube should be treated the same as the decision to remove a ventilator; others disagree.

The decision to discontinue feeding or fluids is particularly difficult because of the cultural meanings of feeding and nourishment. Some argue that feeding always constitutes ordinary care and hence must be given; others emphasize not the issue of feeding but that of the balance of benefits over burdens for the person's life.[45]

If a patient is in a persistent vegetative state and presumably unable to experience anything, the patient can neither be benefited nor burdened.[46] Health professionals are thus not *obliged* to treat, and they may even be morally constrained from treating. In the case of a demented patient—of whom one can question the benefit of a life of pain, discomfort, dimmed consciousness, and loss of communication—the burden of life would so overwhelm the benefits that there would seem to be no obligation to sustain life.[47] If the staff cannot agree upon appropriate treatment, an institutional ethics committee should be consulted. If your hospital does not have an ethics committee, consider whether such a committee would benefit the critical-care patients in your hospital. Ethics committees should be composed of members of various disciplines, including nursing. In the absence of an institutional ethics committee or other moral mechanisms within the hospital, the unhappy alternative is to request judicial intervention and to ask that these cases be settled in court. This is time consuming, inefficient, and an unnecessary burden for patients, family, and staff.

The nurse's motivation is to promote the patient's best interests, to be beneficent, to do what that person would do if he or she were in a position to decide. The ones who best know this are the family and staff who care for the patient. How could a judge know as well?

Appeals to the court may not always be motivated by what is best for the patient, but rather may represent an attempt to protect professional staff from charges of negligence or homicide. Appeals to the court, not beneficently motivated, place too much burden on the patient.[48] They are not for the patient's good, but for the staff and hospital's good. More reasonable and humane measures need to be put in place to help us when making decisions. The ethics committee may provide a forum in which these different issues may be discussed and decided, leading to our goal of the better good: beneficence.

The difficult dilemmas that arise in situations in which life and death decisions are made make it vital to develop ways to help nurses deal with them. The courts are not the appropriate place. Ethics committees are a possible solution to providing a forum for nurses to discuss these issues.

Whatever process is used, what must be stressed is that nurses must have a recognized role in discussions with the patient and family members relative to withholding and withdrawing life-sustaining treatments. It is the nurse who will continue to care for the patient after these decisions have been made.

Once decisions for withholding or withdrawing treatments are made, nurses face an added dimension of concern: which nursing intervention should be withheld or withdrawn? How frequently should the patient be turned or suctioned? What type of mouth care should be given to a patient in whom food and fluids have been withdrawn, or should mouth care be given at all? These issues, during consideration of withdrawal of ventilators, food and fluids, and antibiotics rarely surface except in the minds of nurses as they deliver care.

How can the nurse deal with these issues? How can the nurse assure that beneficence really occurs? Decisions about which nursing interventions will occur to support the patient's comfort, relieve pain, and allow for as natural a death as possible must be shared between the patient and family and the nursing staff. Nurses can then feel confident that the most good is being done.

We know that the nurse maintains an obligation to care for the patient when cure is no longer possible. Clearly nurses will need to provide human support to these patients; what will these be? The staff of each critical care unit must address these issues so that a satisfactory policy of care that is consistent with the patient's and family's wishes and with competent nursing practice may be achieved. The Code for Nurses makes it clear that nurses are responsible for affirming patient rights of privacy and self-determination. When sustaining these rights means that life-sustaining treatments are withheld or withdrawn, nurses continue to have a responsibility to that patient. Discussions about these issues should occur before nurses are actually involved in the case so that approaches to the patient and family members can be made in a conscientious, deliberate manner assuring individually desired outcomes. For it is our hope, as it was in medieval France: "to cure sometimes, to help often, to comfort and console always."

Notes

1. Hippocrates: Epidemics, vol 1, Jones WH (trans), pp 164–165. Cambridge, Harvard University Press, 1923
2. Nightingale F: Notes on Hospitals (London, 1863), facsimile ed. Philadelphia, JB Lippincott, 1957

3. Jonsen A, Siegler M, Winslade W: Clinical Ethics, 2nd ed. New York, Macmillan, 1986
4. Beauchamp T, Childress J: Principles of Biomedical Ethics, 2nd ed, p 148. New York, Oxford University Press, 1983
5. Ibid, p 148
6. Ibid, p 149
7. Frankena W: Ethics, 2nd ed, p 47. Englewood Cliffs, Prentice-Hall, 1973
8. Brewin TB: Truth, trust, and paternalism. Lancet 2:490–492, 1985
9. Duff RS, Campbell AGM: Moral and ethical dilemmas in the special care nursery. N Engl J Med 289:894, 1973
10. ANA: Code for Nurses with Interpretive Statements. Kansas City, MO, ANA, 1976
11. International Council of Nurses: Code for Nurses. Geneva, ICN, 1973
12. Keyserlingk EW: Sanctity of life or quality of life, in the context of ethics, medicine, law (study paper for the Law Reform Commission of Canada). Ottowa, Minister of Supply and Services, 1979
13. Englehardt HT: The Foundations of Bioethics, p 75. New York, Oxford University Press, 1986
14. Ibid, p 81
15. Mill JS: On Liberty. Collected Works of John Stuart Mill, 4th ed, vol 18. Toronto, University of Toronto Press, 1977
16. Faden R, Beauchamp T: A History and Theory of Informed Consent, p 7. New York, Oxford University Press, 1986
17. Beauchamp, Childress, op cit, p 141
18. Hume D: A Treatise on Human Nature. Oxford, Clarendon Press, 1964
19. Shelp E (ed): Beneficence and Health Care, p vii. Dordrecht, D Reidel, 1982
20. Abrams N: Scope of beneficence in health care. In Shelp, op cit, pp 183–198
21. Thomson JJ: A defense of abortion. Philosophy and Public Affairs 1:1, 1971
22. Singer P: Famine, affluence, and morality. Philosophy and Public Affairs 1:3, 1972
23. Beauchamp, Childress, op cit, p 148
24. Kant I: Good will, duty, and the categorical imperative: Fundamental principles in vice and virtue. In Sommers C (ed), Abbott TK (trans): Everyday Life, p 95. Reprint, San Diego, Harcourt Brace Jovanovich, 1985
25. Buchanan A: Philosophical foundations of beneficence. In Shelp, op cit
26. Frankena W: Ethics, 3rd ed. New Jersey, Prentice-Hall, 1982
27. Smith SJ, Davis AJ: How much risk is duty for the health care practitioner? Medicine and Law 5:32, 1906
28. Beauchamp, Childress, op cit, p 157
29. President's Commission for the Study of Ethical Problems in Medicine and Biomedical and Behavioral Research: Deciding to Forego Life-Sustaining Treatment. Washington, DC, Government Printing Office, 1983
30. In re Conroy. 436 A.2D 1209 NJ Super Ct, 1985
31. In re Quinlan. 70 NJ 10, 355 A2d 647, 1976
32. Ibid, p 664
33. Ibid
34. Ibid, pp 671–672
35. Barber v Los Angeles County Supreme Court. 195 Cal Rptr 484. Cal Ct App October 12, 1983

36. President's Commission, op cit, p 152

37. In re Conroy, op cit

38. In re Barber, op cit

39. In re Dinnerstein, 6 Mass App Ct 466, 380 NE 2nd 134 1978

40. In re Eichner (Fox), 73 App Div 2nd 431. 426 NYS 2nd 517 1980

41. Bartling v Superior Court of Los Angeles, 163 Cal App 3rd 186, 209 Cal Rptr 220: 2 Civ No B007907 1984

42. Ibid

43. Ibid

44. Bouvia v Superior Court of Los Angeles 179 Cal App 3d 1127; Cal Rptr 220, April 1986

45. Jonsen, Siegler, Winslade, op cit, p 110

46. Ibid

47. Ibid

48. Bayley C: Who should decide? In Doudera AE, Peters JD (eds): Legal and Ethical Aspects of Treating Critically and Terminally Ill Patients. Ann Arbor, Health Administration Press, 1982

Chapter 6

Fidelity and Veracity: Questions of Promise Keeping, Truth Telling, and Loyalty

Mila Ann Aroskar

Moral concerns about health care in the 1980s focus on assurance of individual autonomy and equitable distribution of the benefits and costs of health services in an era of cost containment. Economic and financial constraints, rather than patient needs, seem to dictate patient care decisions. Families and patients fear that the need for medical care along with inadequate insurance coverage will result in financial catastrophe. At the same time that we focus on situations in which principles and values of patient autonomy, patient safety, and justice conflict, nurses must not lose sight of other moral concerns that are at stake in many patient care situations that require difficult moral choices. Two of these moral concerns or principles are fidelity and veracity. This chapter presents perspectives on fidelity and veracity in the nurse-patient relationship, illustrated by a case study in which fidelity is seriously compromised. Sections on conflicting loyalties of nurses, veracity and other moral principles, critical care environments, and institutional mechanisms for enhancing fidelity will enlarge upon the basic material.

Critical care nurses find themselves in a variety of patient care situations in which their fidelity or primary loyalty to patients is jeopardized or seriously compromised. For instance, nurses work in intensive care units where they feel patient safety is jeopardized, or information about a patient's condition is withheld from the patient by well-meaning health professionals or family members in an attempt to protect the patient. Patients, families, and staff sometimes disagree about treatment options such as not starting a procedure on a seriously ill newborn or withdrawal of treatment for a hopelessly ill patient. In some instances, a physician concerned about the legal ramifications of "do not resuscitate" (DNR) orders will not write such orders for a patient who requests them.

Nurses in critical care units may find themselves questioning their fidelity to a patient when life-sustaining technologies seem to add to the patient's suffering. Critical care nurses have stated their fear of "torturing" patients when benefits of medical intervention are marginal or in some situations clearly futile.

Adequate informed consent also elicits questions of the critical care nurse's fidelity to patients. For example, hopelessly ill patients or their families do not always have the information necessary for informed decision making about experimental procedures or medications used as a last resort. A patient's goals and values in major decisions about treatment may be ignored. This occurs even when patients have discussed their wishes with family members or have included them in advance written directives (the living will) to be followed if they are unable to make decisions because of coma, medication effects, or any other reason. Nurses, as patient advocates, raise questions about the meaning of fidelity (1) when they have promised patients to make their position known to family members and health professionals when there is disagreement about a treatment protocol or (2) when there is a possibility of withdrawal of treatment.

Nurses are often caught in the middle in such situations and question their duties and obligations to patients, families, themselves, and others. Duties and obligations may conflict even when they can be identified. For example, nurses may identify their obligations to patients to reduce suffering—yet they also have an obligation to carry out physicians' orders for treatments that are often very painful. The moral principle of fidelity or faithfulness to patients is at stake in such situations.

Perspectives on Fidelity

Fidelity has received little attention in nursing ethics literature. Most often, one uses the term *fidelity* in talking about marriage relationships. Yet, without fidelity to commitments such as promise keeping, a moral community cannot exist. Fidelity as faithfulness to patients, with promise keeping as one aspect, is as fundamental to the nurse-patient relationship as it is to the wider community and the human relationships that comprise that community.[1]

Ramsey, a prominent theologian in the field of bioethics, argues that fidelity as faithfulness among individuals is the single foundational moral principle. It is the moral bond or covenant between people.[2] A covenant may be viewed as a special kind of contract that emphasizes moral bonds and a spirit of fidelity and trust. From a theological perspective, fidelity as promise keeping expressed through a relationship of faithfulness is morally fundamental and ought to govern social relations in the community widely and more narrowly in communities such as a hospital. The obligation to commitments makes possible such a moral community.

Think for a moment about the critical care unit where you practice. What if every nurse on the unit were no longer committed to her or his patients and their families? What would be the consequences for patients, for families, for other care givers, for the hospital? Refusal of the nurses in a newborn intensive care unit to be faithful to their commitment to the practice of nursing would mean that the unit as a system or "community" could not function reliably. Think about a situation in the pediatric intensive care unit in which parents, who were in desperate need of sleep, could not depend on the nurse who said that she would notify them during the night if their child's condition became significantly worse. Or think about the patient in a bone marrow transplant unit who was promised by a nurse that he would return in a few minutes to assist the patient with needed mouth care, and an hour later had not returned or communicated with the patient.

If situations like this were commonplace, patients would probably think that nurses' promises were meaningless and that they could not be depended on to keep their word. At the same time, it is important to keep in mind that making a promise is voluntary. Whereas respecting a person's autonomy to make a treatment decision when the person is competent and adequately informed is generally morally obligatory, making a specific promise to a patient is generally considered to be voluntary, not obligatory. Yet, promises such as these are in keeping with nursing's commitment to caring.

While nurses may encounter situations in which they are unable to keep a promise made to a patient, it would be disastrous if the nursing profession as a whole could not be depended on to keep promises *made implicitly* to society about obligations to care for the sick, to practice competently, and not to abandon patients in need of nursing. There may be situations in which the consequences of breaking a promise made to a patient would have beneficial long-term consequences for that individual. However, the breaking of a promise that has been made in good faith requires special justification that a reasonable person would understand and accept. The voluntary nature of making promises reminds us that promises should be considered *before* they are made and that a principle of fidelity rests on the idea of *keeping* promises, not making promises.

One might argue that fidelity as faithfulness to patients and promise keeping speaks to the commitment of the nursing profession—that there is an implicit promise or contract to provide nursing care to those who need it. Promise keeping is implicit in a nurse's practice as well. Fidelity might be viewed as the "glue" that holds the nurse-patient relationship together in a moral sense.

Not all philosophers agree with Ramsey's position that fidelity is a fundamental principle.[3] They argue that fidelity is a rule derived from what are considered to be more fundamental moral principles, such as autonomy and beneficence.

In this chapter, fidelity is considered to be integral to the nurse-patient relationship. In nursing, fidelity may be interpreted to mean faithfulness and loyalty to patients as a primary foundational aspect of the professional relationship. Fidelity to patients says that nurses will not abandon individuals, groups, or communities that need nursing care. This places considerations of fidelity to patients as "more than" simply the application of ethical principles in a decision-making situation. Fidelity is placed squarely in the center of the individual nurse-patient relationship and the relationship of the nursing profession to patients and to society through its social contract of the promise to serve those who are sick. Those who are sick must be able to trust that the promise will be kept. When individuals become nurses, they participate in the inherent promises and obligations of the nursing profession.

Faithfulness and loyalty to patients may be demonstrated in a variety of ways. One way is by using a reflective thinking process prior to making difficult choices in

81

patient care in which principles such as enhancing patient self-determination in treatment decisions and reducing suffering are considered. This can be viewed as the practice of preventive ethics in clinical situations to prevent or modify ethical crises.

Documents of the American Nurses' Association (ANA) state positions that are expressive of fidelity to patients. The ANA Code for Nurses (1985) talks about respect for individual clients and commitment to safety and welfare as fundamental principles of the nursing profession, and it is an inherent part of the profession's contract with society.[4] Such a social contract is expressed clearly in the social policy statement that says that in moving to a more health-oriented system of care, ''. . . care of the sick remains a basic responsibility.''[5] This basic responsibility cannot be discharged adequately if fidelity to patients as the foundation of the nurse-patient relationship is altered. Fidelity as faithfulness in the nurse-patient relationship involves strict adherence to promises that have been made and to the fundamental commitments of the nurse. In critical care nursing, commitment to expert and humane nursing care of seriously ill patients such as those on life support is one such commitment. These patients are unable to meet even their most minimal needs by themselves and must be able to trust others to meet those needs. They are totally dependent on others, primarily nurses, for their safety, welfare, and their very lives in many instances. Nurses with support of nursing administration and other hospital departments provide the care on an around-the-clock basis that is necessary in an absolute sense for such a patient to survive.

Fidelity implies that nurses will be steadfast in meeting their obligations to patients in critical care units. At the same time, those duties and obligations, particularly when they conflict, are often unclear. Fidelity implies that nurses will use a reflective thinking process, that is, the nursing process incorporating ethical aspects, to reach the most ethically adequate decisions possible on which to base their actions. Nurses must also realize that some moral ambiguity may still remain.

Think about a situation in which you had promised to control a patient's pain with medication—and then found that the patient's medical status did not allow for adequate dosages to relieve the pain. The analgesics that could be administered were life-threatening when given in sufficient dosages to achieve effective pain control. In this case, you had to make a decision about what to do in light of the conflicting obligations to reduce suffering and to avoid harm.

Fidelity in a Patient Care Situation

Brenda Hewitt died in a critical care unit in a New York hospital, after eight years of an "almost continuous, unimaginable pain." She was a poet and an editor whose dying in an intensive care unit has been powerfully described by one who loved and cared for her for those eight years.[6] She died, surrounded by and subjected to the most sophisticated technologies, including full resuscitation. She had adamantly rejected these interventions in her handwritten living will, drawn up by an attorney and notarized. In a lengthy, pain-filled account of her last hours in critical care, the author has described his frustrated efforts to have Hewitt's voice and values heard in the many decisions that were made by the medical staff. Some of those decisions to act were clearly of no medical benefit to her and added to her suffering.

There is no mention or evidence of any meaningful nursing response, no mention of any nursing support for the person authorized by Hewitt to speak for her (the writer), and no mention of any basic nursing *care*.[7] In fact, the account describes Brenda Hewitt's condition in such a way that one can only conclude that the most basic nursing care needs did not receive attention.

One could argue that this disturbing account can be balanced by the positive accounts one hears about nursing care provided in many hospitals. At the same time, deeply troubling questions are raised about Brenda Hewitt's treatment. They are raised for the nursing profession as a collective body of practitioners with an implicit social contract to provide competent and humane nursing care. They are also raised for individual nurses who embody this social contract or negate it in their daily practice. Profound questions about fidelity or loyalty of nurses to patients are raised by such an account of inattention to a patient's expressed wishes and the lack of any informed consent for procedures that had no benefit for the patient. Nurses, as moral agents and as patient advocates, should be concerned that some human beings are without necessary nursing care and support.

The personal account of Brenda Hewitt's treatment was (as reported) a negation of the promise inherent in the social promise of nursing and society and in the nurse-patient relationship. At the same time, patients must be able to trust in that promise that has been made by the hospital as a moral community, to individual patients. The hospital makes an inherent promise that patients will receive the nursing care necessary for their safety and well-being often in circumstances in which the patient is totally dependent on others for decision making and subsequent actions. Implicit promises of the nursing profession were apparently not kept to Brenda Hewitt. Moral principles of autonomy, nonmaleficence, beneficence, and justice were seemingly ignored in the haste by health care professionals to "err on the side of life." They made their own decisions about what doing good meant in a situation in which the patient had taken care to assure that her voice would be heard. Yet her voice was not heard as the available technologies were overused and inappropriately used, completely disregarding her wishes. Nurses as moral agents and patient advocates in critical care units must realize that they are committing themselves to an often difficult and controversial role particularly in areas of the hospital where high-tech medicine prevails.

Reiser and Anbar, editors of *The Machine at the Bedside*, have said that while technology allows us to improve a patient's quality of life, it ". . . also allows us to sustain life under conditions of great suffering".[8] The stress of maintaining the technologies of patient care may also distance care givers from patients. Nurses in a coronary care unit have been heard to talk about "taking care of the machines." Practitioners, including nurses, must never avoid responsibility for consequences of the use of technology in patient care. It has been said that it is not only what we do that is affected by the use of machines, but also how we think about ourselves and our relationships. The use of machines in patient care does affect the nature of the nurse-patient relationship, including fidelity as faithfulness to patients. Understanding the relationship of care givers, patients, and machines is not easy. Little attention has been given to this area in the nursing literature.

Use of technology has created many ethical questions with regard to whether it should be used and for whom it should be used. Clearly this was an issue as Hewitt lay dying. According to Reiser, the respirator has become the symbol of advanced technological capabilities, and ambivalence toward the use of ventilators raises questions about obligations of health professionals to sustain life and relieve suffering.[9] Often these two obligations conflict and nowhere more clearly than in critical care, where so often "there is always one more treatment to try" as one neonatologist asserted when discussing ethical questions that arise in newborn intensive care.

Critical care nurses are often the ones asked by patients and families why certain technologies are started or why the patient's suffering is allowed to continue. Requests that treatment be withdrawn or that "something be done to end my suffering" are often directed toward the nurse rather than the physician. Nurses are, then, caught in the middle of conflicting obligations and responsibilities as moral agents. Nurses who experience some of the greatest moral conflict are those caring for the "newly dead" who will be organ donors and those caring for patients who are "living." Fidelity to patients in high-tech care units may require that nurses question the use of specific technologies for a specific patient or even the admission of a hopelessly ill patient, for medical technology, to such a unit.

Conflicting Loyalties

While fidelity as faithfulness or loyalty to patients and clients may be considered a primary and foundational principle in the nurse-patient relationship, other competing loyalties may inject conflict into nursing practice. These conflicting loyalties may include loyalty to oneself and one's personal principles and values, loyalty to physician and nurse colleagues, and loyalty to one's employer. Loyalty to patients may conflict with loyalty to one's personal and professional values. Nurses may care for patients with end-stage cardiac disease who continue to smoke whenever they have a chance. The nurse values individual autonomy and freedom of choice for patients; at the same time, the nurse values a smoke-free environment. Loyalty to patient safety may conflict with loyalty to other health professionals. An example would be the nurse who values friendship with a colleague who insists that she will never allow her drug dependency to put patient welfare in jeopardy. Loyalty to patients and to one's employer may conflict when hospital policies such as reimbursement for organ transplants conflict with a patient's future welfare. At the same time, the nurse realizes that the hospital's survival depends on effective cost containment efforts.

The principle of an informed consent is viewed by Ramsey as a primary expression of fidelity in the patient-physician relationship as it expresses the bond between consenting persons. Nurses may find the obligation of fidelity to patients in conflict with other obligations or loyalties when, after careful patient assessment, they determine that the patient has signed a consent form for surgery but is not adequately informed about a procedure that will have profound consequences for the patient's welfare or significant risk. The obligation of fidelity to the patient conflicts with political realities and loyalty to the physicians who are responsible for obtaining adequately informed consent. Yet, the nurse has a duty to the patient to assure adequate and correct information. The nurse must intervene.

Fidelity to patients as a foundational principle includes the moral requirement that we never treat patients solely as means, but always as ends in themselves. For example, it would be difficult, if not impossible, in the above situation to justify morally a resident physician's use of a terminally ill patient to practice a particular surgical procedure when that procedure will provide no known benefit to the patient. This would be an example of treating a patient primarily as a means to someone else's end. This becomes a particularly critical moral test when patients are potential organ donors or participants in experimental research protocols.

Talking about fidelity as promise keeping and faithfulness to patients may seem too vague to be of much guidance to nurses in dealing with conflicting loyalties in complex critical care situations. At the same time, the recognition that fidelity to patients is at stake and is taken into explicit consideration in decision making increases the likelihood that decisions will be more ethically adequate.

Veracity in the Nurse-Patient Relationship

Veracity is an important moral principle to consider in the nurse-patient relationship. Nurses in critical care areas find themselves caught in the middle when someone else has not told a patient the truth about her or his condition. Technically accurate information that is deliberately misleading sometimes is given to a patient. In other instances, major treatment decisions are made for a critically ill patient without the patient's adequately informed consent. In other cases, a nurse may be concerned about the situation when the family requests the patient not be told the truth about his or her condition; at the same time, the patient has told the nurse that he or she wishes to know all the facts to get affairs in order—"just in case." Patient autonomy and veracity or truth telling are two principles that are at stake in these and the following patient situations.

Parents make choices for a child without determining whether that child has the capacity or wish to participate in certain treatment decisions. Or nurses hear physicians "lie" to patients, give patients partial information, or exclude what nurses consider to be critical information for decision making. Nurses sometimes find themselves caring for competent terminally ill patients when they have information that the patient does not have because the physician or family withheld "painful information." Sometimes, competent patients do not know that they have been placed on DNR status because care givers or family disagree about whether the patient can handle participation in this decision. The last exemplifies strong paternalism in which others decide for a competent patient what they consider to be in that patient's best interests—whether or not that patient would agree.

Nurses may be aware of errors in procedures or treatments that increase a patient's length of stay in intensive care. Patients and families are not always told about such mistakes. At the same time, nurses think that the affected patient and family ought to know that the error has occurred because it may influence their ability to make adequately informed decisions about future treatment. While one might decide that this knowledge would do more harm than good to the patient, it is difficult, if not impossible, to justify ethically the withholding of information that may impede reasoned decision making and patient autonomy.

The preceding examples preclude informed decision making by patients and freedom of choice with regard to decisions that have a profound effect on patients. Freedom of choice includes provision of options, noncoercion by others, and the ability of the individual to consider the available options, make a choice, and act on that choice. Negating freedom of choice for a competent individual is difficult to justify ethically and puts a burden on a care giver who makes such a decision.

Nurses question what to do when events occur that negate the possibility of informed decision making by patients and their families. Such events are often life-threatening situations or those in which a patient's long-term physical and emotional health are seriously in jeopardy. Events that preclude informed decision making by patients or their families jeopardize the integrity of the nurse-patient relationship because nurses may feel that they are colluding in a situation in which important personal and professional values are at stake. These values include trustworthiness, honesty with patients, and the advocacy role as part of nurses' faithfulness to patients. Thus veracity as truthfulness in the nurse-patient relationship is an important element in the enhancement of fidelity to patients in the moral community of the hospital.

Consider the consequences of deception. Imagine living in a society or working in a hospital in which you could never count on verbal or nonverbal communication. You could ask a question but could never count on the accuracy of the answer. Your words and those of others would be worthless. You would never know if an individual's words were truthful or deceptive. What would it be like to make decisions and take action under such conditions? Some level of truthfulness is necessary for society to exist.[10] Hospitals and critical care units could not continue to provide services without the practice of a high level of truthfulness in their day-to-day operations. The foundations of human relationships would be seriously undermined.

Lying to patients is one part of the larger issue of patient deception. Lying is making a statement that is intended to deceive. Lying, according to philosopher Sissela Bok, causes harm to the person who lies, to the person lied to, and to the fabric of society.[11] Thus, one can argue that lying causes harm to the nurse who lies, to the patient who is lied to, to the hospital as a moral community, and ultimately to society. When patients are deceived or lied to, they are being manipulated. They can only make choices based on faulty information. Their freedom of choice is seriously negated. Altruistic reasons such as protecting a patient from tragic news or trying to do some defined good through lying requires that the care giver, in this instance the nurse, provide ethically adequate justification for such actions. This is difficult to do in most situations.

Often, the problem of what to tell patients arises when those with professional and technical knowledge, such as physicians or nurses, are not sure of the accuracy of their information or of its meaning to them or to patients. While health care professionals generally assume that patients will tell the truth, they do not always feel bound to answer patients' questions completely. It has been argued that while a physician may withhold the truth, what a physician tells the patient must be accurate. It has also been argued that while the patient has a right to the truth, the duty of the physician to provide it is suspended if the truth will do harm rather than good.[12] This is a paternalistic stance that would require justification by the health care professional who makes such a judgment. One example might be a teenage patient in a critical care unit who has been under psychiatric care as a known suicide risk and has just been diagnosed as having a terminal illness that probably will be fatal within a very short time. One general rule of thumb in the past has been for physicians to tell as little as possible consistent with maintaining hope and cooperation in treatment.

If the prognosis of a terminally ill patient were certain, there would still probably be disagreement about whether, what, and how a patient should be told. Prognosis is never known for sure, and no one, including physicians, can put an exact time on a patient's remaining length of life. Research studies show that physicians generally perform poorly in predicting how long a specific cancer patient will survive except when death is clearly imminent.[13] How one responds under conditions of uncertainty will depend partly on the position one takes regarding one's basic moral principles and values. If one values patient autonomy over avoiding harm, then one would share one's uncertainty with the patient.

Fidelity and Veracity in Nursing

One question that has been asked in nursing ethics literature is whether the disclosure of diagnosis and prognosis is solely the domain of the physician or also proper to the practice of nursing. According to Yarling this is a question of professional dominance or ". . . the professional control of information."[14] Professional, legal, and moral issues are involved in answering this question. Patients have a recognized moral and legal right to information in order to give adequately informed consent for any procedure. There is no recognized corresponding obligation to know.

Yarling argues that honoring the patient's right to information is not solely a medical obligation but also a moral obligation.[15] While medical questions require medical knowledge for answers, moral questions require the recognition of individual rights and obligations. Moral obligation is nontransferable and transcends lines of institutional authority. Other professionals in the patient care community are moral agents with moral obligations to patients. Professional medical or nursing expertise does not automatically include expertise in the moral realm.

Several problems arise in patient care with regard to veracity. Nurses in critical care should be aware of these problems and issues as they impinge on fidelity to patients by nurses individually and the nursing profession collectively. Denying information to terminally ill patients (or any patient) denies that person's freedom of choice and self-determination. The so-called benevolent lie is a second problem; that is, the idea that one lies to a patient in order to do good. For example, nurses might say that they were doing good by telling some patients that they were being given pain medication when they were actually being given placebos alternately with pain medication to prevent addiction.

Yarling also points out that nurses are often in triple jeopardy when they lie to patients.[16] They not only lie to patients, but also *for* the physician, and they live day after day with the knowledge of that lie. One can argue that physicians in some instances delegate to the nurse the responsibility for deception of patients when they ask nurses to tell families that they are not on the unit because they don't want to be "bothered" by a particular family. Have you ever been asked to lie to a child—for example say something would not hurt—to gain his or her cooperation to carry out a procedure? Such deception seriously affects the level of trust with which a health professional's words are taken the next time.

Nurses do not have a clear legal right or obligation to disclose information in most states. At the same time, the argument has been made that in respecting a terminally ill patient's right to information, nurses have a moral right—and in some instances a moral obligation to do so. This is based on the duty to provide information and patient education in a sensitive and skilled manner. These disclosures should be made competently and collaboratively with the full knowledge of colleagues and rapport with the patient.[17] A moral right to disclose information to a patient does not automatically establish a moral obligation to do so. Under specific conditions the obligation to disclose arises along with the right to disclose. Both are rooted in the patient's exercise of the right to know.

Though nursing and medical practice overlap, the issue of right versus obligation cannot be resolved on grounds of medical knowledge alone, but requires a moral decision. The underlying premises to this conclusion are as follows: the patient has a moral right to know; legal rights and obligations ought to be a reflection of moral rights and obligations; and the legal situation of the nurse is sufficiently ambiguous that it is open to precedent-setting interpretation.[18] Needless to say, serious attention to nurses' rights and obligations requires changes in the power/authority relationships of nurses, physicians, and patients and the social structure of hospitals.

In summary, veracity in the nurse-patient relationship is clearly linked with fidelity through the implicit social contract and covenant that binds care givers and patients in the moral community of the hospital. The patient's trust in nurses individually and collectively to consider patient welfare first is at stake.

Fidelity and Ethical Principles of Autonomy, Beneficence, and Justice

Major ethical principles of autonomy, beneficence, and justice are involved in expressing fidelity as a fundamental dimension of the nurse-patient relationship. The ethical principle of autonomy or self-determination claims that individuals should have the freedom to make determinations about what happens to their person. This principle is grounded in respect for persons, which means that each individual is treated as a person of moral worth and moral agency. Interference with an individual's goals and life plans requires adequate justification.

Critical care nurses who consciously incorporate the principle of patient autonomy in the nursing process to enhance fidelity to their patients would realize that failing to do so jeopardizes nurses' faithfulness and accountability to persons who in many instances are dependent on them for meeting fundamental needs and even for survival. Ignoring a competent patient's wishes in making treatment decisions or failing to determine to the greatest degree the best interests of a patient unable to participate in making such decisions are examples of such failure.

The principle of beneficence or doing good has four elements. Beneficence requires that one should not inflict harm or evil, that one should prevent harm, that one should remove harm, and that one should do or promote good.[19] The duty that one should not inflict harm (known as nonmaleficence) overrides the other three aspects of beneficence if they conflict. If nurses in a critical care unit determine that a procedure, such as repetition of resuscitative procedures on hopelessly ill patients who said they did not wish to be resuscitated, is inflicting harm or "torturing" those patients, they have an obligation to question the benefit of the procedure. They also have an obligation to assure that the patient's wishes are known to the health care providers involved in the patient's care. Even if the patients had not requested nonresuscitation, the issue would still arise if patients were unaware that they had a choice.

Administrators or physicians might argue that doing the procedure in question would contribute to the greater good of a community hospital by assuring that the physicians could not be accused of abandoning patients or would contribute to the education of a medical resident for the benefit of future patients. However, fidelity to these patients requires that nurses consider patient interests first. Actions taken to avoid inflicting harm are implicit in the contract of the nursing profession with society, that is, to *care* for the sick.

The principle of justice is basic to the structure of society and to structures for delivery of nursing and health care. Justice can be individual, distributive, and social. Both individual and social justice are involved in issues of fair allocation of societal resources to health care and the fair distribution of health care resources to individuals who live in that society. Distributive justice in health care has to do with the distribution of the burdens and benefits of health care in society where resources are limited. Burdens or costs are not only financial but also psychological, emotional, and spiritual.

While fairness in the distribution of health and nursing care is an overall goal, there should be a way to ethically justify treating people differently. Nurses in critical care know that not all patients need the same amount or type of nursing care. Is need a morally relevant difference that justifies treating individuals differently in critical care? What other competing ideas are used to justify treating individuals differently?

Competing ideas to justify different treatment of individuals include contracts (such as health insurance coverage), individual effort, societal contribution, merit, and the idea of equal shares of whatever is being distributed (such as access to critical care beds).[20] Different rationales are used to distribute benefits in different societal institutions. In our society, *need* is used to do so. Need is used as the basis for welfare payments while achievement and merit are used to distribute jobs and promotions.

Individual patient need is used most frequently by the nursing profession to justify the distribution of nursing and health care services. Recognition of individual need is invoked in the ANA Code for Nurses (1985) in statements such as "The need for health care is universal, transcending all national, ethnic, racial, religious, cultural . . . economic difference."[21] Using individual need as the basis for distribution of nursing and health care presents some problems.

Who defines need is a major question in relation to preferences and wants. A fundamental need can be defined as something without which a person will be harmed—such as emergency or critical care. This definition of a fundamental need makes it easier to justify distribution of critical care as taking precedence over other kinds of nursing and health care. However, if people are also using social worth or some other criterion on which to base distribution of nursing and health care benefits, there will be disagreement about using need as the most compelling argument for distribution of health care resources.

Committees that were convened in the late 1960s to determine who should get renal dialysis when not enough machines were available became uncomfortable when they realized that social worth was being used as a criterion. Need was recognized by the federal government as a more compelling criterion. Thus the passage of the Social Security Amendments in 1972 assured that individuals with end-stage renal disease would have access to renal dialysis. The issue of social worth related to allocation of dialysis resources was resolved with this legislation.

In the 1980s, criteria such as social worth, contract, and individual effort seem to be reemerging as criteria for distribution of health care benefits. Consider federal decisions to cut social and health care benefits to vulnerable population groups, such as the poor, elderly, and children. Critical care nurses undoubtedly have their fidelity to patients jeopardized when hospitals do not allocate adequate resources to provide necessary and safe care for those in intensive care units. Nursing's social contract to care for the sick is in jeopardy in such circumstances.

At the same time that the federal government is cutting health care benefits, the President's Commission for the Study of Ethical Problems in Medicine and Biomedical and Behavioral Research did not focus on individual rights to health care in their report on access to health care. Instead, the idea of ethical obligations was used in concluding that society has obligations to ensure that all citizens have equitable access to an adequate level of health care without excessive burdens.[22] The ANA Code for Nurses (1985) does not limit equitable access solely to citizens, but states that ". . . nurses have an obligation to promote equitable access to nursing and health care for all people".[23]

Justice issues may seem very distant to nurses working with critically ill patients. Yet they impinge directly and indirectly on the care that nurses are able to provide and are an inherent part of decisions made by individual nurses and nursing administration about allocation of nursing expertise to and within critical care units and other areas of a hospital. Brenda Hewitt's treatment in the critical care unit raises questions about the fair and adequate allocation of nursing expertise. These are the issues that cause nurses to question whether or not they wish to remain in nursing when they are unable to provide safe and competent care due to institutional constraints. Nurses' fidelity to patients is undermined in circumstances in which institutional fiscal interests take precedence over patient interests in a hospital. Nurses and others may feel that they are working in an "ethical wasteland" under such circumstances.

In summary, the ability of critical care nurses and others to take serious account of the principles of veracity, patient autonomy, beneficence, and justice in decision making, planning nursing interventions, and acting can only enhance fidelity to patients as an inherent dimension of the nurse-patient relationship.

Fidelity and the Critical Care Environment

Whether or not nurses generally, and critical care nurses specifically, are able to honor the duty of fidelity to their patients is partially a function of the practice environment and the fact that nurses do have multiple and often conflicting loyalties and obligations. The question has been raised as to whether or not nurses can be ethical in their practice given the organizational and institutional constraints in hospital environments.[24] An important question for individual nurses and for the nursing profession collectively is whether or not the principle of fidelity to patients inherent in the nurse-patient relationship can be expressed in a practice environment that is primarily bureaucratic, authoritarian, and paternalistic. Yarling and McElmurry have argued that "nurses are often not free to be moral" in institutions such as hospitals where there are actually disincentives to responsible action and where the integrity and wholeness of nurses is in jeopardy if they seriously seek to practice in an ethically responsible way.[25]

A look at some aspects of the critical care environments in which nursing care occurs is essential to this discussion of fidelity. Both internal and external environments are important to consider. The nurse's own perspectives are a part of the internal environment, that is, the individual's own inner world or reality. That world includes mind sets about health and nursing care delivery systems. The social, cultural, and physical environments of the hospital and the critical care unit are considered to be part of the external environment that influences nurses' fidelity to patients. This external environment also includes the mind sets of the persons involved in giving or receiving care.

Internal and external environments of individuals interact and are interdependent with institutional policies and the broader society. Hence they are the context for the conflicts and tensions nurses experience as they seek to be faithful to their patient care commitments. The recognition that external environments, such as the economic environment, profoundly influence the practice of nursing may leave little time or energy to devote to considering the internal environments of nurses and other health professionals. They are at least of equal importance because they influence if and how individual nurses and the nursing profession deal with fidelity to patients. They also interact powerfully with nurses' professional knowledge and values.

Three possible mind sets of nurses and others about health and nursing care will be examined here briefly.[26,27] They are (1) health care as medical activities (nursing is subsumed under medicine) with cure of disease as the major goal, (2) health care as a commodity to be sold in the marketplace like anything else, and (3) health care as the promotion, maintenance, and restoration of health within a caring community.

The first mind set is illustrated by the critical care nurse who considers the role of nursing mainly as the carrying out of physician orders. The physician becomes the primary client of nursing services rather than the patient. Nurses' primary loyalty and accountability are to physicians and their activities. All other activities are subsumed under those of the physician, and nursing activities are designed solely to meet medical goals for the patient rather than a combination of medical, nursing, and patient goals. Fidelity to patients would necessarily be jeopardized or possibly nonexistent when primary accountability and loyalty of nurses are to physicians and their goals.

There are hospitals in which nursing administration has this view as a predominant mind set. It is obvious that such a mind set, whether that of individuals or of a hospital, would create a particular type of environment for nursing practice and the establishment of institutional policies dominated by medical paternalism. Historically, this is the view of the hospital as the "doctor's workshop."

Nurses who have other perspectives will undoubtedly feel uncomfortable about the ways in which major treatment decisions are made for patients and will experience negation of their own personal and professional fidelity to patients. Mitchell has argued that the nurse who experiences the competing claims of different models of health care "either seeks to salvage individual integrity by quitting or stays and sacrifices integrity."[28] This view also negates the role of the nurse as patient advocate and the current ANA Code for Nurses, which emphasizes nursing accountability to patients as primary and assumes that the nurse is a competent professional with specific obligations to individual clients and society. The view of the nurse as physician extender in this mind set is not adequate to the complex roles and decisions required of nurses in critical care, and is clearly inadequate for nurses as both professionals and moral agents.

The second mind set of health care as a commodity, to be sold like anything else in the marketplace, means that medical care and nursing care are offered for sale with the patient as a customer. This is a pervading view in the 1980s. Physicians, who have traditionally been outside contractors, find their turf challenged by hospital administrators who have increasingly more decision-making power and control over the function of the institution. Critical care nurses find themselves competing for shrinking resources and spending more time trying to justify the need for adequate resources to provide nursing care to those patients who are acutely ill and need particular kinds of nursing expertise. Institutional interests for financial profit or survival take precedence over competing professional privileges of physicians, and seemingly over the interests of patient welfare.

Critical care nurses who hold this view may consider nursing care primarily as a package of services to be sold to patients rather than as provision of necessary individualized services to all patients in need of nursing care. Furthermore, these nurses as employees have chosen to be accountable primarily to the hospital rather than to patients. This approach conflicts with the traditional patient-centered ethos that has permeated medical and nursing care in the past, and commits the nurse to providing care that meets individual patient care needs.

The utilitarian perspective would argue that the greater good will be achieved in this instance through actions and policies that promote institutional survival to meet the health care needs of the greatest number of people. Nurses with this view will probably not question how this influences their fidelity to patients; nursing practice that is congruent with hospital goals will be consistent with what those nurses value as right and good.

The view of health and nursing care as a commodity to be sold in the marketplace negates the idea that there is something special about health care as a service to society. The President's Commission argued that the special importance of health care lies in the mission of health care in society to promote ". . . personal well-being by preventing or relieving pain, suffering, and disability and by avoiding loss of life."[29] Further, individuals do not choose their genetic heritage, that is, their predisposition to certain diseases, or their socioeconomic circumstances. Thus they experience inequalities of opportunity and access to health care. Provision of health care also has special interpersonal significance as an expression of the bonds of empathy and compassion in important life events such as birth and death—that is the idea of a covenant or fidelity. According to the Commission, ". . . a society's commitment to health care reflects some of its most basic attitudes about what it is to be a member of the human community."[30]

Nurses in critical care are in a crucial position to question this view of health care. They deal daily with issues such as the allocation of the scarce resources of nursing expertise and beds for patients who need intensive nursing care. Sensitive staff nurses and administrators question this predominant view as they struggle with the conflict of fidelity to individual patients and institutional interests of well-being in a competitive health care marketplace.

The third mind set is expressed by critical care nurses who seek to enhance a decision-making process in which all participants' goals and values for treatment have an opportunity to be heard. This includes the patient, family, and health professionals caring for the patient. While the interests of the patient are uppermost, such a process implies respect for all the individuals who are involved in or affected by major care and treatment decisions. Nurses would be active participants in the decision-making process along with patients, families, and physicians. Because nurses are the health professionals who are involved with the most intimate and ongoing care of patients in critical care units, it is impossible to justify ethically their not participating in (or being excluded from) important patient care decisions.

An unpublished study of nurses and ethical dilemmas in intensive care units in one teaching research hospital asked nurses several questions about the decision-making process.[31] The intensive care units included those for infants, children, and adults. Seventy-eight percent of the respondents felt that patient care decisions involving ethical dilemmas should be based primarily on ethical principles, rather than on the law or on simply doing everything possible. Ninety-nine percent felt that nurses should have input in the decision-making process because they are a source of information/clarification and support to patients and families. They also have the closest continuing contact with patients and families as the primary care givers. Half of the respondents felt that nurses should have the authority to speak on behalf of patients and families in conferences and so forth. One third also felt that they should have the right to be listened to and respected as professionals by other members of the health care team.

The majority of the respondents indicated that when there was disagreement about treatment decisions that the patient's decision should be determinative. The most important criteria for making decisions were the patient's physical condition, prognosis, and future. The most important reasons for including the family in the decision-making process was that they lived with the consequences of such decisions economically, socially, and psychologically.

However, one must remember that ethically sensitive decisions must be made in situations in which political, legal, and economic realities often dominate the decision-making process. While this third mind set is not a panacea for all hospital problems, it does result in concern for a different order of questions and concerns about availability and access to medical and nursing care. This view is more congruent with the Code, with the special significance of health care, and the Commission's advocacy of shared decision making by patients and health professionals.

If the mind set of the hospital as a caring community prevails in critical care units, nurses' fidelity to patients can only be enhanced. This mind set suggests a more ethically adequate scheme for decision making in patient care units, and suggests more participative kinds of input for hospital policy making. This mind set might also seem hopelessly idealistic. Yet, such a perspective, incorporated with ethical imagination and attention to political realities, has the potential for altering some of the ways in which patient care decisions have been made in the past and for modifying paternalistic and authoritarian hospital structures. Nursing leadership in support of this mind set is essential to carry out adequately the nursing profession's contract with society.

Institutional Mechanisms and the Enhancement of Fidelity

There are no ready-made solutions to the way in which the nurse's fidelity to patients can be undermined in critical care units and hospitals where political, economic, and ethical realities co-exist. Nurses have been able to identify some mechanisms that illuminate ethical problems and provide assistance in efforts to develop more ethically adequate practice, that is, provision of patient care that is more humane and compassionate. Taking action even in the face of seemingly insurmountable odds and hospital tradition has given some nurses a positive sense of power and energy to be used in the struggle for more ethical patient care and the integrity of nurses and nursing. The tragedy of Brenda Hewitt and others like her does not have to happen. Ethically sensitive nurses can work to prevent such events from occurring in critical care units. Nurses' sensitivity to the practice of anticipatory ethics is one way to accomplish this.

Nurses have found a variety of actions helpful in dealing with patient care environments that undermine their fidelity to patients. While systematic study of mechanisms that are supportive of more ethical patient care environments is just beginning, anecdotal information from intensive care, pediatric, and oncology units reveals hopeful developments in this area. Something as simple as talking with nursing colleagues about the moral implications of practice has provided support for nurses and the stress that they experience in dealing with the ethical aspects of patient care. This author is aware of nurses in one intensive care unit who practiced preventive ethics by including an assessment of potential ethical problems for a patient entering their unit. In addition, the availability of regular group meetings on a patient care unit and patient care conferences that include ethical issues and concerns has been supportive. Development of both multidisciplinary and intradisciplinary ethics rounds in patient care units has been useful. Nursing practice committees in some hospitals have taken responsibility to pay attention to the ethical concerns of nurses. Some nursing services include ethical aspects of decision making in orientation of new staff.

More formal institutional mechanisms include development of nursing ethics committees and multidisciplinary institutional ethics committees that provide education and consultation for ethical problems that cannot be resolved on a patient care unit or that require review of existing policies or development of new hospital policies. The ANA has developed guidelines for nurses' participation on these committees and serves as a resource to state nurses' associations that are working to assist nurses with ethical problems encountered in practice.

Enhancement of the fidelity of nurses to patients, collectively or individually, requires action. Individual nurses can take steps to develop more ethically adequate practice through examining their own mind sets about nursing and health care and taking leadership to develop mechanisms on their own patient care units to deal with ethical problems and conditions that undermine nursing's fidelity to patients.

The achievement of long-term goals related to enhancement of fidelity in the nurse-patient relationship can only be achieved with the active assistance of other nursing colleagues who see the reform of the practice environment as essential to humane and compassionate nursing practice. This requires political and ethical nursing action.

Notes

1. The discussion of fidelity is drawn from Veatch RM: A Theory of Medical Ethics, pp 214–226, New York, Basic Books, 1981, and Ramsey P: Patient as Person, New Haven, Yale

University Press, 1970. The author takes full responsibility for the interpretation of their work in this chapter.

2. Beauchamp TL, Childress JF: Principles of Biomedical Ethics, 2nd ed, p 237. New York, Oxford University Press, 1983

3. Ibid, p 238

4. ANA: Code for Nurses with Interpretive Statements. Kansas City, MO, ANA, 1985

5. ANA: Nursing: A Social Policy Statement, p 5. Kansas City, MO, ANA, 1980

6. Schucking EL: Death at a New York hospital. Law, Medicine and Health Care 13:261–268, 1985

7. Greenlaw J: High tech nursing at its worst. Law, Medicine and Health Care 13:278, 1985

8. Reiser SJ, Anbar M (eds): The Machine at the Bedside. Preface. Cambridge, Cambridge University Press, 1984

9. Reiser SJ: The machine at the bedside: Technological transformations of practices and values. In Reiser, Anbar, 1984, op cit, p 14

10. Bok S: Lying: Moral Choice in Public and Private Life, p 19. New York, Vintage, 1978

11. Ibid, pp 24–28

12. Veatch 1981, op cit

13. Brody H, Lynn J: The physician's responsibility under the new Medicare reimbursement for hospice care. N Engl J Med 310:921, 1984

14. Yarling RR: Ethical analysis of a nursing problem: The scope of nursing practice in disclosing the truth to terminal patients. Part I. Supervisor Nurse 9:45, 1978

15. This discussion of veracity or truth telling in nursing is drawn from Yarling RR: Ethical analysis of a nursing problem: The scope of nursing practice in disclosing the truth to terminal patients. Part II. Supervisor Nurse 9:30, 1978

16. Ibid

17. Ibid, p 33

18. Ibid

19. Frankena WK: Ethics, 2nd ed, p 47. Englewood Cliffs, Prentice-Hall, 1973

20. Ibid, pp 172–173

21. ANA 1985, op cit

22. President's Commission for the Study of Ethical Problems in Medicine and Biomedical and Behavioral Research: Securing Access to Health Care, vol 1. Report, p 4. Washington, DC, Government Printing Office, 1983

23. Ibid, p 16

24. Davis AJ, Aroskar MA: Ethical Dilemmas and Nursing Practice, 2nd ed, p 63. East Norwalk, CT, Appleton-Century-Crofts, 1983

25. Yarling RR, McElmurry BJ: The moral foundation of nursing. Advances in Nursing Science 8:63–73, 1986

26. These mind sets were adapted from Newton LH: To whom is the nurse accountable? A philosophical perspective. Conn Med (suppl) 43:7–9, 1979

27. Aroskar M: Are nurses' mind sets compatible with ethical practice? Topics in Clinical Nursing 4:22–32, 1982

28. Mitchell C: Integrity in interprofessional relationships, p 176. In Agich GJ (ed): Responsibility in Health Care. Dordrecht, D Reidel, 1982

29. Ibid, p 16

30. Ibid, p 17

31. Aroskar MA, Schlesinger D: Unpublished research report. Nurses and Ethical Dilemmas in Intensive Care. University of Minnesota, 1983

Chapter 7

Justice and the Allocation of Scarce Nursing Resources in Critical Care Nursing

June Levine-Ariff

The critical care unit of a major teaching hospital has just been informed that two patients from the emergency room require admission. One patient is a policeman, wounded in the line of duty. The other patient is a 70-year-old gentleman with severe gastrointestinal bleeding. There is one bed available and no additional nurses scheduled to absorb any admissions.

It is 3:00 A.M. The neonatal intensive care unit has just received a call to transport a one-hour-old infant with a diaphragmatic hernia. Immediate surgery is necessary to save the child's life. Yet, no one is readily available for transport. The nurse assigned to transport has to give a report on her patient. The nurse responsible for assuming that child's care is in the middle of a chest tube insertion. The senior resident scheduled for transport is placing the chest tube. The only other physician available is an intern.

It is 7:00 A.M. and the charge nurse of the ICU is receiving a report. Two patients were admitted since 5:00 P.M. the day before. The patient in the operating room received a gunshot wound while attempting robbery. Two patients in the hospital are scheduled for surgery; both will need postoperative admission to the ICU. There are no available beds in the unit.

These situations, replayed over and over in critical care units across the country, provide examples of what scarce resources mean to the critical care nurse. In these cases, like others, decisions are ultimately made, though sometimes by default. Most patients receive the care they need—or do they? Beds never appear to be available when needed. Nurses are always in short supply. Criteria used to make these decisions are often based on personal value systems, medical politics, institutional directives, patient need, or insurance coverage. Critical care nurses involved in these decisions often feel uneasy about the way resources are distributed.

A few years ago, before the proliferation of medical technology, the pervasiveness of medical insurance, and the restrictions on health care reimbursement, constraints on the availability of health care resources were largely unheard of. Until recently, our country's health care delivery system emphasized making the highest quality of care accessible to all, regardless of the costs. This philosophy has changed. Although quality and access remain important, cost efficiency has become a crucial component.

If cost containment measures involved only cutting unnecessary health care services, without unfairly targeting specific individuals or groups, they would pose no moral problem. Because of the rising costs of medical care and the meager gain in the general national health, questions are being asked by government and private insurers. Which technologies should be covered? Should more dollars be given to preventive care, acute care, or long-term care? Which diseases or disabilities should receive more dollars than others? The concerns are being raised not only in relation to the payment of services for patients, but also when allocating dollars for research and education. How will decisions about allocation be decided, and who will decide them?

The principle of justice helps us examine these dilemmas in light of the circumstances that lead up to specific social policy decisions. How these positions are translated into allocation decisions in the ICU affects every critical care nurse. Nurses, physicians, and hospital administrators view these issues differently. It is these differences that can pose conflicts at the bedside. Strategies for nurses involved in allocation decisions are the focus of the closing comments in this chapter. For the moment, let us turn our attention to health care economics: payment for health care is being viewed as a scarce resource. The decisions about distribution of these resources are of national concern and are felt acutely by the critical care nurse. In 1950 Americans spent 4.5% of the gross national product (GNP) on health care compared to 9.1% in 1978.[1] Today, health care comprises one of the largest industries, consuming $425 billion or approximately 10.7% of the GNP.[2] There is an expectation that this figure could increase to approximately 14% of the GNP by the year 2000, even with current spending constraints.[3]

The development of new technologies, the proliferation of health care workers, and the increased size of the aged population have all contributed to the escalation of private and public costs for current and new health care resources.

Technology

Technological development, aided by federal funding, has provided miraculous breakthroughs in the fight against death, disability, and disease. Bypass surgery, joint replacement, dialysis, microsurgeries, laser surgery, and organ transplants are but a few of the technological innovations of the last two decades. Concurrent with these advances, there has been a development of invasive and noninvasive monitoring equipment that makes many critical care units look like NASA's mission control center. Techniques developed since the 1970s have extended life and relieved pain, but at enormous costs. Years ago, no one would have thought to ask if we could afford the latest technological achievement. For third-party payors today, it becomes the central and pervasive question. For health care providers, the questions relate more to the perceived benefits and burdens that technology imposes on patients and families. For the patient, the use of sophisticated medical technology remains synonymous with better health care.

Manpower

As technology grew, so did the generalized manpower to manufacture, use, or repair it. Within the hospital, a large diversification occurred among the types of health care workers. Tasks traditionally associated with nursing, and seen as an expense, became a source of revenue when assumed by respiratory therapy, physical therapy, occupational therapy, and pharmacy, adding to the overall costs of providing service. It is no wonder that the ratio of hospital employees to patients has increased about 70% every 10 years since 1960.[4] The health care industry has been shown to be one of the most labor-intensive systems in this country. In addition, the passage of the revision to the National Labor Relations Act in 1974, allowing hospital workers to unionize, contributed further to health care's rising costs.

The Aging Population

As we reflect on the hospitals of the 1950s and 1960s, we see a large number of beds being occupied by young, healthy individuals. When Medicare began in 1965, the elderly accounted for approximately 10% of the population. Current population trends indicate that for the year 1995 individuals over the age of 75 will have increased by 30% from the 1980s and will be mostly comprised of women living alone with severe chronic disease.[5]

It is a well-known fact that individuals over the age of 65 spend over two and one half times as much on medical care as those between the ages of 19 and 64.[6] Yet Medicare as the primary health provider for the elderly covered only 44% of their total health care costs in 1978.[7] The increases in the amounts of co-deductibles and decreases in the types of benefits have lowered this figure further. It is anticipated that the population of the 21st century will be largely composed of the young and the old. It will be the first time in history that those contributing to the country's financial resources will be smaller in number than those who depend on those resources. As the aged population has increased in size, along with the rising costs of providing services, there has been an increased recognition of the rights of adults to determine their own health care needs. Patient autonomy is thriving as concern for the allocation of resources rises.

Growth in Spending

Before 1950, health care was available to those who could afford to pay. The 1950s saw an expansion of health care resources, with services centered largely in hospitals. Aided by the Hill Burton Act of 1948, hospitals received construction dollars in exchange for guarantees of care to the poor. The increasing expansion of hospital beds promoted increased utilization of services, which in turn promoted further expansion. Open access in the availability of hospital resources for all individuals was the policy of the country. The rise of private third-party payors and government entitlement programs that fostered the consumer and provider noninvolvement in health care costs spurred an algebraic increase in demand for services that few anticipated.

The decade of the 1960s was characterized by intense national spending for hospitals, technology, research, and the education of doctors and nurses. Titles 18 and 19 of the Social Security Act, Medicare and Medicaid, were enacted. It was a time of social sensitivity to the health needs of the aged and the poor. There was a belief that these federal programs would meet the needs of the country's citizens for many, many years. The health planning policies of the 1950s and 1960s supported the traditional economic view that increasing the supply would increase the access and decrease the costs. Yet at the time of Medicare's enactment, policy makers seemingly forgot that the 75 million individuals born between 1946 and 1964 would one day grow old.[8] Furthermore, expensive technology now in use was not yet being dreamed about.

Cost Containment

Cost-based reimbursement had fueled the enormous growth in hospital bed capacity, intensity of care, and the development of technology. The medical cost component of the consumer price index rose from 2.1% in 1965 to 6.5% by 1967.[9] By then, Congress was already amending Medicaid to reduce cost overruns. From 1962 to 1973 the number of intensive care units increased by 2225, while the number of acute care hospitals increased by only 146.[10] "Between 1979 and 1983, the number of ICU beds rose by 30%."[11] In 1983 there were 6900 intensive care units with approximately 81,000 beds in 6300 hospitals.[12] Retrospective reimbursement gave incentives to physicians and hospitals to perform and to provide as many procedures and services as possible. In fact, such reimbursement offered no encouragement to use resources efficiently; it actually facilitated overutilization.

The decade of the 1970s was an era of increasing regulations designed to control increasing expenditures for health-related programs. The availability of technology, coupled with the concerns of malpractice suits, resulted in the proliferation of overuse of expensive diagnostic procedures. As the government's share of expenses in health care continued to increase, national health policy shifted from one of guaranteed access to one of cost containment.

The 1980s saw an even more economically stringent approach to health care spending. In 1981 major cuts in the Medicare program were made for the first time. In March 1983 Congress approved a Medicare prospective pricing plan for most inpatient services, which mandated a change from retrospective payment for hospital service to a predetermined prospective payment rate for a specific diagnosis. Diagnostic related groupings (DRGs) became the buzzword of the industry.

The strategy behind the current federal changes is to contain costs and to allow private enterprise to respond to the consumer's health needs. It is believed that encouraging competition among providers will ultimately force the elimination of excesses and duplication of goods and services. Certainly, each hospital makes a decision about the range of services to be offered. These decisions should relate to assessed community needs, availability of services in the area served, the hospital's ability to provide the service (personnel, equipment, space), and the financial viability of the service. However, the latter may supercede all other needs. The full-service hospital of the past is defining its "product lines" and eliminating some financially draining services. A competitive surge among health care providers has indeed occurred, but hospitals are competing for the "private" health care dollar. Patients reimbursed by Medicare and Medicaid, or those without any insurance, are usually sicker and consume more resources. The double-edged sword, however, is that private insurance companies are negotiating with providers for cost breaks in charges in return for their customers' use of the hospital's services. The proliferation of preferred provider organizations (PPOs) and health maintenance organizations (HMOs), promising low costs for the consumer, are adding competition for the private dollar in an already highly competitive market. Thus, the sicker and more financially at-risk patients are being seen in greater numbers in teaching and publicly supported hospitals. The disproportionate burden these institutions are experiencing is not being compensated. Other hospitals, in a better position to balance high and low cost patients, can be more economically competitive.

Cost containment and eligibility requirements have become the major focus of federal health programs. As of 1975 over 6 million people below the poverty line were ineligible for Medicaid, and in 1978 nearly 8% of the American population had no health insurance at all.[13]

Allocation of Services

Who pays the bill usually determines which health benefits are covered. Third-party payors, whether they be Medicare, Medicaid, Blue Cross, or an HMO, decide which services are covered. Many large corporations are becoming self-insured because of the dramatic increase in premiums charged by regular insurers. These corporations are making independent decisions as to which services are covered. Concerned with the "indiscriminate use" of covered benefits by consumers, government, private, and corporate insurers have increased co-insurance payments and deductibles. This was initially seen as a way to improve the consumer's decisions about which health care services to use. The result, however, has been a decrease in utilization of services for less acute illness, and an exacerbation of both chronic and acute health needs that require more immediate treatment. In fact, the costs of providing services may actually be greater—a variable that is difficult to measure. The elderly, hit hard by Medicare's increases in deductibles and decreased coverage options, without a like percentage increase in Social Security benefits, have often waited until their symptoms became so severe that they could not be treated as outpatients.

Decisions on how the government plans to spend its dollars for health care resources often set precedents that private insurers follow. Priorities are being determined as to, for example, whether heart disease will receive more money than heart transplants; whether prevention will receive a larger dollar outlay than chronic disease. Will more dollars be used to aid victims of disabling diseases such as arthritis or terminal illnesses? Finally, will everyone who has arthritis be given the same access to available therapies?

According to Roger Evans, federal law and insurance companies allocate dollars that lead to societal limits on the distribution of resources at the health care program level, that is, they make macroallocation decisions. Such rationing further implies decision making at the individual patient level, that is, microallocation. Thus, macroallocation decisions usually precede microallocation or institutional or unit rationing decisions.[14] For example, in the early days of kidney dialysis, the federal government allocated a specific amount of money for this purpose. It was up to the clinicians at the bedside to decide who should receive this scarce resource.

Although the American public deplores rationing in health care and openly defends the concept of equal access to health care services, as will be discussed later, the rationing of health care services has occurred and still does so; in fact, it is accepted and widely used. The principle of justice helps us look closely at the ways health care resources are allocated at both the macro and the micro levels, thus clarifying why concerns of the nurse differ from those of other health care colleagues.

Justice

The principle of justice has three major areas of application. *Retributive justice* is concerned primarily with punishing someone for wrongdoing. The word *retribution* comes from this concept. *Procedural justice* focuses on fairness in how things are done. Following procedural justice does not guarantee a just outcome. A guilty person may receive a procedurally fair trial yet be acquitted. *Distributive justice* focuses on the allocation of goods and services, *usually* in situations of scarcity. It is justice as it applies primarily to the distribution of health care resources and will be the focus here.

The fundamental premise of justice simply proclaims that like cases should be treated alike and that those that are different should be treated differently, taking into account their ethically relevant differences.[15] This has been called the formal principle of justice. The difficult issue is to determine what constitutes a relevant difference between individuals that allows some to get a specific health care resource and others to be denied it. The basic principle does not specify what constitutes relevant differences. How can society make such distinctions?

Described below are five commonly held ideas for the distribution of limited resources. Public policy and institutional decisions have ultimately derived from the acceptance of one or another of these material principles of justice.[16,17] All these specifications of the relevant differences presume and further define the basic principle.

1. Distribution to each person according to effort/merit
2. Distribution to each person according to societal contribution
3. Distribution of an equal share to each person
4. Distribution to each person according to need
5. Similar treatment for similar cases

Distribution Based on Merit

This approach bases access to services on amounts of energy expended (effort) or kinds of results achieved (merit). In some areas one can exert little effort, and achievement can be great. There are individuals who spend just a few hours studying and receive high grades on examinations. Others exert much effort for no rewards. This allocation method would distribute health care services on the basis of the personal achievement of individuals with regard to their own health. It asks whether a specific person *deserves* care. Merit is an appropriate consideration in job promotion and the granting of college degrees. It is difficult, however, to use merit as a relevant factor in the allocation of health care resources. How could a health professional determine the merit of an individual? Such decisions are often based on highly particular value systems. Health care crises often occur for uncontrollable and unpredictable reasons. They befall all people without regard for a person's past or present achievements or style of living. A newborn baby, a child, or an adult with severe handicaps does not deserve discrimination based on inability to achieve health through his own efforts.

Yet, while some individuals need health care because of circumstances beyond their control, others are victims of their own choices. There are those who argue that the voluntary nature of using drugs, alcohol, and cigarettes should limit these individuals' access to health care services needed because of these vices. Thus, a person who smokes and has emphysema might not be entitled to the possible advantages of the respiratory intensive care unit. Alcoholics who need liver transplants might be denied or given lower priority. Obese individuals who had a weight-related heart attack might not be admitted to the coronary care unit. Taking this concept further, individuals choosing a certain line of work, like professional football or race car driving, may become victims of their own choices if job-related disease or disability were to strike. Accident victims might not be treated if they were known to have caused the accident. However, the same people who argue from this perspective would not deny health care services to sedentary professors or corporate executives with type A personalities whose life styles also contributed to certain diseases. Those with overtly socially unacceptable traits or behavior are often targeted by this position.

Distribution Based on Societal Contribution

This perspective essentially looks at the social worth of individuals. Thus, the socially disregarded, such as the elderly or the very young, may be automatically ruled out as health resources are distributed. The young, not yet having had an opportunity to contribute to society , and the old, whose previous years of giving have been forgotten, are not perceived as current contributors. Another limiting factor is the unequal opportunities people have to contribute to society. Physical ability, intelligence, and socioeconomic status are limitations that can be beyond a person's control. Although it has been said that ours is a land of opportunity, ''. . . the overwhelming power to hold most individuals in their social place cannot be ignored.''[18]

Demand plays a large part in what society views as a contribution. Athletic stars are rewarded and idolized; city parking enforcement personnel are not. Values also change; those who were not looked upon to have social worth in one period of history may deserve resources in another. Computer programmers were once considered to be strange and to contribute little to society's productivity. Today they are viewed as one of our country's greatest resources. In 1953 the much-publicized Seattle selection committee for dialysis used factors such as church membership and scouting leadership to assess a person's right to dialysis. The fact that most recipients were male, married, employed, and between the ages of 25 and 45 contributed to the uneasiness in the country when these facts were made public.[19]

Distribution Based on an Equal Share

While traditional notions of equality of access to health resources continue to be espoused, some of the most difficult questions facing society deal with the reality that equal access may not be possible. Historically, society has underwritten much of the economic costs of health professional education, research, and service delivery, believing that a function of social policy is to balance inequities. The right to health services appears in many references and public opinion polls throughout the 19th and 20th centuries. Studies by the American Hospital Association in 1983 and 1984 demonstrate the American public's aversion to rationing health care and its preference for equal access.[20] However, this inclination is not matched by society's willingness to supply the financial resources to underwrite these services. Some physicians refuse to see Medicare and Medicaid patients, government priorities do not reflect health care, and some hospitals limit access to emergency services to those who can pay.

Central to the issue is the question: is health care a right or is it a privilege? A right evokes entitlement—things people must have, not just prefer or wish to have. Thus these rights cannot be denied. An equal access principle supports the assumption that the rich cannot buy health services that are not also equally available to the poor. This concept is anomalous as we look at other sectors of society. Housing, education, legal assistance, and transportation are not distributed equally; yet in all those areas society has attempted to provide a decent, fair minimum standard. Most philosophers would agree that a decent, fair minimum standard for the distribution of health care resources must be established. Many favor providing government coverage for basic and catastrophic health needs and asking private insurance to provide other health care needs. Charles Fried, a noted philosopher, has specified that a decent minimum should incorporate maternal and child health programs.[21] It is obvious that in discussions of a decent minimum standard no one has yet resolved what the specific aspects of care should include. Because discussions of the distribution of health care resources virtually strike at the heart of one's own existence, the definition of a decent minimum standard is understandably difficult.

Proponents of the concept of equal access suggest that if we do have limited resources for health care, perhaps technology should not be used at all, or should be used minimally, since increased costs prohibit its use for everyone. Nurses who work in critical care units know that disease and disability know no income barriers or sociocultural lines. Feelings of fear and despair often accompany certain diseases and disabilities. Good health is considered to be essential to what one wants to do during a lifetime. Nurses firmly support the concept of equal access. That belief often places nurses in an adversarial role with physicians and institutions when decisions about the allocation of nursing resources are made. The Code for Nurses states that "the need for health care is universal, transcending all national, ethnic, racial, religious, cultural, political, educational, economic, developmental, personality, role, and sexual differences."[22]

Distribution Based on Individual Need

The definition of a health care need is a difficult one. In general, to say a person needs something is to say that he/she will be harmed if they do not get it. In this perspective, the relevant difference between individuals, then, is need. However, there are problems inherent in the determination of needs: (1) Differentiating between a need and a desire, (2) deciding what needs should be met, and (3) deciding what level of need will be met. Beauchamp and Childress have used the term *fundamental need* to describe a situation in which a person may be harmed when a need goes unmet. They believe health care to be a fundamental need.[23] For example, patients needing medication equally should have equal access to medication. Gene Outka has differentiated between universally basic health needs, such as food and shelter, and essential needs, such as health care. He claims that basic, universal needs can be planned for appropriately, while essential health needs are arbitrary. They arrive unplanned for and uninvited. Patients should thus receive health care services on the basis of a natural lottery, such as first-come, first-served.[24] Finally, as with any resource, what does one do when need outstrips availability? Currently, due to rising costs, availability has been limited as the need increases.

Within nursing there is general agreement that allocating resources on the basis of merit and societal contribution is not acceptable. While distribution based on need is supported, nursing fails to define what constitutes a need and further fails to differentiate medical and nursing needs. Equal access is, as previously discussed, a basic concern. Equal access gives everyone the same opportunity to obtain treatment, yet recognizes the limitations of certain services.

Similar Treatment for Similar Cases

According to Outka, this concept "may be construed so as to guide actual choices in the way most compatible with the goal of equal access."[25] The difficulty rests with deciding which diseases or disabilities should be treated before others or which should not be treated at all. Outka has stated, "All persons with a certain rare, noncommunicable disease would not receive priority, let us say, where the costs were inordinate, the prospects for rehabilitation remote, and for the sake of equalized benefits to many more."[26] This is a decision society as yet has failed to make.

Age, health status, autonomy, and notoriety have also been utilized for allocating services. Age has certainly been a determining factor for resource allocation. The Seattle dialysis committee did not recommend anyone over the age of 45, and most heart transplant centers do not take anyone over the age of 50. Individuals whose zest for life has not been hampered by age and who have the funds to pay for an organ transplant are frustrated and scared about their life prospects. Consider this excerpt from an editorial in *Heart and Lung:*

> When the physician explained that an age of 57 years precluded a transplant, the patient said, "I worked hard all of my life. My wife and I have been able to save some money over the years and we are more than willing to spend those savings for an operation that would allow me to live longer. If I am willing to take the risk, and I have the money to pay for the surgery, why can't I get a new heart?"[27]

Health status also has been a determining factor in allocation decisions. Restraints in the application of heroic measures for the dying have been advocated. Beginning in 1975, the Los Angeles County Burn Center has offered patients a choice between maximal therapy or palliative care with burns of a severity known to be without precedent for survival. Fifty percent of the patients, all of whom died, chose palliative care.[28]

Autonomy has recently begun to play a role in the allocation of health care resources. With the economic crunch, many more physicians and hospitals are willing to let individuals, in terminal or ventilator-dependent states, choose to withhold or to withdraw futile technology. Allocation decisions are being made on a technologies potential for enhancing the patient's quality of life. One would like to believe that this sudden support for a patient's rights had a moral impetus rather than an economic emphasis. The Code for Nurses states this as a basic tenet of the profession.

> Clients have the moral right to determine what will be done with their own person; to be given accurate information, and all the information necessary for making informed judgments; to be assisted with weighing the benefits and burdens of options

in their treatment; to accept, refuse, or terminate treatment without coercion; and to be given necessary emotional support.[29]

In the last few years, as organ transplantation became more successful, notoriety has determined allocation decisions. During 1985, President Reagan became involved in a search for an adequate donor for 14-month-old Ryan Osterman from Gainesville, Florida. The president asked the then secretary of the Department of Health and Human Services (DHHS), Margaret M. Heckler, to publicize the child's need as well as the needs of all children like Ryan. An organ donor was found and a successful operation was performed.[30] Newspaper headlines that describe the plight of a young child in need of an organ transplant grab the emotions of most readers.

Organ Transplantation

Notoriety, need, lack of resource availability, and cost have spurred the national debate over organ transplantation. The criteria for distributing organs are varied and reflect many of the resource allocation concepts previously discussed. Thus, we can view organ transplantation as a model for allocation of any scarce resource, such as critical care nursing. Two questions are central to these concerns. The first is whether the benefits of the transplant outweigh its costs. The second is how decisions are made for the distribution of this scarce resource. There are neither national nor state guidelines that aid in the selection of transplant recipients. Each transplant center uses its own discretion in establishing criteria. These vary from age and tissue match to issues of "need," chance of success, ability to comply with postoperative care, absence of psychiatric illness or drug abuse, and presence of familial support. Others use a first-come, first-served basis. The criteria followed by centers in a national transplantation study emphasized familial support, an understanding of the risks, and an ability to comply with treatment plans.[31] Lately, there has been increasing concern that prominent foreigners have received cadaver organs before citizens. Citizenship is surfacing as an allocation criterion for transplantation.

With all the recent attention, controversy over organ transplantation is not new. After much public debate about the use of social worth as a criterion for kidney dialysis, Congress, in 1972, unwilling to define specific criteria for this scarce resource, authorized an entitlement program to extend Medicare benefits for renal dialysis to virtually all U.S. citizens with kidney failure or end-stage renal disease. The economic consequences of this decision were staggering. "In 1985, more than 80,000 patients with chronic kidney failure accounted for Medicare expenditures in excess of two billion dollars."[32]

In 1976, 24 heart transplants, 14 liver transplants, and approximately 4000 kidney transplants were performed. In 1984, these numbers had jumped to 325 heart transplants, 300 liver transplants, and 6900 kidney transplants."[34]

The costs for transplantation are high and depend to some degree on which center performs them. For example, the cost for a heart transplant can range from

$57,000 to $110,000 per operation, depending on the patient's condition and the institution where the transplant surgery was performed."[35]

Third-party payors vary in their coverage for transplants. Some states are considering legislation that prohibits insurance companies from denying coverage of any procedure. The federal government now pays for the cost of all kidney transplants and the cost of liver transplants for some children. In June 1986, DHHS Secretary Bowen announced that Medicare would begin to cover heart transplants, but only at centers that meet preestablished criteria for personnel, equipment, and experience. The DHHS estimates that in the first year of coverage, approximately 65 transplants will occur at a cost of roughly $5 million. These estimates do not include payment for immunosuppressant drugs. The current cost estimate for a year's supply of cyclosporin use is $5,000 to $10,000. This area is currently under study.[36]

Despite increased willingness to pay for organ transplantation, cadaver organs are in short supply.

> There are probably 14,000–15,000 people in the population who could potentially benefit from heart transplantation. If we use very, very stringent criteria, that number may be more on the order of 2000, but in any case, we have more candidates than hearts. There are currently between 500–1300 heart donors available each year.[37]

With all the talk about scarcity and money, "it is predicted that by the year 2000, organ transplantation will be common. Public demand will encourage this despite ethical and economic concerns. However, the issue of who decides who is to receive this scarce resource has not been answered."[38]

Now, as we turn our discussion to the critical care unit, we must keep in mind the economic conditions, in society and within the hospital, that cause questions to be raised about the utilization of critical care services. Yet, amidst these concerns there continues to be a movement to promote the growth and utilization of critical care beds. The critical care nurse must practice in this climate. What forces are at play that cause nurses to compromise the care they deliver to patients? How do nurses decide who receives what aspects of nursing care? The utilization of nursing as a resource constitutes the remainder of our discussion.

The current economic conditions of health care in the United States pose an ethical dilemma for the distribution of resources by placing the principles of beneficence and nonmaleficence at odds. It's a challenge to do good and not inflict harm. The economics of the 1980s have required hospitals to redefine the services that are offered and to market these services to physicians and patients. In an attempt to attract the private-pay patient—in which case the reimbursement for intensive care is still greater than for other hospital beds—intensive care units of 4 to 8 beds are being built. In hospitals vying for obstetrical services, for example, NICUs are being opened. The development of pediatric intensive care units follows, since pediatricians caring for patients in the NICU would prefer to have all their patients in one hospital.

The opening of an intensive care unit is usually considered to be a great event. Technology and the "pleasant" environment of colors and private rooms are displayed. Usually the business of assuring a staff of competent nurses is last on the list; thus the inevitable often happens. Physicians become upset that they cannot admit a patient to the unit; after all, there is a vacant bed. Sometimes, the economic pressures force a nursing administrator to hire LVNs or nurses' aides. This is not the place to discuss the quality of care differences. Let it suffice to say that nursing care has been compromised. It is easy to believe that the nursing administrator could have held firm and assured patient safety while denying admission when nursing staff is not available. Unfortunately, the burden falls not only on nursing administration but also on the nursing profession because it allows itself to be compromised in order to get the job done, sometimes in direct violation of its own code of ethics. Most physicians and hospital administrators view the necessity of a critical care unit admission as a need for technology and close observation. *Actually, the need for a critical care nurse who does the observation and operates the technological devices is the reason patients are admitted to the unit.* In the discussion of nursing resources, this issue will be explored further. Another interesting point is the antithesis to the expansion of critical care beds that we touched on initially. Questions are being raised about the efficacy of such units. In a study published by Knaus and colleagues, it was found that approximately 25% of critical care therapy goes to patients who are either too low risk, or too severely ill, to benefit. Critical care therapy was felt to provide greater short-term correction, but there is little evidence of improved survival or quality of life from the use of critical care.[39] In other studies, data are demonstrating that the benefits of admission to the unit may be overestimated in patients with exacerbations of chronic, irreversible diagnoses such as congestive heart failure or chronic obstructive lung disease.[40-42] Many articles are critical of physicians' lack of knowledge about, and involvement with, reviewing the outcomes of patients discharged from such units. Coronary care units and surgical, medical, and neonatal intensive care units are being screened for the efficacy of the care provided. Authors note that little has been done to set clearer standards for admission and discharge from the unit and that methods have not been developed to compare treatment results from one unit to another.[43] Because critical care consumes approximately 20% of hospital costs, these issues must be taken seriously. In the light of scarce resources, patients who do not benefit from intensive care should be excluded from it. One study emphasized that "for nearly half (49%) of the admissions and during two-thirds (65%) of the nursing shifts, the emphasis was on close nursing care and observation, not intensive care."[44] This is the crux of the dilemma for the nurse. In the AACN position statement of 1980, the organization describes the patient to whom the critical care nurse offers care. "The critically ill patient is characterized by the presence of real or potential life-threatening health problems and by the requirement for continuous observation and intervention to prevent complications and restore health."[45] It does not necessitate that technology be used or that cure be a desired outcome. Nurses practicing in critical care must begin to define nursing admission and discharge criteria, lest the medical profession prevail in its efforts to admit only those patients who will benefit from medical diagnostic or treatment interventions and deny admission to those patients in need of critical care nursing. Studies must be developed by nursing that define the outcomes of intensive nursing care. Nursing care hours on noncritical care units are too few to be able to provide the intensive observation and intervention that patients requiring admission to the critical care unit need. Perhaps the future hospital will house two different intensive care units, one offering high-tech medical intervention and one offering very intensive nursing care. In either case, the skills of a critical care nurse will be needed.

Discussions in the literature about the allocation of critical care services focus not only on admission criteria but also on the efficacious use of technology—both of which are factors in high hospital costs. Should a specific technological intervention be used when the benefits to the patient are questionable? Certainly, this issue is also of concern to the nurse as we consider the allocation of nursing resources. One aspect of the use of technology that, although discussed in the ethical literature, refuses to focus on its impact on nursing is how new technology is introduced into the ICU. New technology often results in new procedures and practices that have implications in terms of cost, quality of care, exclusion of other services, and human resources. For example, to begin offering extracorporeal membrane oxygenation (ECMO) in the NICU requires more than enthusiastic physicians and appropriate equipment. Because ECMO requires a lot of space for equipment and supplies, the hospital must be willing to support the unit, lest other space requirements be compromised. Patients require a 2:1 nurse-to-patient ratio. Are there enough nurses available to support this resource intensive program? What about the impact on other children who need the care offered in these units? How will decisions be made if the number of children who are admitted exceeds the availability of nurses and backup equipment? Will the educational process of nursing personnel be condensed so that more children can be taken care of sooner? It has always been interesting to note how quickly physicians, and nurses themselves, are willing to compromise thorough educational preparation if it means having a nurse at the bedside sooner. Nursing must ask these questions early and receive answers that assure patient safety and quality of care. Nursing and medicine must function collegially, for it is certain that without the cooperation of both disciplines, such a program cannot be safely implemented. Nursing need not assume a passive role when nursing resources and the operation of the unit are in question.

Because technology is expensive, equipment to be used by nurses at the bedside must have both nursing and medical concurrence before purchase. Too often, equipment is brought into a unit without input from nurses. When nurses point out a flaw that makes adaptation to bedside care impossible or difficult, they are usually told that "the dollars have been spent—do the best you can." The cost increases in nurses' working hours are never accounted for in productivity reports, yet they contribute significantly to the increased waste of a vital resource—nursing care. A nursing product evaluation committee whose goals are to maintain quality of nursing practice and care, minimize duplication of supplies, and decrease costs would be an asset to any institution. Those products that require medical input would receive it, and the cooperative effort with the hospital's purchasing department would go far in curtailing wasted money and human resources. This concept fits well with the proposals in the literature that advocate cautious evaluation of technology in light of its effectiveness, safety, patient benefit, and cost. The concern for nursing resources ought to be regarded as part of the cost.

Policy decisions that enhance the physical facility, increase the level of available medical technology, improve research, and provide for medical education—and yet fail to focus on inadequate bedside equipment, staffing levels, and staffing skill—create dilemmas for the nurse as she or he is expected to assume responsibilities greater than professional conscience can allow. It is the nurse who must cope hourly with the impact of others' decisions, who often feels no power to deal with the ramifications, and who sees the patient and family as the center of concern.

Nursing offers an essential health service. Nurses affirm the right of all individuals to these services. The pragmatics of meeting multiple and competing needs can place nurses in difficult situations. When nursing resources are scarce, the patient's need for nursing care and his ability to benefit from that care are the criteria most often used by nursing.

Certainly, some patients need more care than others. Defining care in medical terms of mortality and morbidity obscures the contribution nurses make toward a patient's health care. A patient who requires close nursing observation after neurosurgical intervention may have little, if any, technologically sophisticated equipment at the bedside, nor be in immediate life-threatening danger. Yet the need for close observation and monitoring of vital systems certainly requires the skill and staffing levels of a critical care nurse. Nurses must be careful not to consider themselves only as operators of technological machines and purveyors of physicians' orders, lest they be replaced by LVNs or physicians' assistants who focus merely on parts of the patient's care.

It is vital that nursing develop acuity tools that have been tested for validity and reliability to measure a patient's nursing needs. These acuity tools must be standardized if nursing is to become less the whim of actual time studies and be based more on what practice should be. It is then that nursing can demonstrate the patient criteria for nursing care needed for admission into the ICU.

The current concern for limited health care resources has caused philosophers, such as Veatch, to write eloquently about the burden imposed on physicians who may be asked to set standards for a "decent minimum" of medical care.

Veatch said, "Asking physicians to be cost-conscious, however, would be asking them to abandon their central commitment to their patients. In effect, they would be asked to remove the Hippocratic Oath from their waiting room walls and replace it with a sign that reads, "Warning all ye who enter here. I will generally work for your rights and welfare, but if benefits to you are marginal and costs are great, I will abandon you in order to protect society."[46]

Veatch should also be this eloquent about nurses. The commitment of the nurse to her or his patient seems to be laid aside when priorities need to be shifted to accommodate another admission, when others replace the registered nurse at the bedside, or when other department staff members go home, leaving nursing to fill in the gaps. Recently, in a major teaching hospital, a message flashed across the computer screen in the ICU: "Attention, Physical Therapy is short staffed today. Only the priority patients will have treatments done. Nursing will have to assume all others." The irony is that in some institutions nurses would be expected to assume all these responsibilities, and the nurses would not protest. After all, someone has to do it. No one seems to be paying much attention to, and certainly not putting much value on, the fact that patients may be denied essential nursing services. Unless nursing begins to affirm the rights of patients to nursing care, set standards for what that care is, and decide what constitutes essential nursing needs, nursing will not be able to defend itself as an essential resource.

In today's economic environment, values deemed important for cost effectiveness must be balanced with the values necessary for the delivery of adequate critical care nursing services to patients and families. Price-driven decisions that compete with professional values generate unavoidable ethical dilemmas for nursing. The movement by all third-party payors to lower their expenses has motivated hospitals to review high cost areas. Because labor is the most expensive part of any hospital budget and nursing constitutes the largest portion of those dollars, nursing has become an unfair target for cost containment measures aimed solely at dollar savings. In deciding how to allocate nurses, decisions must be made that can clearly identify those necessities of nursing practice that must be provided for all ICU patients. The benefits to patients receiving these services must be viewed against the potential harm that could occur should these services not be available. Benefits and harms must be thought of in both immediate and long-term effects. Once identified, these services can be tailored to individual patient needs. Policy decisions concerning the macroallocation of nursing services must be made by nursing administration, so that the nursing staff will not be thwarted in microallocation decisions. The department of nursing must take a position of how to allocate nursing resources that is congruent with nursing's code of ethics. Environments that support and encourage nursing allocation decisions at the bedside utilizing consistent standards will assure that patients receive essential nursing care.

The current economic climate forces nursing to recognize itself as a valuable resource. Patients who need admission to a critical care unit must be assured of that service. The principle of justice reminds us that in situations of scarcity resources must be allocated fairly. Nurses must be the ones to say which patients receive critical care nursing services and the kind of nursing care they should receive.

Notes

1. Herrell JH: Health care expenditures—the approaching crisis. Mayo Clin Proc 55:705, 1980
2. American Hospital Association: Hospital Week 22:31, 1986
3. Currents, Hospitals, p 24. July 20, 1986
4. LaVioletta S: Staff growth may be cut abruptly. Modern Health Care, p 48. January 1983
5. Blendon RJ: Health policy choices for the 1990s. Issues in Science and Technology 2:65, 1986

6. US Bureau of the Census: Statistical Abstract of the US: US Dept of Commerce Table 150, Washington, DC, 1979

7. Harrington C: Policy options for Medicare. Nursing Economics 7:187, 1983

8. Friedman E: 50 years of US health care policy. Hospitals, p 102. May 5, 1986

9. Ibid, p 96

10. Knaus WA, Draper E, Lawrence DE et al: Neurosurgical admissions to the ICU: Intensive monitoring versus intensive therapy. Neurosurgery 8:438, 1981

11. Richards G: Critical care under pps: Hospitals 59:66–68, 1985

12. Ibid

13. Arras JD: Health care vouchers and the rhetoric of equity. Hastings Cent Rep 11:29–39, 1981

14. Evans RE: Health care technology and the inevitability of resource allocation and rationing decisions. JAMA 249:2208–2219, 1983

15. Beauchamp TL, Childress JF: Principles of Biomedical Ethics, 2nd ed, p 186. New York, Oxford University Press, 1983

16. Ibid, p 187

17. Outka G: Social justice and equal access to health care. The Journal of Religious Ethics 2:13, 1974

18. Veatch R: Voluntary risks to health—the ethical issues. JAMA 243:50–56, 1980

19. Beauchamp, Childress, op cit, p 206

20. Friedman E: Rationing and the identified life. Hospitals, p 65. May 16, 1984

21. Fried C: Equality and rights in medical care. Hastings Cent Rep 6:32, 1976

22. ANA: Code for Nurses with Interpretive Statements, p 3. Kansas City, MO, ANA, 1985

23. Beauchamp, Childress, op cit, pp 189–190

24. Outka, op cit, pp 22–23

25. Ibid, p 24

26. Ibid

27. Dracup K: Editorial. Heart Lung 15:1, 1986

28. Zawacki BE: Personal conversation, September 1986

29. ANA, op cit, p 2

30. Heckler NM: Exciting new era of organ transplantation progress poses numerous ethical questions. FAH Review 18:19–20, 1985

31. Christopherson L: Heart transplants. Hastings Cent Rep 12:19, 1982

32. Evans R: The heart transplant dilemma. Issues in Science and Technology 2:92, 1986

33. Heckler, op cit

34. American Hospital Association: Will success spoil the stock hunter? Hospital Ethics 1:7, 1985

35. American Hospital Association: Hospital Week 22:27, 1986

36. Evans RW: Transplants Force Larger Payment, Access Issues (Interview by Emily Friedman). Hospitals 60:62–63, 1986

37. Blendon, op cit, p 65

38. Knaus WA, Draper EA, Wagner DP: The use of intensive care: New research initiatives and their implications for national health policy. Milbank Mem Fund Q 61:563, 574, 1983

39. Thibault GE, Mulley AG, Barnett GO et al: Medical intensive care: Indications, interventions, and outcomes. N Engl J Med 302:938–942, 1980

40. Chassin MR: Costs and outcomes of medical intensive care. Med Care 20:2, 1982

41. Cullen DJ, Ferrara LC, Briggs BA et al: Survival, hospitalization charges, and followup results in critically ill patients. N Engl J Med 294:982–987, 1976

42. Knaus WA, Wagner DP, Draper EA et al: The range of intensive care services today. JAMA 246:2711–2716, 1981

43. Ibid, p 2711

44. AACN: Position Statement: Scope of critical care nursing practice. Newport Beach, CA, AACN, 1980

45. Veatch RM: DRGs and the ethical reallocation of resources. Hastings Cent Rep 16:32–40, 1986

Chapter 8

Duties to Self: Professional Nursing in the Critical Care Unit

Andrew Jameton

When working at the hospital, one sometimes hears a nurse or physician tell a non-compliant patient, "You really owe it to yourself to try harder." Or, "You are the one who will have to live with this." The phrasing suggests a moral teaching: the practitioner is saying that the patient has obligations in regard to himself or herself and that the patient is primarily answerable to himself or herself for these obligations. Practitioners address themselves similarly. A nurse who makes a mistake may hear an internal voice reflecting, "I let myself down," or, "I promise myself I will do better." The philosophical rubric under which such judgments are usually discussed is *duties to self*.

What specific duties do critical care nurses have to themselves? An important one to consider is a duty to develop one's competence and to strive for excellence. Basic competence raises questions of personal integrity at least as important to the nurse as the actual impact of nursing care on patients. But, what does this duty involve? To what extent do nurses have a duty to spend private time developing new skills through continuing education? If the level of nursing care is threatened by budgetary limitations, do nurses have a duty to themselves to make a public protest? Another duty to consider is that of taking care of oneself. To what extent should nurses make personal sacrifices or undertake risks to provide better patient care? Or, a nurse may have an important ethical objection to a plan to discontinue care, but the decision seems to have been made by others. Does the nurse owe it to herself or himself to speak out, perhaps at some personal risk, on the issue? Or, patients in critical care units tend to experience a high level of control by nurses and physicians. The margin of error for the staff is also narrow. To what extent should nurses force or manipulate themselves to uphold standards of conduct that may or may not be comfortable for them personally?

Philosophers have differed strongly over the importance and meaning of duties to self. Thus, before discussing specific duties of critical care nurses to themselves, it is important to develop the basic concepts involved in a more general way. First, *mo-*

rality will be defined. Then, since some philosophers think that one's concern for self is not an ethical matter, morality will be distinguished from *prudential concerns*. Also, basic moral standards will be distinguished from ideals or aspirations, since these concepts affect the reasoning behind claims of duties. *Duties to self* will then be defined and interpreted as covering three distinguishably different areas of ethical concern: identity, self-regarding duties, and integrity. Selected cases drawn from critical care settings will be discussed under each of these three headings. Professionalism strongly shapes how we perceive our duties to ourselves and thus shapes much of the discussion. Thus, some final comments will discuss nursing professionalism and autonomy in respect to self-regarding duties.

Ethics and Duties to Self

Morality sets normative or prescriptive standards and expresses ideals for each of us in relation to other individuals, to society, and to the social institutions around us.[1] Important functions of morality are to identify our duties or obligations and to explore our personal relationship to those obligations. Given that we can identify our obligations, many questions can still be raised about how we should deal with them. Such questions regard our intentions or motives in acting, as when we say, "Dagwood did the wrong thing but he sincerely meant to do his best." We may also struggle within ourselves to meet what we see as moral expectations: we are subject to phenomena such as temptation, bad faith, and weakness of will. We may also be more or less unable to act competently and responsibly when we lose our mental faculties or become intoxicated. Our relationship to obligations is a ripe source of inner dialogue with our internalized judges and our "ideal selves." Two important distinctions in identifying our obligations and finding our relationship to them arise in discussions of duties to self:

Standards Versus Aspirations

First, we need to distinguish between basic normative standards and ideals or aspirations. In my internal dialogue, a voice may persist in criticizing me for not being the absolutely perfect nurse or philosopher even though I may be functioning clearly above a basic standard. When one fails to meet the basic expectations of society, one may be called to account by others, but one's failure to make work meaningful or to perfect oneself is often only of personal concern. The aspirational aspects of morality can be regarded as generally more self-regarding and more involved in obligations to oneself than the basic standards of morality.

Moral Versus Nonmoral Expectations

Second, when I assess my conduct in relation to social norms, not all norms, expectations, and ideals are of moral importance. Being beautiful, handsome, strong, rich, and smart are often regarded as desirable, but no one is immoral for failing to be any of these. Typically, practical, nonmoral concerns about myself and others are termed *providential* concerns.

The distinction between providential and moral concerns is not precise. Although there are many treatises on ethics and morality, few philosophers have offered a thoroughgoing statement on how to distinguish distinctively moral values from nonmoral ones. The importance of this distinction to the concept of duties to self is that some people regard duties to self (such as staying healthy) as merely providential concerns while others regard them as moral duties. Because my relationship to myself is not like a social relationship between two people, and morality is strongly concerned with relations among people, it is hard to distinguish the moral elements, if any, in concerns regarding only or primarily myself. Indeed, some philosophers deny that it makes sense to talk of duties to self at all.

Paradoxes and Distinctions in Duties

Sturdy denials that it is meaningful to talk of duties to self can be found among important philosophers. John Stuart Mill, for example, had defined a realm of self-regarding behavior into which obligations should not extend: "The only part of the conduct of anyone, for which he is amenable to society, is that which concerns others. In the part which merely concerns himself, his independence is, of right, absolute."[2]

Aristotle denies that it is possible to be unjust toward oneself.[3] Marcus Singer draws attention to some of the paradoxes in the concept of duty to oneself. He notes that if I have a duty to someone then that person has the power to release me of that duty, but I lack that power toward myself. He has concluded: "What are called 'duties to myself' are either not genuine moral duties at all, or, if they are, they are not duties *to oneself.*"[4]

Others note that if I have an obligation to others, they are entitled to force me to meet my obligation, but it is not meaningful to talk of self-coercion.[5] For instance, Kurt Baier had argued:

> Clearly, one cannot be literally under an obligation *to* oneself. . . . It is paternalism for society to exert moral pressure to get people to treat themselves well. Societies cannot create valid rules like "Develop your talents" or "Don't commit suicide." This is meddling in people's own affairs.[6]

Whatever one concludes about the validity of these objections, it is nevertheless at least psychologically possible and indeed common for people to think in terms of obligations to themselves. Most people experience some level of internal conflict, internal dialogue, and mixed objectives in life so that it is possible to think in terms of making impositions on oneself, struggling to hold to principles, to develop oneself as a moral being, to treat oneself well.

Many philosophers assert the meaningfulness of speaking of duties to oneself. Kant, for instance, works within a tradition of ethical thought that makes a major division between duties to self and duties to others. Under the heading of duties to self, he discusses concerns such as self-respect, self-love, self-mastery, suicide, care of the body, sexual impulses, sex crimes, wealth, luxury, greed, thrift, honor, and ambition.[7] More recent philosophers touch on concerns such as arbitrary limitations of one's personal liberty, self-degradation, displaying pride or envy, self-deception, causing oneself unnecessary suffering, treating oneself unjustly, selling oneself into slavery, or knowingly harming one's own health.[8,9]

Philosophers who accept the ethical validity of internal dialogue defend the concept of duty to self in a number of ways. There are three important lines of argument: analogical, instrumental, and universal. Making promises to oneself, although not identical to making promises to others, is at least analogous to it. It may be possible to release oneself from one's promises to oneself at any time, but it can still be meaningful to speak of "answering" to oneself for that release. The psychological phenomena of guilt, self-rebuke, and shame that accompany the internalization of social obligations can also occur in relation to conduct only of concern to oneself. Thus, one may promise oneself to be more prompt in the future, and have to reckon with oneself when one is not.

Duties to oneself may be instrumental in supporting one's duties to others. For instance, to meet my work obligations, I need to maintain my health. I may see maintaining my health as a duty to myself, but the basis of the obligation is in its importance to meeting my obligations to others. It is evidence that I take my obligations to others seriously and that I assume duties to myself that support these obligations.

Perhaps the most important way in which moral philosophy supports the concept of duties to self is through the concept of universal obligations. Basic moral obligations—such as not harming people—apply to everyone. Because I am a person, I owe the same fundamental duties to myself that I owe to others. Most ethical theories count all people as fundamentally of the same worth. To regard everyone else as worthy and not to count myself as worthy in the moral scheme would be servile and unassertive to the point of moral fault.[10]

If, as in one theory, the moral goal of action should be to maximize the overall happiness of people, it is perfectly appropriate to include myself in that count. Alan Donagan uses a universal moral principle to defend the concept of duties to self: "that each human being has duties to himself follows immediately from the fundamental principle; for if it is impermissible not to respect every human being as a rational creature, it is impermissible not to respect oneself as such."[11]

Aspects of Duties to Self

When we started, we stated that duties to self have three distinguishably different areas of ethical concern; self-regarding duties, integrity, and identity. When people talk about duties to themselves, they are often underlining, highlighting, or calling attention to the importance of some aspect of their relationship to moral obligations. Three aspects are important to a discussion of ethics in critical care settings. (1) The speaker may be calling attention to the content of the duty and emphasizing that the duty largely involves personal concerns. This is the self-regarding aspect of duties to self. (2) The speaker may be emphasizing that he or she will have to account to himself or herself for the fulfillment or neglect of a duty. This is the aspect of answerability or accountability and is associated with integrity. (3) The speaker may be emphasizing the importance of his or her identification with or acceptance of these duties. These duties play a role in his or her identity. Duties to self thus need to be understood partly in relation to the concept of the self.

Self-regarding duties: The content of a self-regarding duty refers to a realm of activities and effects that concern primarily oneself—one's health, talents, life, dignity, and so forth. Professional competence, for instance, can be viewed as primarily having an impact on oneself, that is, as self-regarding. After all, the effects of health care on patients are often uncertain, while one's knowledge of whether one acts according to standards is immediate. In the long run, incompetent practitioners, though undetected by others, may suffer continuing self-criticism and low self-esteem.

Integrity: The second aspect of duty to self that can be emphasized is that of integrity. If I take patient care seriously, besides saying that I have a duty to others to maintain good patient care, I may also say I owe it to myself. I make myself answerable for the quality of patient care and must judge myself in regard to meeting this obligation. The practice area perhaps most associated with this notion is that of dedication to patients. To what extent am I obligated to take risks and to extend myself on behalf of those under my care? This question is a basic one of professional integrity and cannot be answered without some attention to the concept of duties to self. For, in placing my patient's welfare in opposition to my own, I am creating a tension between my duty to care for myself and my duty to care for others.

Identity: Who is this self who both acts and makes demands? Who am I in relation to my obligations? This is a question of personal identity. The process of internalizing obligations to others involves evaluating, accepting, and internalizing some obligations; I can act autonomously on these values and think of them as obligations to myself as well as others. I may reject other obligations, and if they are imposed on me, I can be said to be acting on principles that are heteronomous, external, or alien to myself.

The practice and spirit of professionalism raises a variety of interesting questions of identity. Professionalism carries with it a set of professional values and principles that are limited in application to the work setting and to some degree independent of one's personal and private life. If I become a professional, I am in danger of dividing my conscience into personal and professional spheres. It is, however, meaningful to ask sometimes whether I am acting in my role as a professional when at work or whether I am stepping out of that role to express a personal opinion. How should my personal conscience affect my professional work?

There are thus three important aspects of duty to self—self-regarding duties, integrity, and identity—that are expressed in ethical concerns in critical care units.

119

In the next section, we will take three areas of professional practice —competence, dedication, and individual judgment—and discuss each of them primarily in relation to one aspect of duty. Thus, we shall discuss individual judgment and identity, dedication and integrity, and competence and self-regarding duties. Although these pairings are somewhat artificial, a discussion of them should help to delineate some of the concerns indicated by references to duties to self. It will be most convenient to start with identity.

Identity

Professional identity can be well integrated with one's personal identity. If one has strong ideals of service and an interest in meaningful work, the right professional placement can produce an integrated expression of these personal goals. Yet, it is possible to be alienated from one's profession, either because of personal conflicts with its standards, or because of practices in a particular setting. Achieving a professional identity is an aspiration, however, since all that is required by professional standards is that one practice the profession within the limits set by the ethical codes and standards of practice. Let us consider four cases that touch on the borderlines of professional practice and personal life.

> **Case 1:** Mary Ann North worked closely for several weeks with a 77-year-old man who was dying of squamous cell carcinoma of the lung at Memorial Hospital. He seemed to be very angry at being ill and was often uncooperative with therapy. During his hospital stay, he survived a cardiac arrest and suffered multiple rib fractures during resuscitation. While on the ventilator, he seemed angry, struggled to remove tubes, and then became increasingly obtunded. His kidneys failed precipitously. A case conference was held among staff. It was decided not to institute dialysis because of his poor condition and because of his opposition to therapy. North personally disagreed with this decision. She felt that his anger showed a great deal of vigor and will to live, even though it was negatively expressed. She felt that her own private moral views called for at least a trial with dialysis. However, she felt that the decision of the group represented professional ethics, and so she decided not to air her private moral opinions. Should she have said something?

The bottom-line answer to this question is yes; one should generally express one's opinion. This is not derived from a simple claim that one's personal moral views should always dominate professional views, or that the profession should strive to reflect the moral values of the community. Indeed, the profession may be called on at times to act in conflict with the moral values of the community, as a nurse might who provides care for a criminal or outcast spurned by others. However, professional values should be seen as connected with broader moral principles; they are intended to express a conception of humane care that is consistent with broad moral principles. They are not autonomous principles. Because health care is involved in such basic human themes as birth, death, suffering, and community, there is room for disagreement as to what is appropriate care. Professional ethics continues to develop through conscientious interpretations of principles by individual professionals.

The duty to self involved here is authentic expression of one's own moral viewpoint. There is also an obligation to others to bring one's own moral viewpoint to an ongoing dialogue. Absence from the dialogue hardly interferes with care, but participation would be an important part of one's aspiration to make work meaningful.

Case 2: Sherry Edwards was a member of a small evangelistic church called the "Apocryphytes." She carried a small supply of Apocryphyte pamphlets in the pockets of her lab coat. She gave them to patients who had questions about the meaning of their suffering, on which the Apocryphytes have much to say. Spreading the word (drawn largely from the Apocrypha of the Bible) was a major tenet of her moral convictions. In fact, she said that "Nursing is just a means to bring people to God." Community Hospital, where she was on staff, asked her politely, but with the hint of a threat, not to mix religion with nursing. She wondered whether to take a stand on the issue.

Surely, health care practice is consistent in specific situations with missionary work. However, there are limits to this consistency. First, professional principles deserve some respect on their own. Thus, in saying, "My nursing practice is just a draw; I am really here to bring patients to Christ," Nurse Edwards degrades nursing, which is in itself a service and to which as a nurse she has obligations. Second, proselytizing should be limited by the setting. If the hospital or practice has an open commitment to missionary work, it can be assumed that patients are aware of the nonhealth objectives of the setting and reasonably expect exposure to religious exposition. But where practice is explicitly religiously neutral, as in a state institution, it is only when a patient requests help of a religious nature, or where it appears that such help may be both appropriate and well received, would it be justifiable to introduce religious doctrine to patients.

Integrating one's religious identity with one's professional identity can appropriately integrate one's personal and professional aspirations. Minimal professional standards can neither prohibit nor require religious expression, since the health professions are multicultural in scope. Either conducting or refraining from evangelizing could be seen as a duty to oneself insofar as it is part of forming a coherent identity based on religious commitments.

Case 3: It was a bad day at King Memorial Hospital. Maggie Smith spent the day working intensely with a ventilator patient in a vegetative state who had specifically and competently refused therapy many times previously and who had even come into the hospital with a living will pinned to his shirt. A resident prescribed ten times too much digoxin. When Smith suggested a correction, ironically saving the life of her patient, the resident suggested she would be happier coaching a baseball team. Before the surgeon examined the patient's surgical scars, she had to remind him to wash his hands, and another scene ensued. Then a medical student attempted to do a lumbar puncture. The student was having a lot of trouble placing the needle. Smith overheard the resident tell the student that "It won't make any difference to the patient, but it will be a good learning experience for you."

Evil events take place in the world every day. We have the potential to identify with all who suffer worldwide. This is a temptation for health professionals, who are often "fixers." The problem for the professional is to set balanced priorities in dealing with the evils of the world. This is a question of personal identity in that it involves setting limits to our participation and connectedness with others. My duty to self would be to form a consistent identity with respect to handling the evils and errors of others.

The minimal standards of the profession require nurses to be concerned, for the sake of their patients, with some of the wrongs committed by others. This duty is expressed in major codes of nursing ethics. "The nurse takes appropriate action to safeguard the individual when his care is endangered by a co-worker or any other person."[12] "The nurse acts to safeguard the client and the public when health care and safety are affected by incompetent, unethical, or illegal practice of any person."[13] "Caring requires that the nurse represent the needs of the client, and that the nurse take appropriate measures when the fulfillment of these needs is jeopardized by the actions of other persons."[14]

Nursing professionals must therefore be involved where they encounter harmful or inept care for patients, where one is involved in performing the procedure itself (for instance, administering an unwisely prescribed medication), or where one is physically present as a witness (of, for example, a break in sterile technique). Greater danger to the patient weighs in favor of acting, using whatever effective mechanisms the institution offers. The duty to be self-involved is partly that of keeping morally "clean hands." Failure to act is complicity. When one makes authentic choices, one has responsibility to take seriously the moral weight of one's commitments. If one's moral viewpoint is regarded as an entirely individual matter, there would never be a reason to exert power in the world or to disagree with others. However, it is the point of an obligation to involve others, and thus self-respect and a notion of duty to self require action on moral judgments. Duties to self thus form an important means of defining one's personal identity.

> **Case 4:** It has been a hard week in the neonatal intensive care unit at King Memorial. The death rate has been high. A new high-frequency ventilator is being tried without much success. The two attending physicians on service this month keep giving contradictory orders. Nurse Finley is performing another heel stick on Kathy, who has been in the unit five months and is still on a ventilator. Even if Kathy makes it home, her poverty-stricken fifteen-year-old mother will be hard put to care for her. Her developmental prospects are uncertain but almost certainly poor. She squirms and cries at the expected jabbing pain, and Finley knows she is becoming increasingly inconsolable as it becomes more difficult to keep her comfortable. Finley is thinking, "Why am I doing this? What am I doing here?"

It is sometimes easy in an ICU to feel that one is in a dubious battle. Where cases appear hopeless, patients and families are suffering, and only the machines are in working order.[15] Indeed, ICUs can give the impression that they are not so much dedicated to a moral aim, service to patients, but that they are controlled by a technological imperative to do all we can.

> Not for the good that it will do
> But that nothing may be left undone
> On the margin of the impossible.[16]

Like the problem of complicity, this is a problem of engagement in practice to which one feels opposed. The question, however, is about objectives rather than about ethical commitments. Are the common aims of work in this unit meaningful? Do they really serve people, or are they to some degree under the control of other professional aims, such as individual achievement, teaching, or technological advancement?

As health technology rapidly advances, nurses become involved in questions of personal identity. Do they see themselves primarily as technologists, or as providers of personal and intimate care to patients? Can one do well in both realms? Is the nursing profession becoming "medicalized" by its involvement in high-tech procedures? And if it is becoming medicalized, is this a regrettable trend? Nurses frequently disagree in their answers to these questions. The duty to self involved here is not to avoid these questions, but to give some thoughtful response to them; otherwise, nursing work is likely to become meaningless and unrewarding.

Duties to self, regarded as formation and maintenance of a personal moral identity, are very much shaped by professionalism; that threatens to divide the self into personal and work-related moral realms. The preceding cases indicate that maintenance of personal identity is not an isolated concern uninvolved with the practices of the profession; to the contrary, duties to self require active participation in moral judgment regarding the work setting and its relationship to a broader moral sphere.

Self-Regarding Duties

Self-regarding duties have a content that affects or applies to oneself primarily. To consider a simple paradigm, brushing one's teeth is a self-regarding action. One does it to oneself; it affects oneself primarily. A duty to brush one's teeth would be a self-regarding duty.

Professional competence is a major self-regarding duty. There is no problem in seeing competence as a duty to self for two reasons. First, competence speaks to the integrity of the practitioner. Competent work is necessary to self-esteem as a professional and to the meaningfulness of work. Second, the practitioner is answerable for the quality of his or her work. It is one thing to be criticized by others, another to take criticism to heart and to listen to the voices of self-criticism.

But, these reasons do not make competence a self-regarding duty. Nor would it be enough to see competence as primarily governing one's own behavior rather than the behavior of others, for *all* obligations involve control of one's own conduct primarily, rather than controlling the conduct of others. In some sense, one needs to be seen as the object of the duty, the recipient of one's own attentions. If we follow a perspective approximating that of Kant's, it is possible to see competence in the following way. (1) Competence can be seen as part of one's personal self-development. Kant sees people as having a duty to develop and increase their "natural perfection."

> Man owes it to himself (as a rational being) not to leave idle and, as it were, rusting away the natural dispositions and powers that his reason can in any way use. . . . It is . . . a *duty* of man to himself to cultivate his powers . . . and to be . . . equal to the end of his existence. . . . Man has a duty to himself to be a useful member of the world, since this also belongs to the worth of humanity in his own person, which he ought not to degrade.[17]

Competence is seen primarily as an attribute of self to be cultivated, and secondarily as a means of affecting patients. For some, maintaining minimal professional competence requires perfection of natural capacities; for the more talented, self-development moves nurses toward high achievement. (2) Insofar as one is perceived as competent, one's status and respect from others is affected. By establishing one's competence with others, one defines one's own place in a society or institution. (3) Maintaining competence requires virtues of character that are largely personal and self-regarding. One needs to maintain health, alertness, and vigor for stressful critical care shifts. (4) One of the major duties to self identified by Kant is the duty to be one's "own innate judge."[18] To continue to improve competence, nurses must become objective and honest judges of their own work. No one else is in as good a position as a nurse carrying out a procedure, to witness the full process and details of performance. Self-judgment regarding competence echoes Kant's discussion of the ethical significance of being one's own judge of moral principles. To practice autonomously, one needs to be able to adopt and apply standards of competence to one's own work. (5) Nursing, as a practice, provides a set of "internal" goods that are satisfying in themselves. Internal goods are the intrinsic excellences of good nursing practice, as distinguished from external rewards such as salary, the gratitude of patients, and so forth.[19] The existence of intrinsic conceptions of excellence makes it possible for nurses to regard development of competence as a matter of self-development rather than simply a matter of achieving external rewards through affecting others.

The three cases that follow develop some aspects of competence as a self-regarding duty.

Case 5: Susan Marsh is crying in the hall bathroom. She injected Mr. Sweet with an overdose of insulin. He is OK now, but he nearly died. People won't figure out what happened either, since Mr. Sweet isn't her patient this evening. She was absorbed in thinking about a problem with a philosophy paper she was writing. She just did not notice she went into the wrong room, but she is sure no one was around when she went in. She knows she should be getting more sleep. Marsh is wondering whether to report the incident and if they will tell Mr. Sweet what happened. He is such a pleasant and trusting man; she is afraid he will be disillusioned with her.

It has been suggested that the best approach by a surgeon to the family after the surgeon has clumsily killed the patient on the table is to say, "We did everything we could to save him, but he was just too far gone for us to help him." This exemplifies a maximally *prudential* approach to the problem of competence. Indeed, in circumstances like the preceding some professionals would be careful not to disclose information about the mistake to patients. They would not do so because they feel that knowledge of the professional's mistake would damage the patient's confidence in therapy. Other professionals favor admission of errors, since it shows honesty on the part of the staff. Patients are often unable to judge competence and are much more interested in and more responsive to the character of their care givers. Thus, the trust of patients may well be increased by an admission of errors. This is not to say that the patient is to be used as priest-confessor. Professionals need to realize that patients often have a different view of errors. An error of great significance to the professional may be of little concern to the patient and vice versa.

Marsh's case is not exactly about competence; it is about the appearance of competence. The notion of duty to self focuses Marsh's attention on herself as judge of her work and away from the issue of what others think of her. Self-assessment is crucial to the internal rewards of nursing and its meaningfulness. Moreover, the case involves Marsh in the duties to self required for maintaining competence: honest assessment of one's own capacities and an adequate level of self-care. Moreover, in order to derive satisfaction from relations with patients, it is important to feel that one is offering a genuine and honest service. If by not admitting an error I judge that I am in a dishonest position in regard to a client, then it is more difficult for me to experience rewards from my work.

> **Case 6:** King Hospital is trying to keep costs down due to federal DRG requirements. It is laying off staff in many departments, including nursing. In spite of fewer admissions, the pace of work is increasing. There is less time for talking with patients. The error rate is going up. The social work department has been cut so far back that it is virtually impossible to make out-of-home placement arrangements. Respiratory therapy, in order to handle its staff cuts, has turned some of its procedures over to the nursing department, and this is increasing the nursing work load. When the patient load gets high, the hospital calls in nurses from a registry. So far the hospital is just barely meeting state-mandated staffing requirements, but the state health department is considering adjusting these requirements downward under pressure from the local hospital association. When they get a spare moment to think about it, some of the nurses are wondering whether they have an obligation to protest the situation.

Staff reductions limit the amount of work that can be done; if severe enough, reductions must eventually lead to cutting corners on essential services and eliminating less necessary ones. Combined with concrete modes of evaluating the quality of care, staff reductions tend to diminish the humanistic aspects of care—communication with patients, control of care by patients, individualized therapy plans, rest, and so forth. Instead, a pretense of humanism is shifted to hospital advertising and public relations departments (billboards scream, "We Care!").

Reduced staff interferes with the competent work of individual nurses. Moreover, a collective threat is posed to nursing as a profession. The "self" concerned here is global and collective; the duty to self is a duty to a collective self. The ANA Code expresses a professional assumption of a duty to be involved with issues of staffing: "The nurse participates in the profession's efforts to establish and maintain conditions of employment conducive to high quality nursing care."[20]

Viewed as a duty to self, the analogy between the collective and individual responsibilities is not exact. Individual nurses can have duties to each other and to the profession as a whole. Unlike with the self, it makes sense here to speak of duties to the profession as a whole, to each other, and to themselves. Some discussions of duty to one's self are intended partly to foster inner harmony, and similarly, the concept of a duty of the profession to itself is intended to foster harmony on significant professional issues. As with Marsh's case, an element of autonomy in judgment is also suggested by the collective responsibility of the profession: it must also take responsibility for judging when it thinks the level of nursing care has fallen below an acceptable level.

> **Case 7:** Sabrina Matthews has been nursing on staff for close to ten years. In the last three years, she has shown increasing signs of alcoholism. She was moved from the intensive care unit to a floating position, and since then nursing administration has ignored the situation despite complaints from her colleagues, who were having to cover for her errors. Finally, things were brought to a head when Matthews misappropriated some narcotics prescribed for patients. She was told in clear terms by administration that she must undergo a treatment program or she would be fired. She underwent treatment and is obviously recovering. She wants to resume work in the ICU, and administration told her that if she underwent therapy she would be reinstated in the unit. Does the unit have to take her back? Some of the staff feel that she is still too high a risk for a critical care area.

Impairment, more than simple incompetence, can be seen as a problem of a duty to oneself. This is because impairment has a global impact on the life and welfare of a professional. We are no longer thinking of specific mistakes or even general problems restricted to the work setting, but of global repercussions interfering with love, family, health, and enjoyment, as well as work.

The impaired professional also encounters a struggle for power with the pattern of abuse itself. To recover, the professional may have to become a patient. As a patient, the professional acquires the duties of patients. The duties of patients with regard to recovery are self-regarding duties. The duties of patients to themselves include maintaining virtues such as fortitude, hope, and trust.[21] They also involve duties such as taking care of oneself insofar as possible, cooperating in therapy, and striving to recover.

When it is a question of reporting someone else who is impaired, complex questions of loyalty arise. Duties of friendship may conflict with duties to patient care. Insofar as friendship is important to the identities of many people, a duty to maintain friendships can be seen as a duty to oneself.

Impairment also raises questions of the utility and moral wisdom of punitiveness with regard to failures of people to meet their obligations. If impaired professionals are simply punished and go without therapy, potentially useful and rewarding workers may be lost to the world. Moreover, excessive self-blame can interfere with therapeutic processes, which require a high level of love and support. Thus, unless the problem has become utterly intractable, the first direction to take with regard to impaired professionals is therapy and support with an offer of loyalty from staff working with the individual.

Integrity

The concept of integrity has many facets.[22] It can be regarded as wholeness of character. One's wholeness is primarily one's concern, not that of others, and so is an obligation to oneself. Many of the preceding issues could have been discussed in terms of integrity. But integrity is especially stressed when the self, divided by professional and personal concerns, faces conflicting duties to self. This most often arises when professional activities require a level of dedication threatening to the welfare of one's personal life. As one nurse reflected:

> My family is my first priority. Yet sometimes I make life difficult for my husband and children in order to get work done. I will stay up late at night working on something. I do this because I am conscious of what people think of me. I spend a lot of my life pleasing others. I am very conscious of this. I put my family through hell in order to get through graduate school. And yet I really put my family first. I make my husband take care of the children to get space to work at home. I think part of this is being a type A personality.

It is historically interesting to note that when Isabel Hampton Robb called on nurses to be obedient, she was directing new nurses not to devote themselves excessively to work but to obey their supervisor's instructions to go home:

> Thus, it not infrequently occurs that a head-nurse directs a probationer to leave the ward at a certain hour; the probationer, however, finding there is still much work to be done, probably out of mistaken kindness, or from a desire to help, takes it upon herself to remain beyond her time, until she is finally ordered off with a gentle reproof or the request to do only what she is told.[23]

Work in the critical care unit offers extensive opportunity for open-ended dedication. There is always a patient worse off than the nurse, in great need, and for whom enough cannot be given. It has been suggested that the intense residency of medical students is designed to wear out, and thereby limit, the empathy of students for patients to protect them in their professional life from personally costly dedication

127

to patients. The more dedicated professional can be seen as exceeding the minimal expectations of the profession and assuming a duty to self to devote more to patient care than is required.

While the professions call for dedication to the welfare of patients, it is an ordinary duty to take care of oneself. This is a duty expected of patients, and it is generally a duty of all persons able to do so. In this sort of case, there is a conflict of duties to self: one to dedicated care, the other to self-care. This conflict is well exemplified by the existence of both principles in the Canadian Nurses' Association Code of Ethics:

> Caring demands that the needs of the client supersede those of the nurse, and that the nurse must not compromise the integrity of the client by personal behavior that is self-serving. Caring commands fidelity to oneself, and guards the right and privilege of the nurse to act in keeping with an informed moral conscience.[24]

The struggle to care for self and others at the same time is not simply one between duties to self and duties to others; the concept of duties to self emphasizes the internal nature of the struggle as one between two commitments, both of significance to oneself. The problem for the professional is to strike a consistent balance between these two competing duties; however, there is no official method or statement indicating how that balance should be struck.

Case 8: Rick's primary nurse, Ellen Emerald, told her husband that she loved Rick from the very start. "There are just some babies you care for more than others. I can't stand to do heavy procedures on Rick. It is easier with the ones who have less of an identity for me." Rick was born prematurely, and as a result of respiratory complications, he became a chronic NICU infant. He was in the nursery for eight months before he went home, on a respirator, to his parents' tiny apartment. As the primary nurse, Emerald was involved in every conflict, every decision, every issue of Rick's care. Although many people—including his parents, who came in almost every day—took care of Rick, Emerald was the one steady person always there for him. She was both exhilarated and grief stricken when Rick finally went home. She did not feel she was Rick's mother, but she never felt satisfied that Rick's parents could take as good care of him as she did. She is afraid to take on any more infants as their primary nurse, since it is still too painful to think of little Rick.

This is a good case of conflict between the needs of the patient and the needs of the care giver. The needs of the infant for consistent care are real; the family is also highly anxious, suffering, and in need of consolation and education. It is very difficult for patients to make transitions, especially frequent transitions, to different care givers during such an ordeal. At the same time, the commitment of eight months of deep caring to Rick was costly to Emerald.

The emotional integrity of professionals depends in part on their ability to limit and define their relationships with patients; but chronic care invites deeper long-term commitments. The potential for tragedy is great. When staffing for chronic infants, it is possible to protect the nurses themselves by rotating primary nurses. But, where better continuity is called for, it is important to maintain a high degree of voluntariness for nurses to undertake such work, and it is important to recognize clearly the level of personal commitment involved. It is appropriate to offer nurses who choose to undertake the care of a chronically ill infant support, rest, and assistance with grief after the infant has left the unit. Another option is to set up a small team of primary nurses to work closely with such an infant.

> **Case 9:** Mr. Viper is in King Hospital for a pacemaker operation. He smokes a lot in the hospital. This contracts his veins and makes access difficult. He is often angry and irascible. When in a good mood, he yells bawdy remarks, tells dirty jokes, and grabs and pinches the nurses. In a bad mood, he makes loud racist and anti-Semitic remarks. Whenever he detects a problem, he threatens to sue. He often uses the call button for trivial requests and is angry if he does not get immediate attention. He never says thank you for anything and seems completely unappreciative of the care he gets.

Mr. Viper poses quite a different problem from that of young Rick. He does not impose risks; instead, he fails to provide many of the relational and emotional benefits that clinical work usually offers nurses. Influenced by the tradition of providing even-handed care to all patients, some nurses respond to Mr. Viper by trying to treat him just like other patients. But, this is not necessarily required by health care ethics. An element of reciprocity is expected in the practitioner-client relationship. This is expressed, for instance, by the statement of patient responsibilities included with the American Hospital Association statement of patients' rights:

> A patient is responsible for following the treatment plan recommended by the practitioner primarily responsible for his care. This may include following the instructions of nurses and allied health personnel as they carry out the coordinated plan of care and implement the responsible practitioner's orders, and as they enforce the applicable hospital rules and regulations. . . . The patient is responsible for being considerate of the rights of other patients and hospital personnel and for assisting in the control of noise, smoking, and the number of visitors.[25]

It would be appropriate to hold that Mr. Viper is failing to meet some of his responsibilities as a patient. Thus, he should not expect to receive the extra measure of devotion that some patients receive. However, there are important considerations that mitigate any impulse to punish him or to deprive him of any benefits of care to which he is entitled.

First, health professionals are expected to undergo a certain amount of emotional strain in caring for patients. They are partially compensated for this by salary, status, and interesting work, and they are rewarded by acquaintanceship with and gratitude from patients, solidarity with other professionals, and so forth. In the balance, of benefits over costs, a nurse may receive a high level of these rewards and indeed may even receive more than patients as a group receive from the nurse. Difficulty with one patient may be well balanced by the rewards of courageous, interesting, and thoughtful clients. It would be inappropriate to calculate this balance too carefully in a particular case; Mr. Viper should not have to bear the entire burden of maintaining a rewarding professional career for the nurse.

Second, Mr. Viper is ill. Being ill, he may be excused for *some* of his behavior. Parsons, for example, has developed the social importance of illness as an excuse for not fulfilling ordinary responsibilities.[26] But, Mr. Viper is not entitled to a blanket excuse for everything, only mitigation of some responsibilities. "Some persons think that when they are ill enough to require a physician and watchers, they may be excused from all effort at self-government, and all consideration for others. . . . The trials of nursing are increased by such unreasonable conduct."[27]

Some nurses may be comfortable working with him as they recognize that his terror, denial, and need to assert himself compound his less enduring traits of character or personality. Third, he is not dangerous physically. If his assaults are sufficiently degrading, he may be dangerous to a nurse's sense of self-respect and dignity. Nurses should defend themselves from such acts, out of a sense of duty to self not to be degraded. Otherwise, his unpleasantness should not be confused with physical dangerousness.

Fourth, even if he deserves punishment, individual clinicians do not have a responsibility to act as a moral police, judge, court, or jail. Complaints about him can be adjudicated by involvement with security (if he is dangerous) or with administrative staff (if his problems are so flagrant that they require administrative action). One of the most delicate balances in ethics is to be able to attribute responsibility without anger or blame.

> **Case 10:** Brian Sprain is a nurse in the ICU at King Hospital. He has been assigned to care for an AIDS patient, Roger Quale, one of the first to appear at this small Maine hospital. Although he is familiar with infection precautions, Sprain does not want to take care of Mr. Quale. Sprain himself is gay. He fears that he is already at risk for AIDS and is worried about increasing his exposure. Other nurses do not want to take care of Mr. Quale either. They think that since Sprain is gay, he has a greater responsibility to take care of Mr. Quale, and they are not anxious to accept the perceived risk themselves.

This is intended as a case that challenges nurses' sense of dedication in the face of exposure to personal health risks. The judgment of risk is complicated by common uncertainty about the communicability of and immunity to AIDS. Moreover, the actual health risks created by Mr. Quale's illness may be exaggerated in some nurses' minds by the negative feelings and judgments regarding homosexuality.

It is standard for health professionals to take health risks in caring for patients. These involve risks of infection, radioactivity, or injury. Part of the compensation to health professionals should be payment, insurance benefits, and recognition for taking these risks. At the same time, *precautions are obligatory where risks are undertaken*. If adequate precautions are possible, risk can be reduced to the level incurred by those in non-health-care occupations. A key question for this case is the following one. Is the risk of caring for Mr. Quale probably greater than risks commonly encountered by nurses? If it is, then taking care of the patient should be considered a heroic or supererogatory act, rather than one that is obligatory.

If Sprain is particularly vulnerable to the disease for some reason (more frequent exposure does not by itself increase the probabilities), then it would be appropriate to consider that a reason for selecting other nurses for the work. This would be comparable to permitting pregnant nurses to avoid work with radiation.

Does he have a special obligation to undertake this work? In the ethics of human subjects, it has been argued that risky experiments may be performed on children, only if, among other considerations, the experiment benefits children as a class. Thus, being a member of a class likely to benefit from experimentation is regarded as a reason for assuming some risks to support experimentation. However, participation is voluntary. Thus, it may be praiseworthy for Sprain to take this risk, but it would not be obligatory. He need not assume this responsibility. It is important that heroic risks be undertaken meaningfully. This requires that they have significant benefit to others. It also requires that they be necessary and that all precautions have been taken. Moreover, it requires that a high level of voluntariness be maintained, and that risks be distributed equitably. *Voluntariness* means that nurses need to be informed of the risks and, when possible, have the opportunity to volunteer or to refuse. Equitability means that no particular staff member is favored with special protection or special burdens.

It may be difficult to organize a process by which both voluntariness and equitability are maintained. For instance, different staff roles involve different levels of risk and obligation to the patient. Moreover, if the process involves drawing straws and those who get the short straw then refuse, equity and voluntariness are not well balanced. Instead, a pool of volunteers, from which staff members are randomly selected is needed.

The question of integrity and dedication is the balance between one's personal risks in undertaking professional work and the duties to clients. Again, this is an internal struggle between the meaningfulness of dedication versus the intensity of self-care.

Case 11: Charley McGhee is providing care for an ICU patient, Mrs. Mary Liu, who is over 90 and quite frail. On many occasions, she has expressed a wish not to be maintained by artificial means. She has explicitly requested that she not be resuscitated in the event of an arrest. She has a good understanding of what this means and has written a short essay for the newspaper on the subject. In the article she cites such ethics sages as Fry, Davis, Aroskar, Fowler, and Kant. Partly because they respect her wishes, and partly because they feel that she is too frail to survive resuscitation, the team has decided to write a no-code order. Unfortunately, the order does not meet the requirements of hospital policy. Policy requires that death be "imminent" and the condition "irreversible." McGhee believes this to be what current case law also requires. Although she believes it is ethical to write a DNR order, she is sure that it is also illegal. She is wondering whether to go along with the order or to press the staff to act in consistency with the law.

The prospect of malpractice or even a criminal charge can be regarded as a risk to self and other staff. In this respect, the legal questions raise much the same questions as the preceding cases of personal risk-taking on behalf of patients. If after due conscientious consideration one determines that the law is out of line with what professional practice requires, then the issue of self-protection is the only one that counts against immediate violation of the law in order to protect patients.

On the other hand, the law is meant as a guide and teacher. Many of the most interesting moral questions in health care have been thoroughly discussed in the courts. And there is something to be said for the point of view of the law that situations that would permit discontinuing therapy should be limited. It may even be argued (often weakly) that following a patient's decision to discontinue care when the prospects of recovery are relatively good gives too much credit to the patient's discouragement and hopelessness.

Thus, legitimate moral considerations are raised by the law in this case. We are returned to a case much like Case 1 above. The nurse has a personal moral reservation in regard to a staff judgment. In this case it involves both considerations of the patient's welfare and the nurse's duty to protect herself from legal jeopardy. There is every reason to bring up a discussion of the issue, even if the final decision is to write a no-code order.

Professionalism and Ethics: Past and Present

Appealing to the concept of duties to self serves to underline the dignity and importance of individuals as moral agents. It focuses obligations and the responsibility of making moral judgments on individuals rather than on the authority of tradition and institutions. It does not identify duties as originating in individuals, but it places the individual at the center of identifying and interpreting moral rules. Moreover, it emphasizes the ability of the individual to think morally and to make choices, even self-regarding choices, on the basis of moral principles rather than simply on perceived self-interest or selfishness. Instead of subordinating choices regarding self to self-love or nonmoral impulses, it embraces these within moral principles that include self among others.

This principled approach is important to the nursing profession. For, as nurses take an increasingly important role in making health care decisions, the profession needs to distinguish autonomy of nurses that serves personal and professional idealism, from autonomy conceived simply as power in one's own interest. For nurses to participate actively in the moral dialogue regarding patient care, it is important that they not violate duties to self—the need to be self-respecting, not servile—and not give up autonomy unnecessarily. Victorian notions of virtue that shaped early nursing practice by defining nursing ethics in terms of external requirements of womanhood must be set aside and replaced by a morality more strongly based on personal autonomy.[28]

Concepts of professionalism both help and hinder this development. As a practice, rather than an institution, the nursing profession includes, as part of its definition, positive ideals that resist the corruption of hospitals and other health care agencies.[29] Professional responsibilities can be assumed by individual nurses as duties to themselves. However, as a limited part of a person's activities as a whole, the nursing profession cannot define those responsibilities that nurses have to themselves personally and that supersede or encompass professional obligations. For instance, it is one thing to aspire to professional ideals; it is another to sacrifice oneself to them.

Those notions of duty to self that see the reflexive duties as providing primary guidelines for the treatment of others indicate how duties to self may be used to reduce the conflict between self and work raised by professionalism. It is important, morally, to treat oneself well. This means treating oneself as an autonomous individual and not placing oneself into degrading situations, not depriving oneself unduly, and not forcing or coercing oneself to obey meaningless demands. When the nurse learns how to avoid these sins of self-treatment, she or he has begun to develop a character able to respect the dignity and needs of others. Thus, the development of character in respect to self can be a primary source of principles for the treatment of others in professional practice.

Notes

1. For most of this chapter I have used *ethics* and *morals* equivalently, although it is appropriate to reserve *morality* for the existing codes, practices, and commitments of a society and *ethics* for general theories about morality. Neither have I distinguished *duty* and *obligation* here.
2. Mill JS: On Liberty (1859), reprint, p 13. New York, Bobbs-Merrill, 1956
3. Aristotle: Nichomachean Ethics (Ostwald M, trans), bk 5, chap 11, 1138117–20, pp 143–144. New York, Bobbs-Merrill, 1962
4. Singer MG: Duties and duties to oneself. Ethics 73:133–142, 1963. See also Singer MG: On duties to oneself. Ethics 69:202–205, 1959. For a discussion and refutation of this paradox, see Kant I: The Doctrine of Virtue: Part II of the Metaphysics of Morals (Gregor MJ, trans), p 79. Philadelphia, University of Pennsylvania Press, 1964
5. For a review of other arguments, see Gewirth A: Reason and Morality, pp 333–334. Chicago, University of Chicago Press, 1978
6. Baier K: The Moral Point of View: A Rational Basis of Ethics, pp 217, 230. Ithaca, Cornell University Press, 1958
7. Kant I: Lectures on Ethics (Infield L, trans), pp 116–191. New York, Harper & Row, 1963. The concept of duties to self does not originate with Kant, but he is the first whom I can identify that gives the concept a central role in characterizing moral virtues. He uses the concept to form the most broad and basic division of virtues in Part II of The Metaphysics of Morals (see Kant 1964, op cit). Duties to self can be found in the British moralists of Kant's time, such as Richard Price:

   > There is, undoubtedly, a certain manner of conduct terminating in ourselves, which is properly matter of *duty* to us. . . . If it is my duty to promote the good of *another*, and to abstain from hurting him, the same, most certainly, must be my duty with regard to *myself*.

   Price R: A review of the principal questions in morals [originally 1758, cited from 1787 ed] in Raphael DD (ed): British Moralists 1650–1800, vol 2, pp 178–179. Oxford, Oxford University Press, 1969. John Locke refers to them in an early work: ". . . all that men owe to God, their neighbour, and themselves." See Locke J: Essays on the law of nature in Raphael, op cit, vol 1, p 166. Hume has mentioned them:

> That we owe a duty to ourselves is confessed even in the most vulgar system of morals; and it must be of consequence to examine that duty, in order to see whether it bears any affinity to that which we owe society. . . . [and whether] the approbation attending the observance of both is of a similar nature, and arises from similar principles . . . [Hume D: An enquiry concerning the principles of morals. In Selby-Biggs LA: Enquiries, 2nd ed, pp 322–323. Oxford, Oxford University Press, 1902

St. Thomas Aquinas also discusses the problems of self-referential moral concerns:

> . . . strictly speaking, we do not have a friendship for ourselves, but . . . man possesses unity, which is something more than union. Accordingly as unity is presupposed to union, so our love for ourselves is the model and root of friendship, for our friendship for others consists precisely in the fact that our attitude to them is the same to ourselves. (Aquinas T [Batten RJ], trans]: Summa Theologiae, vol 34, p 91. New York, Blackfriars and McGraw-Hill Book Company, 1975)
>
> Homicide is a sin not only because it is contrary to justice, but because it is contrary to that charity a man owes to himself. Considered in this way, suicide is, therefore, a sin. [Aquinas, op cit, vol 38, p 33]

The British moralists of the 18th century heavily debated the role of self-love and related sentiments as motives of moral action. Kant's concept of duty to self helps resolve some of these problems by putting self-regarding concerns in terms of rational (as opposed to feelings) duties (as opposed to motives) to self. The "self-love" of Hume and other British moralists is replaced by "duty to self." Kant's notion of duty to self is highly strict, ascetic, and aspiring to moral perfection. This is representative of the Protestant asceticism characteristic of the Reformation and Enlightenment (See Weber M [Parsons T, trans]: The Protestant Ethic and the Spirit of Capitalism. New York, Charles Scribner's Sons, 1958)

 8. Eisenberg PD: Duties to oneself: A new defense sketched. Rev Metaphysics 20:602–634, 1967

 9. Jones H: Treating oneself wrongly. J Value Inquiry 17:169–177, 1983

10. "Servility manifests the absence of a certain kind of self-respect. The respect which is missing is not respect for one's merits but respect for one's rights. The servile person displays this absence of respect not directly by acting contrary to his own rights but indirectly by acting as if his rights were nonexistent or insignificant." From Hill TE Jr: Servility and self-respect. The Monist 57:87–104, 1973

11. Donagan A: The Theory of Morality, p 76. Chicago, University of Chicago Press, 1977

12. International Council of Nurses: Code for Nurses (1973). In Jameton A: Nursing Practice: The Ethical Issues, p 300. Englewood Cliffs, Prentice-Hall, 1984

13. ANA: Code for Nurses (1976). Ibid, p 300

14. Canadian Nurses Association: CNA Code of Ethics: An Ethical Basis for Nursing in Canada (1980). Ibid, p 312

15. See Duff RS: Counseling families and deciding care of severely defective children: A way of coping with "medical Vietnam." Pediatrics 67:317, 1981:

> Nursery policy is shaped by two main forces, neither rooted consistently in the values of families. The first is medical opinion which in a minority of instances represents a rigid "moral entrepreneurship.". . . These leaders emphasize the appealing ethics of the crusade against disease and death and point out their obligation to observe homicide laws. This avoids controversy and protects institutional license and finances and jobs. . . . If nursery policy is rigid, life for nurses and physicians is difficult, for social workers it is miserable, and for families it is a nightmare.

16. Eliot TS: The Family Reunion (Agatha). New York, Harcourt Brace Jovanovich, 1939
17. Kant 1964, op cit, pp 110–112
18. Ibid, p 103
19. MacIntyre A: After Virtue: A Study in Moral Theory. Notre Dame, University of Notre Dame Press, 1981
20. ANA: Code for Nurses (1976) in Jameton, op cit, p 307
21. Lebacqz K: The virtuous patient. In Shelp EE (ed): Virtue and Medicine, pp 275–288. Dordrecht, D Reidel, 1985
22. Mitchell C: Integrity in interprofessional relationships. In Agich GJ (ed): Responsibility in Health Care, pp 163–184. Dordrecht, D Reidel, 1982
23. Robb IH: Nursing Ethics: For Hospital and Private Use, p 58. Cleveland, JB Savage, 1901
24. Canadian Nurses Association: CNA Code of Ethics (1980) in Jameton, op cit, p 312
25. Joint Commission for the Accreditation of Hospitals: Rights and responsibilities of patients. AMA/86: Accreditation Manual for Hospitals, p xiv. Chicago, JCAH, 1985
26. Parsons T: Illness and the role of the physician: A sociological perspective. Am J Orthopsychiatry 21:454–460, 1951
27. A Lady: The Young Lady's Friend (improved stereotype ed), p 88. Boston, American Stationers' Company, 1837
28. Benjamin M, Curtis J: Virtue and the practice of nursing. In Shelp, op cit, pp 257–274
29. Ibid, p 259

Chapter 9

Values: The Cornerstone of Nursing's Moral Art

Diann B. Uustal

Value conflicts and ethical dilemmas increasingly confront nurses in critical care practice settings on a daily basis and add to the stress of their changing roles and responsibilities. What are the major issues you face in your practice? How effectively were you prepared to resolve conflicts in the clinical arena? Are you able to identify personal and professional values and ethical principles that can help you examine and resolve these confusing issues? Do you ever ask yourself, "Did I do the 'right' thing?" This chapter will increase your ability to deal more effectively with the demanding issues you face as a nurse by introducing you to ways that will help you identify, analyze, and put into action those values that can serve as frameworks for your decision making. It will get you thinking about the moral art of nursing, the value-related aspects of the nurse-client relationship, the nature of values, the theories of value formation, and the importance of identifying your values. It will give you plenty of opportunities to identify, examine, and clarify your values by completing the strategies at the end of the chapter.

Your mind is reeling. Just today you have been dealing with timeless ethical questions as well as others seemingly generated overnight by technological advances that apparently threaten to suspend life almost indefinitely. You find yourself raising questions about the "quality" of life and wondering about the "quantity" of life as you care for a 17-year-old comatose boy who can be expected to live for years because of the available life-support systems. "Is it a life-support system," you think, "or is it a life-prolonging system?" "How do you define 'life' anyway?" you ask yourself.

During the past few years as an intensive care nurse you have watched the courts and the government become increasingly involved in life and death decisions in health care; seen the costs of health care financially, emotionally, and spiritually continue to escalate; and witnessed the confusion generated when a patient refuses treatment and a physician believes everything must be tried. Just today you have emotionally supported a family unable to pay for their child's open heart surgery, and prepared an elderly person for open heart surgery that is covered by Medicare. "Should health care be a right?" "Is it possible to care for everyone who needs it?" Then you recall the youngster who died a few weeks ago because there was no liver available for transplant. What about the lack of clarity in the do-not-resuscitate policy in your hospital? As if these questions were not enough to sort through, you are increasingly uneasy with the "slow code" mentality that seems to be accepted by some 11 of your colleagues without much apparent conflict. What do you value as a critical care nurse? What values does nursing uphold? Do these values help you wrestle with the ethical questions that confront you and your colleagues? As a critical care nurse, how do you decide what to do in the face of such difficult dilemmas?

Are you someone who believes that all life is precious, whatever the circumstances? Are you a nurse who believes that knowingly withholding life support is wrong? What should you do when there are limited resources in the intensive care unit? How do you define euthanasia? Is intentionally withholding treatment active or passive euthanasia? Do you believe patients have the right to refuse treatment, even if it will hasten their death? Do you ever question a physician colleague about the quality of patients' lives as they are struggling to make a decision? In your opinion, which is more important, "quality" of life or "meaningful" life? How do you define these terms? Who should define the quality of life? How do you react when a competent patient refuses treatment that will save his or her life? Does it ever confuse you to attempt to balance the quality of life against the cost of prolonging it? Does a person's age influence how aggressively she or he is treated in your unit? How does age influence the decision you help patients make?

The questions you can raise are seemingly endless and your responses to these questions are based on your values. You are faced with urgent demand to thoughtfully examine health care dilemmas imposed by advancing medical technology, changing health care delivery, and changing medical and nursing practice. However, you are probably feeling, like many of your colleagues, that your education in nursing has poorly prepared you to do this. As a critical care nurse you have an obligation to gather the facts in these difficult areas so that you are more informed. You also have an obligation to reason ethically, which means that you have a working knowledge of ethical principles, ethical theories, and decision-making models. Finally, as a professional nurse you must be willing to voice your opinion about these issues. All nurses have an obligation to help increase the public's awareness concerning the ethical issues related to health care. We need to take action to affect national health policy by making our opinions known in writing and by political lobbying of elected officials in government. There is no greater need in nursing today, both for those who have been in the profession and for those who are entering the profession, than to understand how we are to match the delivery of care in a rapidly changing health care system with those ethical and spiritual values that have defined nursing as a profession.

Before you can respond to these and other ethical questions and dilemmas, it is important to understand what values and value systems are, how values are formed, and what the distinctions between values and beliefs and attitudes, morals, and ethics are. You need to know the effects of your values on your decision making, your behavior, and your ability to care for clients and families in critical care situations. Your values directly influence your ethical reasoning and choices on both conscious and unconscious levels.

The Moral Art of Nursing

Nursing is a moral art because it involves other people, our relationship with those people, and the promotion of a value that we consider to be "good," a person's health. It involves the design and fostering of a healing atmosphere that rests on the creation of a therapeutic relationship and the application of scientific knowledge and skill. As nurses, we agree that a primary goal of the nurse-client relationship is promotion of the well-being and safety of the person. We can also say that we value the patient's safety and seek what is good or in the best interests of the patient.

The primary end value of nursing is the good of the patient.[1] This is a moral end, and therefore nursing is a moral art. We also know that nursing is a science and that our technological skills are the means to meeting the ends that we value. It can also be said that nursing is a ministry that is both a moral art and a science and that focuses on the welfare of each client, the individuality of the recipient of our services, the quality of the nursing care, and the nurse-client relationship. Clients, knowing that their welfare is nursing's central motivating value, can expect to be treated with dignity and respect. The quality and effectiveness of nursing care is a primary value for both nurse and client.

A moral value that I believe is both a traditional and a contemporary one, and that serves as nursing's cornerstone, is that of caring. It is no doubt the most basic of all values in nursing and, in fact, serves as the springboard for the application of all the other values inherent in the nurse-client relationship. It enables another value, that of advocacy, to be operationalized, and encourages the nurse to take on a variety of roles, such as that of care giver, health educator, protector, surrogate, counselor, healer, and a variety of relationships with the patient, such as client and counselor, colleague and colleague, parent and child, and friend and friend.

How do you define caring? Is it a process or a product? What are its components? Take a few minutes right now, before you continue reading, to write (or at least mentally jot) a definition of caring.

Caring is not easy to define or describe, and yet we have all experienced the feeling of warmth, respect or regard, and genuine concern that is a gift of encouragement from those we describe as "caring." Mayerhoff describes caring as "a process, a way of relating to someone that involves development . . . in time through mutual trust and a deepening and qualitative transformation of the relationship."[2] Leininger claims that "caring acts and decisions make the crucial difference in effective caring consequences. Therefore, it is caring that is the most essential and critical ingredient for any curative process."[3]

Caring is the cornerstone of nursing's moral art and is fundamental to a therapeutic nurse-client relationship. Levine comments on caring and states that "the willingness to enter with the patient that predicament which he cannot face alone as an expression of moral responsibility; the quality of the moral commitment is a measure of the nurse's excellence."[4] In nursing we must remember to do what we value, and value what we do. Authentic caring is of value in enhancing the nurse-client relationship. It is a value in nursing, as well as a measure of our commitment as health care professionals to provide distinguished service to people.

Caring is a personal and professional value that serves as the cornerstone for a therapeutic relationship with a patient. This fundamental value entreats us to be humane, compassionate, and sensitive in preserving the person's identity and integrity. We have all professionally "grown up" on value messages that implored us to "treat the patient as a person, not merely as a diagnosis," or to "minister to the whole person," or perhaps you have seen the anonymous quote dating back to the 15th century that says, "Cure sometimes, relieve often, care always." Add to these value messages the one that states, "Good relationships don't just happen," and you realize that caring is a process as well as a product and that it is *a value that serves as a normative guideline* that shapes our attitudes as well as our behaviors toward patients in critical care units.

The literature amply documents that this value of caring has been sharply eroded by the development of the team approach, specialization, and the increasing use of high technology. These three factors are pertinent especially in the physical environments created by most intensive, medically specialized units. Patients charge health care providers with dehumanization and claim that the hospital experience is depersonalizing. Health care professionals themselves have examined the highly institutionalized bureaucracy of modern health care facilities (notice the word "care") and describe these centers as "no-care" societies. A person "becomes just another patient, another disease, another medication order, another name on the daily operating room schedule. . . . He is required to discard his identity as a person and become a 'patient.'"[5] It is not enough to be competent. Although we value competency in professional practice and there are many competent nurses in critical care units, we must also value and be genuinely caring. Competence without caring is hollow and perceived by people as not being "cared for."

The quality of care we offer our clients can also be jeopardized when we forget to honor the person as a unique individual. To diminish a person's identity and sense of self by failing to respect an individual's values is to interfere with the person's healing and to obstruct a therapeutic nurse-patient relationship. It also is demeaning and unethical because the client is not respected as a person. Levine reminds us that caring is best exemplified ". . . when no act diminishes another person, and no moment of indifference leaves him with less of himself."[6] Authentic caring involves being empathic toward another, believing in the dignity and worth of each person, and being sensitive to the meaning of the values, priorities, and choices a client expresses. Before we can be of help (minister) in a significant way to any patient, we must first critically examine our own personal and professional values and identify those clinical situations that might pose value conflicts that cause us to interfere in a patient's autonomous decision making. Pellegrino warns us that "in a matter so personal as health, the imposition of one person's values over another's . . . is a moral injustice."[7] Refusing to respect a client's values erodes the value of caring.

The Nurse-Client Relationship

The nurse-client relationship is the point at which values, morals, ethical principles, and traditional and contemporary philosophies of nursing unite. The nurse-client relationship ideally is an expression of the values, the moral and ethical principles, and the traditional and contemporary philosophies upheld in nursing. It offers its practitioners a specialized relationship with people. This relationship includes implicit and explicit expectations that the nurse will behave in specific ways, such as caring for each person equally and as a unique individual regardless of the person's attributes, social worth, or illness.

What are the legitimate expectations or claims that clients have the right to expect of critical care nurses? What are the values that serve as the foundation for your philosophy and practice of nursing? What moral obligations do we have in the nurse-client relationship based on our values and ethical principles? Curtin says, "Nursing can and should be distinguished by its philosophy of care and not by its care function."[8] What values are the foundation for this philosophy of care and for the practice of the moral art we call nursing?

Before you continue reading, it is important that you take time to identify some values that you feel influence your definition and philosophy of nursing and guide your actions as a professional. Do not rely on the authors of this text to take on the task of identifying values for you. Take responsibility for this personal and professional identification, clarification, and reflection on your philosophy of nursing (Exercise 9-1).

After writing your philosophy of nursing, you would probably agree that nursing is caring experienced between human beings. Nursing acts directly influence the quality of a person's healing, living, and dying. Nursing is concerned with helping people restore health, sustain health, and promote health. It is not only concerned with a person's wellness, but also with wholeness and living to one's full potential, which is highly individualized. Nursing is doing what you value and valuing what you do. Nursing, based on the value of caring, is an expression in action, not just rhetoric, of the nurse's authentic commitment to become involved in a person's healing.

Historically, nursing has been portrayed as a benevolent, one-way relationship between patient and nurse, with the nurse acting on behalf of the patient, based on the physician's orders. In contemporary nursing, caring is still the foundation for a therapeutic nurse-client relationship and the client's best interests are still the primary goals, but the nurse-client relationship, rather than being like a mother-child or care giver–receiver role, is a more mutually responsible relationship.

Nurses today believe that their genuine presence is of value and makes a significant difference in a client's situation and in the healing process. They realize the value of the use of self as therapeutic and that it is the quality of the nurse's being, as well as the caring, that influences the person's healing and health.

Nursing is a behavioral manifestation of the nurse's value system. It is not merely a career, a job, an assignment—it is a ministry. It is a freely chosen human response and involves the nurse's whole being and presence on a personal and professional level. The nurse's willingness to enter into a relationship with a client, at a time when the client is vulnerable, is behavioral evidence of the nurse's commitment to the importance of the nurse's presence and use of self in a therapeutic relationship. We have all had the experience of "being there" for and with a friend who needs our active demonstration of caring. As nurses we know the value of being there for a client and of communicating our genuine interest in the person and willingness to be available. Nursing is beyond a mere "doing" for another; it is an expression of what is or has gone on between the nurse and the client and involves genuine presence, authenticity, communication of emotional support, and commitment to improving the health of another.

The Theoretical Framework of Values

Values are the foundation for ethical practice in critical care nursing. They are the "whys" that give us a sense of meaning and purpose in nursing. Before we begin to identify values we hold in nursing, we first should take the time to define what values and value systems are; to distinguish the differences between values and attitudes, morals and ethics; to identify the effects of values on behavior and decision making; and to explore some theories about how values are formed. This brief discussion will introduce you to the theoretical framework of values, but it is not proposed as a comprehensive review. You are referred to the bibliography at the end of this book in addition to the specific references documented in the text in order to continue your learning.

What Are Values?

The use of the word *values* in everyday speech, and as a term used by a number of disciplines, evokes various connotations. There is little uniform agreement as to the definition and meaning of the concept values or the processes by which values are developed. Educators, psychologists, anthropologists, and sociologists have made contributions to the literature and research and have influenced both definition and theory. According to Kluckhohn, people in these fields consider values as: ". . . attitudes, motivations, objects, measurable quantities, substantive areas of behavior, affect-laden customs, or traditions, and relationships such as those between individuals, groups, objects, and events. The only general agreement is that values some-how have to do with normative as opposed to existential propositions."[9]

There are a number of other scholars who have significantly contributed to the definition and clarification of the concept values. These definitions vary slightly and complement one another. Raths, Harmin, and Simon define values as guides to be-havior that evolve and mature, are seen as worthy, and give direction to life. They use the term *values* to denote "those beliefs, purposes, attitudes and so on that are cho-sen freely and thoughtfully, prized, and acted upon."[10] Values are described as those elements that indicate how a person has decided to use his or her life. Values are not seen as static; rather, they change as the individual matures and changes. The devel-opment of values is seen as a lifelong process.

Raths, Harmin, and Simon are less concerned with the particular values one chooses than with the process one uses to obtain one's values. They feel it is wiser to focus on the process of valuing and describe a series of seven steps that make it clear how they define a value. "Unless something satisfies all seven of the criteria noted . . . we do not call it a value. In other words, for a value to result, all of the . . . seven requirements must apply."[11] They see values as based on the following three proc-esses: choosing, prizing, and acting. These processes are subdivided into seven steps. Collectively, the steps define the process of valuing or choosing values, and the products of this process are called values. An updated and modified version of the valuing process is included for your closer review and use (see Table 9-1). This val-uing process emphasizes that if individuals are to develop values, there must be the crucial element of personal choice and selection from alternatives that are prized and have meaning for the individual. These alternatives must be truly available for selec-tion, and the consequences of each must be fully understood. Based on this process, values are described as personal in nature and involving affective responses.

Kluckhohn states that "a value is a conception, explicit or implicit, distinctive of an individual or characteristic of a group, of the desirable which influences the selec-tion from available modes, means, and ends of action."[12] According to Rokeach, a conception of the desirable is a preference for one mode of behavior over an opposite mode or mode-state lower in one's value hierarchy, or a preference for one state over an opposite end-state.[13] Kluckhohn also states that a value

> implies a code or standard which has some persistence through time, or more broadly put, which organizes a system of action. Value . . . places things, acts, ways of behaving, goals of action on the approval-disapproval continuum. A value is not just a preference but is a preference which is felt and/or considered to be justified— "morally" or by reasoning or by aesthetic judgments, usually by two or all three of these.[14]

Kluckhohn also describes values as personal in nature:

> Values are clearly, for the most part, cultural products. Nevertheless, each group value is inevitably given a private interpretation and meaning by each individual, sometimes to the extent that the value becomes personally distinctive. Some values are directly involved in the individual's existence as a "self." Values which manifest

Table 9–1
The Process of Valuing*

Choosing: Involves the *Cognitive Component*
Includes logical, critical, creative thinking, and moral judgment development. Choices are made:

1. Freely
2. From alternatives
3. After considering the consequences of each alternative
4. As complements to other values one has previously internalized. (This process of internal prioritization is both cognitive and affective.)

Prizing: Involves the *Affective Component*
Includes an awareness of one's position, the expression of one's value, experiencing positive self-esteem.

5. One is proud of and happy with the choice.

Acting: Involves the *Behavioral Component*
Actions result in competence (personal, professional, and academic),and result in resolving conflict.

6. One is willing to affirm the choice publicly.
7. One makes the choice part of one's behavior.
8. One repeats the choice consistently.

* The original version of this theory was presented in Raths L, Harmin M, Simon S: *Values and Teaching*, 2nd ed. Columbus, Charles E Merrill Publishing, 1966

this quality appear to be especially important in many ways . . . are apprehended as part of the "self," . . . such values . . . are constitutive of the person's sense of identity.[15]

According to Maslow, values can be classified as B (being) values and D (deficiency) values.[16] This suggests that values can be ordered along a continuum of lower-to-higher-order values, as is indicated by his theory of motivation.[17] Maslow identifies values with needs and categorizes subsets of values based on his well-known hierarchy of needs: safety, security, love, self-esteem, and self-actualization. These basic needs are common to all humankind, and since needs are seen as values, Maslow believes that values are shared and common to all persons.[18] He proposes that certain values are better, higher and more desirable for psychological fulfillment than others, and believes that evidence supports that there is an ultimate value toward which all people strive. This value has been called "self-actualization, self-realization, integration, psychological health, individuation, autonomy, creativity, productivity, [which] amounts to realizing the potentialities of the person, that is to say, becoming fully human, everything that the person can become."[19]

According to Rokeach, a value is an enduring belief that a certain type of behavior or a certain condition of life is desirable. More specifically, he defines a value as "an enduring belief that a specific mode of conduct or end-state of existence is personally or socially preferable to an opposite or converse mode of conduct or end-state of existence."[20] Rokeach also agrees that values have a strong motivational component as well as cognitive, affective, and behavioral components. He describes the functions of values as standards that serve as principles for conflict resolution and decision making, which have motivational functions, and which have adjustive, ego defensive, knowledge, and self-actualization functions.

Rokeach formulated five assumptions about the nature of human values:

1. The total number of values that a person possesses is relatively small.
2. All men everywhere possess the same values to different degrees.
3. Values are organized into value-systems.
4. The antecedents of human values can be traced to culture, society and its institutions, and personality.
5. The consequences of human values will be manifested in virtually all phenomena that social scientists might consider worth investigation and understanding.[21]

By dividing values into two categories, Rokeach identifies a typology of human values: instrumental values (desirable modes of conduct) and terminal values (desirable end-states of existence). Instrumental values are also referred to as "means" values, while terminal values are labeled "ends" values. Instrumental values are further divided into moral and competence values. Moral values are considered more narrow than the general category values. They categorize mainly modes of behavior that "have an interpersonal focus which, when violated, arouse pangs of conscience or feelings of guilt for wrong doing."[22] Competence values or self-actualization values are not concerned with rightness or wrongness and have a personal rather than an interpersonal focus. Terminal values are also divided into two categories: personal and social. In turn, personal values and social values can each be divided into an intrapersonal and an interpersonal focus. This categorization of values into means and ends values has been recognized by philosophers Hilliard[23] and Lovejoy,[24] by psychologists English and English,[25] and by anthropologists Kluckhohn[26] and Strodtbeck.[27] Still other scholars have focused on either means or ends values. French and Khan,[28] Kohlberg,[29] Piaget,[30] and Scott[31] have concentrated on values as means values or idealized modes of behavior. Woodruff,[32] Morris,[33] Maslow,[34] Allport, Vernon and Lindzey,[35] Rosenberg,[36] and Smith[37] have focused on values as desirable end states.

Definitions of a value are articulated differently by a number of individuals who represent a variety of fields of learning; however, it is possible to identify elements of these definitions that are held in common. Kluckhohn notes that there are three significant elements that are essential to the definition of a value and these elements can serve to organize the similar elements of the definitions identified by Raths, Harmin, and Simon, and by Rokeach.[38] They are the cognitive (conception), conative (selection), and the affective (desirable) components.[39] Steps one through three of the valuing process as identified by Raths and colleagues demonstrate this cognitive component of values.[40] The affective elements of a value are expressed in definitions by Kluckhohn as "a conception of the desirable,"[41] by Raths and colleagues as "prized and cherished and publicly affirmed,"[42] and by Rokeach as a "preference considered to be justified."[43] The conative or selection element of the definition is articulated by Kluckhohn, Raths and colleagues, and Rokeach. These major theorists also agree that values have another component that is a behavioral or action-oriented element associated with values and that it serves as a fourth common element in each of the definitions.

What Are Value Systems?

Value systems are frequently referred to in the literature. According to Rokeach, a value system is defined as "an enduring organization of beliefs concerning preferable modes of conduct or end-states of existence along a continuum of relative importance."[44] It is a learned set of principles and roles organized to help a person choose between alternatives, resolve conflicts, and make decisions.

Raths and colleagues also believe that there is a dynamic interrelationship among an individual's values: "Values seldom function in a pure and abstract form."[45] Judgments are made on the basis of a number of interacting values and by a process of weighing and balancing one's values.

Williams writes that value systems, rather than a single value, guide a person's behavior:

> Particular acts or sequences of acts are steered by multiple and changing clusters of values. After a value is learned it becomes integrated somehow into an organized system of values wherein each value is ordered in priority with respect to other values.

Such a relative conception of values enables us to define change as a reordering of priorities and, at the same time, to see the total value system as relatively stable over time.[46]

Silver believes that a value system is the rank ordering of values in terms of their importance with respect to one another: "A person's value system represents a learned organization of values for making choices and for resolving conflicts between the values."[47]

What Are the Distinctions Between Values and Value Indicators?

The literature often erroneously refers to beliefs, aspirations, goals, and attitudes as values. Distinctions between values and concepts, such as needs, beliefs, goals, and attitudes, have been extensively explored by a number of scholars. According to

Raths and colleagues, *value indicators* are those expressions that do not meet all the criteria of the valuing process.[48] They include goals or purposes, aspirations, attitudes, interests, feelings, beliefs, convictions, and activities. Value indicators are seen as potential values and are important because they indicate expressions that approach values, but are not considered to be values since they do not meet all the criteria of the valuing process. Any belief, attitude, or other value indicator that is chosen freely and thoughtfully, prized, and acted upon consistently is defined as a value.

The terms *values* and *beliefs* are often used interchangeably; however, values and beliefs are also seen as different by Kluckhohn, who states that "a belief refers primarily to the categories 'true' and 'false,' 'correct' and 'incorrect.' Values refers primarily to 'good' and 'bad,' 'right' and 'wrong.' "[49] Rokeach, however, disagrees with the idea that beliefs and values differ. He has identified three types of beliefs, one of which forms a value:

> . . . descriptive or existential beliefs, those capable of being true or false; evaluative beliefs, wherein the object of belief is judged to be good or bad; and prescriptive or proscriptive beliefs, wherein some means or end of action is judged to be desirable or undesirable. A value is a belief of the third kind—a prescriptive or proscriptive belief.[50]

Values and other value indicators are also incorrectly used as interchangeable concepts. For example, values and ideals should be defined separately because the concept of "ideal" does not imply the notion of choice or selections that is inherent in the most frequently accepted definitions of a value.

Values and goals have also been mistakenly referred to as the same concept. Although values are seen as a fundamental component in all aspects of action, they "are not the concrete goals of behavior. . . . Values appear as the criteria against which goals are chosen" and are, therefore, unique.[51]

Values and needs have been described as closely related; however, they are not identical with specific needs of the organism:

> Physiologic deprivations and gratifications may be relevant to a great many values, but do not themselves constitute value-phenomena . . . to put it another way, "value" can only become actualized in the context of "need" but is not thereby identified with need. A value might be considered as "that which continues to be desired . . . after imperious segmental deprivations have been removed."[52]

What Are the Effects of Values on Behavior and Decision Making?

Many theorists and writers discuss values in terms of their influence on behavior. Raths, Harmin, and Simon (1966) discuss the interrelatedness of values and behavior: "Where we have a value, it shows up in aspects of our living. . . . Values tend to have a persistency, tend to make a pattern in a life. . . . The development of values is a personal and life-long process."[53] Persons with unclear sets of values "seem not to have clear purposes, to know what they are for and against, to know where they are going and why." They seem "to lack direction for their lives, lack criteria for choosing what to do with their time, their energy, their very being."[54] It is clear that Raths, Harmin, and Simon identify values as having significant and direct influence on behavior.

Rokeach (1973) also concurs with the control role of values in affecting behavior. He asserts that values serve as standards that guide behavior and lead us to choose particular positions, and help us evaluate, judge, and compare what is of worth. "Values are nevertheless more central than attitudes as determinants of human behavior."[55]

Values have been given a role of central importance as the basis for social action and interaction by psychologists, sociologists, and anthropologists. Parson and Shils (1951) report that "patterns of value orientation have been singled out as the most crucial cultural elements in the organization of systems of action."[56] Everything we do, every decision we make and course of action we take, is based on our consciously or unconsciously held beliefs, attitudes, and values. Decision making and one's actions are directly influenced by one's values.

Moscovice and Nestegard (1980) suggest that a hierarchy of values, or a value system, enables one to resolve conflicts and make decisions. The more important a value is in relation to other values in the conflict, the more it is utilized for the decision-making process and resolution of the conflict.[57]

Theories of Value Formation

There are several different theoretical frameworks that attempt to account for the origin and development of human values. Three of the most common theoretical frameworks for the study of values development are the psychoanalytic, social-learning, and cognitive-developmental theories:

Psychoanalytic Approach. An early explanation of the development of values was derived from Freud's work. The psychoanalytic approach describes the development of values based on the establishment of the super ego. The super ego is seen as the center of moral and ideal standards within the person, and its function is to suppress, neutralize, or divert instincts that, if acted upon, would violate moral values the society holds. According to this theory, a child learns values by identification with the parent and incorporates the parent's values. Psychoanalytic theory holds that values are internalized and established early in childhood and that they are not affected by later influences and identifications.

Erikson (1950) continued the work of the psychoanalytic approach and identified eight stages of ego identity that were described as a series of psychological stages related to physical maturation.[58] These stages begin at birth and continue until old age and define the central concerns and conflicts in values unique to each developmental period. The eight stages are: (1) basic trust versus basic mistrust, (2) autonomy versus shame, (3) initiative versus guilt, (4) industry versus inferiority, (5) identity versus role confusion, (6) intimacy versus isolation, (7) generativity versus stagnation, and (8) ego integrity versus despair.

Social-Learning Approach. The main premise of social learning theory is that values are learned. Social learning as applied to value development is based on stimulus-response learning: values are learned by direct positive or negative reinforcement of behavior.[59] Parents are identified as the crucial figures in the process of social learning since they shape a child's values in three ways: punishment, reward, and modeling.[60] Even though a child's preferences for particular values and behaviors change as a result of age, cognitive development, and importance to the child, this theoretical approach asserts that values and behavior learned early tend to persist.

Cognitive-Developmental Approach. The cognitive-developmental approach to values and value judgment processes was pioneered by Piaget and continued by Kohlberg's research. According to this theoretical approach, moral value development (moral values are a category of values) occurs in stages and sequence. Piaget (1932) demonstrated that moral rules and values become more internalized or "interiorized" as an individual moves through the stages. Values and rules are seen as entirely external by the young child and with cognitive maturation they become a part of the child's internal guidelines. At this point, reciprocity enters into the child's thinking and she or he complies with rules and values because of mutual respect and cooperation and not merely because of external authority. Moral judgment and value selection is then autonomous.[61]

The second major theory of cognitive-moral development is that of Kohlberg (1964).[62] Kohlberg's explanation of moral development, like that of Piaget, is aligned with cognitive development and emphasizes the child's ability to reason about moral problems and to choose values more autonomously. Kohlberg's longitudinal research identifies three levels of moral judgment reasoning: preconventional, conventional, and postconventional. There are six stages into which these levels are divided, two at each level. The stages are categories that are representative of successively more adequate ways of handling moral/value reasoning. For example, the way in which rules and values are conceived changes with each stage of development. First, a child follows rules and values based on external compulsions and punishment (stage 1), and later based on rewards (stage 2), then according to social approval (stage 3), then in relation to upholding some ideal order (stage 4), and finally based on the articulation of social principles necessary for living with others (stage 5), and (stage 6) principled morality. It is not until an individual has matured cognitively to stage 5 that one is truly autonomous in the choice of one's values as guides for behavior, since the need for external approval is so operative at the earlier cognitive maturational levels (stages one to four). Kohlberg has also shown that these arbitrary stages represent organized systems of thought and that these stages are natural steps in one's value development. He claims that all people move through these stages in an invariant sequence and that a person reasons predominantly from one stage. Individuals can progress to higher stages of development by deliberate educational programs and techniques that create cognitive conflict in a person's mind and encourage the person to examine personal values and decision making.[63]

Fundamentals of Nursing: Values

So why is it so important to understand the theoretical framework of values, to identify values, and to recognize their influence on your decision making and behavior? Three reasons spring to mind. First of all, how you perform as a nurse depends on your personal and professional philosophy. Values shape this philosophy and are the basis for your actions. If you are unwilling to take the effort to examine and articulate them, you will not be as clear or conscious of your beliefs and values and the significant impact they have on your choices and behavior. The price you pay for unexamined values is often confusion, indecision, and inconsistency. Your behavior in a difficult dilemma is then reflective of this lack of clarity of your values in relation to the issue. Your values have a direct effect on your nursing actions. Second, the clearer you are about what you value, the more able you are to choose and initiate a response that is consistent with what you say you believe. The quality of your decision making is a direct reflection of a clear vision of your values. Competency and clarity in decison making is valued in nursing. Third, we have experienced controversy as the natural state of applied ethics and decision making in today's rapidly changing health care settings. When you make an ethical decision, it is based on the nature of the dilemma itself, the personal values and ethical principles in conflict, the people involved, the possible outcome of the proposed actions, and the type of decision-making model you choose to resolve the issue. It is easier to sort through an ethical dilemma when your values in the dilemma are clarified and when they have been examined in relation to ethical principles.

In an ethical dilemma, the choice is often between equally unfavorable alternatives, and the people involved often place significantly different value judgments on the actions that could be taken or the consequences that could result from the actions. When we are involved in an ethical dilemma as nurses, we must choose which alternative actions or which consequences are of more or less value. Clearly, this part of ethical decision making rests on prioritizing one's values first and on valuing one of the options more than the others. By first bringing one's values into awareness, examining their importance in relation to alternatives or consequences in the dilemma, the alternatives or consequences can be weighed against each other and the comparative importance of each can be determined. In other words, values directly influence the prioritization that occurs in an ethical dilemma. This critical cognitive step is not clearly stated or emphasized in traditional ethical theories.

Again, it is important to emphasize that your values must be considered in the fuller context of their relationship to ethical principles in nursing. It is not enough to merely identify and then act on one's values. The critical question "Are my values ethical?'' is extremely important and demands personal introspection, reflection, and answering by each of us as a nurse before we take action based on personal or professional values.

By now you know that values education can be broadly defined as the systematic effort to help nurses identify and develop their personal values. Its purpose is to provide an opportunity for us to identify and choose among competing values and to examine the consequences of our choices before we are confronted with value conflicts in the clinical arena. Values education enables us to gain sensitivity to value conflicts and ethical issues and allows us to exercise our capacity for moral judgment. It helps us to focus on our values, feelings, beliefs, and judgments as we attempt to resolve value conflicts. Values education also provides students with tools or strategies, abilities, and skills for clarifying values and making value judgments. It offers written strategies that enhance verbal interaction among colleagues. It also offers opportunities to examine a variety of modes of thinking and analyzing alternatives, and to determine whether their decisions and actions reflect their stated values. Most important, values education attempts to expose each of us to alternatives and encourages us toward free choice in terms of values. This choice is crucial since it is only when individuals begin to choose and evaluate the consequences of their choices that they begin to develop a firm commitment to their values.

You know, too, that values education includes four main components: values identification, values analysis, values clarification, and the development of values. Collectively, these components assist you in identifying and developing personal and professional values and in examining the influence of values on your decision making and behavior. Values education offers you a process for systematic decision making rooted in personally identified and chosen values that can be utilized in resolving values issues and ethical dilemmas. It is a collection of effective, experimental strategies and exercises that are developmentally appropriate for the learner and designed to enhance your personal and professional development and potential.

Personal and professional values must be identified, analyzed, clarified, freely chosen, and utilized in one's process of decision making and behavior before the more abstract and ideal ethical principles are taught and the patterns for decision making are prescribed by a given theory. Both values and ethics education enhance effective decision making, but the sequencing of these educational opportunities is critical. I believe that it is important and developmentally sound to study values, moral judgment development, and then ethics. On the basis of this preparation, the nurse is better prepared to resolve value conflicts and ethical dilemmas that are confronted in critical care nursing.

Summary

This chapter helps you reflect on the moral art of nursing, the value-related aspects of the nurse-client relationship, the nature of values and the theories of value formation, and the importance of identifying your own values. It also provides you with opportunities to identify, examine, and clarify your values by completing the strategies at the end of the chapter.

By now you realize that the purpose of this chapter is to establish nursing as a moral art, and the value—caring—as the cornerstone of nursing's moral art as well as its central motivating value. Caring serves as the springboard for all the values inherent in the nurse-client relationship and is fundamental to a therapeutic nurse-client relationship. Authentic caring is of value in enhancing the effectiveness of the nurse-client relationship and, as a value, serves as the measure of our commitment as health care professionals.

You have read that the nurse-client relationship is the point at which nursing's values, morals, ethical principles, traditional and contemporary philosophies unite. It offers each of us, as nurses, a specialized relationship with people that includes implicit and explicit expectations that we will act in ways that embrace the values of caring for each person equally and as unique individuals regardless of the person's attributes, social worth, or illness. We have continued to answer the question, "What values are the foundation for our philosophy of care and for the practice of the moral art we call nursing?" My hope is that you will continue to address this question long after you have read this chapter.

You have also learned three reasons why it is so important to identify and clarify your personal and professional values. First of all, how you perform as a nurse depends on your philosophy and values and serves as the basis for your actions. In other words, values directly affect your nursing actions. Second, the quality of the decisions you make in difficult situations is a direct reflection of the clarity you have of your values. The clearer you are about what you value, the more likely you are to act consistently on what you say is of value. Third, when your values are clarified it is easier to prioritize ethical principles and to sort through a confusing ethical dilemma. Finally, you now realize that you must take an additional and crucial step past merely identifying and clarifying your values. You know that you must "test" your values in relation to ethical principles and so you ask yourself, "Are my values ethical?"

You have been introduced to many ideas about values and numerous strategies for identifying and clarifying those values that influence your behavior. I hope that you have found this chapter challenging and catalyzing, and that you continue to grow personally and professionally.

Notes

1. Rokeach M: The Nature of Human Values. New York, The Free Press, 1973
2. Mayerhoff V: On Caring, p 1. New York, Harper & Row, 1972
3. Leininger M: Caring: The essence and central focus of nursing. The Phenomenon of Caring: Part V. American Nurses' Foundation, Nursing Research Report, vol. 12 (1), p 2
4. Levine M: Nursing ethics and the ethical nurse. Am J Nurs 8:845, 1978
5. Goldsborough J: Involvement. Am J Nurs 69:66, 1969
6. Levine, op cit, p 849
7. Pellegrino ED: Educating the humanist physician, JAMA 227:1293, 1974

8. Curtin L, Flaherty J: Nursing Ethics: Theories and Pragmatics. Bowie, MD, Brady Communications, 1972

9. Kluckhohn C: Values and Value-Orientations in the Theory of Action: An Exploration in Definition and Classification, p 390. In Parsons T, Shils E (eds): Toward a General Theory of Action. New York, Harper & Row, 1951

10. Raths L, Harmin M, Simon S: Values and Teaching. 2nd ed, p 38. Columbus, Charles E Merrill Publishing, 1978

11. Ibid, p 28

12. Kluckhohn, op cit, p 395

13. Rokeach, op cit

14. Kluckhohn, op cit, pp 395–396

15. Ibid, p 398

16. Maslow A: New Knowledge in Human Values. New York, Harper & Row, 1959

17. Maslow A: Psychological data and human values. In Maslow AH (ed): Towards a Psychology of Being. New York, Van Nostrand, 1968

18. Maslow 1959, op cit

19. Ibid, p 123

20. Rokeach, op cit, p 5

21. Ibid

22. Ibid

23. Hilliard AL: The Forms of Value: The Extension of a Hedonistic Axiology. New York, Columbia University Press, 1950

24. Lovejoy A: Terminal and Adjectival Values. Journal of Philosophy, 47:593–608, 1950

25. English HB, English A: A Comprehensive Dictionary of Psychological and Psychoanalytic Terms. New York, Longmans, Green, 1958

26. Kluckhohn, op cit

27. Kluckhohn C, Strodtbeck F: Variations in Value Orientation. Evanston, IL, Row, Peterson, 1961

28. French J, Kahn R: A programmatic approach to studying the industrial environment and mental health. Journal of Social Issues 18:1–47, 1962

29. Kohlberg L: The development of children's orientations toward a moral order, vol I, Sequences in the development of moral thought, Vita Humana 6:11–33, 1963

30. Piaget J: The Moral Development of the Child (1932). Reprint, New York, The Free Press, 1965

31. Scott WA: Values and Organizations. Chicago, Rand-McNally, 1965

32. Woodruff AD: Personal values and the direction of behavior. School Review 50:32–42, 1942

33. Morris C: Varieties of Human Value. Chicago, University of Chicago Press, 1956

34. Maslow 1959, op cit

35. Allport G, Vernon P, Lindzey G: A Study of Values. Boston, Houghton Mifflin, 1960

36. Rosenberg MJ: An analysis of affective-cognitive consistency. In Rosenberg MJ, Hovland C, McGuire W, Abelson R, Brehm J (eds): Attitude, Organization and Change. New Haven, Yale University Press, 1960

37. Smith MB: Social Psychology and Human Values. Chicago, Aldine, 1969

38. Kluckhohn, op cit

39. Raths, Harmin, Simon, op cit

40. Ibid
41. Kluckhohn, op cit, p 395
42. Raths, Harmin, Simon, op cit
43. Rokeach, op cit, p 5
44. Ibid
45. Raths, Harmin, Simon, op cit, p 27
46. Williams 1968, p 287
47. Silver M: Values Education. Washington, DC, National Education Association, 1976
48. Raths, Harmin, Simon, op cit
49. Kluckhohn, op cit, p 432
50. Rokeach, op cit, pp 6–7
51. Kluckhohn, op cit, p 428
52. Ibid, p 428
53. Raths, Harmin, Simon, op cit, pp 29, 37
54. Ibid, p 12
55. Rokeach, op cit, p 51
56. Parsons T, Shils E: Toward a General Theory of Action. Cambridge, Harvard University Press, 1951
57. Moscovice L, Nestegard M: The influence of values and background on the locus of decision of nurse practitioners. Journal of Community Health 5:244–253, 1980
58. Erikson E: Childhood and Society. New York, WW Norton, 1950
59. Bandura A, Walters R: Social Learning and Personality Development. New York, Holt, Reinhart & Winston, 1963
60. Wright D: The Psychology of Moral Behavior. Baltimore, Penguin Books, 1971
61. Piaget, op cit
62. Kohlberg, op cit
63. Ibid

Values Exercises

Introduction

James Smith said, "Controversy is the natural state of applied ethics." Rarely does one emerge from a values conflict or ethical dilemma without the lingering question "Did I do the 'right' thing?" When you make an ethical decision, it is based on the nature of the dilemma itself, the personal values and ethical principles in conflict, the people involved, the possible outcome of the proposed actions, and the type of decision-making model you choose to resolve the issue.

The exercises in this chapter can help you identify, clarify, and actualize your values, continue your search for excellence in critical care nursing, and gain insight into the megatrends and passages in your own personal growth and professional development. As you use the strategies and questions, and raise your own, you will discover facets of yourself and your values that you have not been aware of. This section of the chapter provides you with situations and questions for reflection so that you can analyze them, name and clarify those values shaping your decision, and enhance your decision-making skills when faced with difficult dilemmas or conflict. You can do any of the exercises by yourself or, if you prefer, they can also be tackled in small group discussions in situations such as team meetings or ethics rounds.

Few of us in our quiet moments do not ask and seek answers to questions such as the following. Who am I? What do I truly believe in and value? What do I stand for? My hope is that you find this section of this chapter both thought provoking and challenging.

Exercise 9–1

My Philosophy of Nursing

What is your philosophy of nursing?

Write a statement reflecting your philosophy of nursing on a piece of paper.

1. Read over your philosophy and examine your statements in relation to the concepts below.
2. Identify the values you hold in relation to the concepts you addressed, as well as those named below.
3. Ask yourself as many introspective questions as you can about your philosophy. Some of the following questions may be useful for you:

   - What distinct concepts did I choose to address in my philosophy? What concepts can I think of now that I forgot?
   - What personal values are reflected in my philosophy?
   - What professional values are reflected in my philosophy?
   - What values can I identify in relation to:

     Humankind—health
     Nursing as an art—patients or client
     Nursing as a science—the health care environment
     Nursing as a ministry—obligations of health providers
     Any additional concepts you want to examine

If you want to explore further:

1. Consider your philosophy in other professional and personal arenas and repeat this exercise. For example, if you are an educator, write your philosophy of nursing education, or adult education. If you are a parent, write your philosophy of parenting and watch your values emerge! (The importance of this exercise is in identifying the values that serve as the backbone of your philosophy. Your philosophy will take on more meaning and provide you with more direction when your values are named, clarified, and prioritized.)
2. Obtain the written philosophy of nursing at your institution, or the written philosophy of education published by the faculty of a local college of nursing. Examine the philosophy for the values positions taken in relation to the concepts you think ought to be included. What concepts are not addressed? Are there concepts and values you disagree with? Agree with?

Exercise 9–2

Childhood Value Messages

By the time we were ten, most of our values had already been "programmed." Remember the values you learned as a child? They were taught to you by family members and friends, through the media, in religious classes, and by observing others. What are the value messages you remember learning as a child? Recall as many of them as you can and write them in the space provided. Here are a few examples to get you going: "Clean your plate—don't you know children in other parts of the world are starving ?'' "Finish your work first, then you can play." "Whatever you do, do well." Now it's your turn to write some of the value messages you heard in childhood.

1.
2.
3.
4.
5.
6.
7.
8.

How many of these values still influence the way you think and act today? Which ones influence you professionally?

If you want to explore further:

1. Next to at least half of the values on your list, write the person's name who taught or modeled that value.
2. Put a star next to those messages that are your values today.
3. Put a check next to those that seem to be liabilities.
4. Talk with your colleagues about the childhood values you've identified and how they influence you today.

Exercise 9–3

Professional Nursing Values

What do nurses value? What do you value as a nurse? Literally hundreds of articles in nursing journals identify, implicitly and less often explicitly, the values nurses espouse. Take the time to complete this exercise before you go on to the other strategies in this chapter.

Identifying, analyzing, and prioritizing one's values can be more challenging than it appears at a casual glance. There are three distinct and demanding components to this exercise. The first is to *identify values* that have importance to you. The second is to *examine* those values *in relation to each other* and to begin to discover which values are more centrally motivating and which are supporting values. Being able to discuss the *relative importance* of your values with your colleagues will provide insight in relation to your choices and will also help you understand your colleagues' priorities whether they are similar to or different from yours.

1. Write your own list of values on a piece of paper. Give yourself plenty of time for reflection. If you want to do this exercise with your colleagues, ask

each person to generate a list of values that are important to her or him. Again, give people plenty of time to do this.

2. Schedule a team meeting where people can share and discuss their lists of values. Next, encourage a public and total group brainstorming session to identify values and write them down on a blackboard or on a newsprint easel. (See the list of values provided if this step is too time consuming.)

3. Next, ask the participants to select those values they think are most important from this total list and to number them in order of priority.

As colleagues, or on your own, address some of the following questions:

1. What value(s) do you seem to rank consistently highest?

2. Can you identify an area of conflict when you feel forced to choose between one or more of the values on your list?

3. What do you think of the idea that a person's behavior is not necessarily an accurate indicator of a person's values?

4. Do you think that two people can act in the same way based on different values?

5. What values do you want to be known for on your unit?

6. What values are especially relevant for critical care nurses to uphold?

Exercise 9–4

Professional Nursing Values

Sometimes, identifying values can be difficult and the task can seem elusive or unimportant, so to help you get started, here are some values most frequently mentioned in my workshops. There are numerous others, of course; they may be similar or different from the ones you and your colleagues have already identified. Select 10 from either List I or List II, do a simple rank ordering of these values, and discuss their relative importance in small groups.

List I

Nonjudgmental attitude
Honesty with patients
Involvement with families
Listening
Patient advocacy
Not prolonging a person's suffering
Dignity of the patient
Sharing self through nursing interventions
Integrity of profession through each nurse's example
Promoting health

Care regardless of ability to pay
Emotional involvement with patients
Patient education
Quality care (physical, emotional, spiritual, social, intellectual)
Individualized patient care
Being knowledgeable
Competence
Empathy
Flexibility
Openness to learning
A patient's trust in me
Functioning as a team
Encouraging/allowing a patient to make his or her own decisions
Reduction of pain (mental and physical)
Therapeutic relationship between patient and nurse
Dependability, accountability for one's own actions
Nurses supporting each other

List II

Being caring, compassionate, humane
Treating the person and not merely the disease or the "patient"
Treating people equally regardless of personal attributes, social worth, or nature
of the illness
Caring for the whole person, physically, emotionally, intellectually, spiritually
Preserving the integrity of the human self in spite of the fragmentation of health
care
A sound knowledge base in nursing
Competence of the nurse
Health care professionals should assist in decision making and respect the
client's decision once it is made
Not to trespass on a person's values—not to replace his or hers with ours and
then trick ourselves into believing that it is what the patient wanted
Helping a person find meaning or purpose in living or dying
Acknowledging that the patient is the center of the decision-making team and
advocating for the choices the person makes
Truth telling
Patient education
Control of discharge planning and coordination of continuing care in the
community
Involving the family and/or significant others
The use of self as a therapeutic tool
Collegiality with other nurses
Active listening

Being acknowledged for achievements, expertise

Collaboration with physicians and other professionals

Respect from physicians for professional competence

Patient as the final decision-making authority in spite of differences with family and/or physician's choices

Informed consent

Confidentiality and patient privacy

One entry level into nursing as a means of strengthening nursing's professional image and competency

Caring for the care giver in order to care for others

Accountability for patient care and for professional judgment and actions

Professional pride

Enhancing nursing's image within and outside the profession

Improving the environments where nursing care is practiced so that high-quality, safe care is delivered

Health—restoring, maintaining, promoting, and health teaching

Exercise 9–5

Megatrends in Nursing

There are two objectives for this strategy: (1) to identify traditional, contemporary, and emerging values in nursing and to compare them with your values, and (2) to determine which values have precedence when they conflict.

1. Write down all the *traditional values* you can think of that nurses were taught. For example, to uphold the reputation of the doctor, not to question authority, to stand when a physician entered the room.

2. Identify all the *contemporary values* you can and jot them down on paper. For example, to advocate for a patient, to give individualized care that meets the client's needs holistically.

3. Next, identify as many *emerging values* as you can. For example, to perform as a competent colleague, to be politically involved as a nurse. What other *megatrends* in nursing values do you think will occur? Next, list all the values in nursing that you personally hold. This is an important step in this exercise since you are often taught to uphold certain ideals, and yet, you may not support them for a variety of reasons. For example, in the past, nurses were taught not to question authority. In contemporary nursing, accountability is a fashionable value; if you embrace it, it will often conflict with the former value of not questioning authority. To advocate for a patient, you may have to question authority, yet another example of conflict between traditional and contemporary values or between what has been taught and what you feel is of value.

4. Examine closely the traditional and contemporary values that conflict. How do you choose between them? How do you weigh the conflicting values? Think of examples when these values might conflict. Which values in each solution tend to emerge as the preferred?

If you want to explore further:

Look again at the list of your values in nursing. "Code" your list in the following ways, using the steps of the valuing process to help you assess whether or not the statements you have made are truly values for you. Put the letters representing the various steps of the valuing process in front of those values on your list that you feel meet this step of the process.

CF: Chosen freely
CA: Chosen from among alternatives
CC: Chosen after considering the consequences
 C: Chosen after recognizing that this new value fits with others you hold
PA: Have publicly affirmed this value
 P: Proud of this value
 B: This value shows up in my behavior
 R: This value shows up in my behavior repeatedly, consistently

Once you've identified some of your values, it is important to assess their significance to you and to clarify your action commitment in relation to each value. By incorporating the eight steps of the valuing process in the following questions you can assess a value's meaning to you or help others more closely examine their values. *The following clarifying questions are organized based on the steps of the valuing process and reflect that theoretical model for decision making.* Use them for yourself and with your colleagues.

Exercise 9–6

Clarifying My Personal and Professional Values

Step 1. Choosing freely

a. Am I sure I've thought about this value and have chosen to believe it for myself?

b. Who first taught me this value?

c. How do I know I'm "right"?

Step 2. Choosing from among alternatives

a. What other alternatives are possible?

b. Which alternative has the most appeal for me and why?

c. Have I thought much about this value/alternative?

Step 3. Choosing after considering the consequences

a. What consequences do I think might occur as a result of my holding this value?

b. What price will I pay for my position?

c. Is this value worth the price I might pay?

Step 4. Complement to other values

a. Does this value "fit" with my other values and is it consistent with them?

b. Am I sure this value doesn't conflict with other values I deem important?

Step 5. Prize and cherish

a. Am I proud of my position and value? Is this something I feel good about?

b. How important is this value to me?

c. If this were not my value, how different would my life be?

Step 6. Public affirmation

a. Am I willing to speak out for this value?

Steps 7 & 8. Action

a. Am I willing to put this value into action?

b. Do I act on this value? When? How consistently?

c. Is this a value that can guide me in other situations?

d. Would I want others who are important to me to follow this value?

e. Do I think I'll always believe this? How committed to this value am I?

f. Am I willing to do anything about this value?

g. How do I know this value is "right"? How do I know? Are my values ethical?

Exercise 9–7

"Voting" on Values Issues

This strategy will provide you with the opportunity to examine where you stand in relation to specific issues in nursing and to what extent you agree or disagree with the questions posed or statements made about the issues. You can complete this exercise yourself, or use it to generate a lively discussion among your colleagues.

Read each of the following questions and determine the extent to which you agree or disagree with the statement. You'll notice the statements are written in very strong terms—so that you will not find it easy to take a middle-of-the-road stand. Use the following letters in the spaces provided in front of the questions to indicate your position.

SA: Strongly agree with the statement or issue

A: Agree with the statement or issue

U: Undecided about the statement or issue

D: Disagree with the statement or issue

SD: Strongly disagree with the statement or issue

Do you believe that . . .

1. Patients have the right to die?
2. A person has the right to refuse treatment, even if it will hasten his or her death?
3. Patients should always be told the truth?
4. People have the right to participate in all decisions related to their health?
5. Slow codes are unethical?
6. Proposals to allow members of the health professions to actively end an imminently dying person's life on his or her request should be opposed by nurses and physicians?
7. You will donate your organs after death?
8. Living wills should be legally binding on health care professionals?
9. Severely impaired newborns should be allowed to die?
10. Children should be allowed to make their own treatment decisions after the age of seven?
11. The therapeutic use of marijuana for pain control should be legalized in all the states?
12. Health care is a right?
13. Quality of life should be the criterion for making a decision concerning discontinuing treatment?
14. Patients have a right to examine their health record?
15. Nurses are professionals?

Now make up your own values voting questions.

Exercise 9–8

Ranking Choices

The process of valuing suggests that we examine alternatives and choose from them when making a decision. How do you prioritize the following alternatives? There is no one "right" way to order these responses. Examine these priorities as you see them and share your feelings with your colleagues about why you chose the way you did. Be sure to identify your values behind each of these choices. Generate other alternatives that may more accurately reflect your responses and priorities.

Each question has a series of responses. Rank these responses based on your reaction to the question. Put a number 1 in front of the response that most resembles your position. Use number 2 for your second choice and so forth. Focus on the *relative importance* of the choices in relation to one another and the *values* that influence your choices.

1. Which is the biggest problem facing professional nurses today?
   _____ Definition of nursing
   _____ DRGs
   _____ Lack of fee for service (paid by client directly to nurse)
   _____ Relatively little power within the system to effect change
   _____ Public's understanding of the nurse's role is minimal
   _____ (Choose your own alternative)

2. Which patient would be the most difficult for you to care for?
   _____ A person who is in a persistent vegetative state
   _____ A person who is refusing treatment for religious reasons
   _____ A person who has AIDS
   _____ Patients who refuse to take responsibility for their own health
   _____ A substance abuser

3. What is the most important quality in a critical care nurse?
   _____ Competence
   _____ Caring
   _____ Loyalty to colleagues
   _____ (Choose your own alternative)

4. What is the most important role of a nurse manager in critical care?
   _____ Promoting collegiality on a unit
   _____ Managing human resources fairly
   _____ Instituting a cost-effective budget
   _____ Encouraging staff to further their education
   _____ Letting staff know their work is appreciated

5. The quality I value most in myself as a critical care nurse is . . .
   _____ I am a good listener.
   _____ I make accurate nursing diagnoses.
   _____ I am a competent practitioner.
   _____ I am a spiritual person.
   _____ (Choose your own alternative)

6. Which death would be the most difficult for you to accept?
   _____ My parent's
   _____ My child's
   _____ My best friend's
   _____ My own
   _____ My spouse's

7. What do you think is the most harmful to your health?
   _____ Ineffective coping patterns
   _____ Smoking
   _____ Stress
   _____ Lack of daily exercise

8. What diagnosis would you fear the most?
   _____ Cancer
   _____ Degenerative disease
   _____ Cardiovascular disease
   _____ Mental deterioration
   _____ Chronic pain

9. What competency is the most important for a critical care nurse?
   _____ Communication skills
   _____ Clinical expertise
   _____ Leadership skills
   _____ Teaching ability
   _____ (Choose your own alternative)

10. Which would be the most difficult for you?
    _____ To testify as an expert witness in your specialty area
    _____ To lobby for political change
    _____ To attend the institution's board of director's meeting to voice your views
    _____ To write a letter to the editor of a newspaper about a health issue in your community

11. What is the primary reason that collegiality is difficult to establish in nursing?
    _____ Mistrust among nursing staff
    _____ Toleration of negative criticism
    _____ Little feeling of loyalty among nurses
    _____ Jealousy among the nursing staff
    _____ Different levels of educational preparation in nursing

12. The most confusing issue I face is
    _____ Distinguishing the difference between quality of life and meaningful life
    _____ Identifying what is "ordinary" vs "extra-ordinary" treatment
    _____ The right to die
    _____ A patient's right to refuse treatment
    _____ Allocation of scarce resources

13. The most difficult ethical dilemma in nursing is
    _____ Conflict between obligations to a patient and obligations to an employer
    _____ Conflict between obligations to a patient and obligations to a physician
    _____ Conflict between obligations to a patient and requests made by the patient's family that differ from the patient's wishes
    _____ Conflict between the needs of the patient and the needs of the institution

14. The most difficult thing for me to do would be
    _____ To admit I don't know something
    _____ To report a colleague for stealing narcotics
    _____ To fire an incompetent colleague
    _____ To fail a student

15. I would most like to change my
    _____ Outlook on life
    _____ Physical appearance
    _____ Judgmental attitudes
    _____ Intelligence
    _____ Spiritual maturity
    _____ Level of self-esteem
    _____ Creativity

Now make up some of your own questions.

Exercise 9–9

A Penny for Your Thoughts

This strategy will help you identify and examine your feelings and values as you respond to the following incomplete sentences. Don't "edit" your thinking. Complete the sentences based on your initial response. Then go back and write down all the values you can identify that are inherent in your responses. If you can, do this exercise with a few of your colleagues and listen for the similarities and differences in values. Have fun!

1. Critical care nursing is . . .
2. As a critical care nurse I feel . . .
3. Two areas in which I have expertise are . . .
4. A quality I like in myself as a critical care nurse is . . .
5. Most nurses . . .

6. The two most important qualities in a critical care nurse are . . .

7. I get pressured when . . .

8. The most difficult part of my being a nurse in critical care is . . .

9. The most satisfying experience I've had as a critical care nurse is . . .

10. Two areas I'd like to master are . . .

11. One of my goals as a critical care nurse is . . .

12. Something I'd like to hear from my colleagues is . . .

13. One thing I enjoy most about nursing is . . .

14. A "good day" to me is . . .

15. As a critical care nurse, I'd like to be known for . . .

Now make up some of your own unfinished sentences and complete them.

Exercise 9–10

Values Issues in Nursing: Where Do You Stand?

Read the list of values issues below and make a brief *statement* describing where you stand. Next, identify *what values* are important to you in each of the issues. You can do this alone or discuss your responses with a colleague.

1. Certification in nursing

2. Credits for self study

3. Understaffing in critical care units

4. Peer review

5. Whistle blowing or reporting of incompetent health care professionals

6. Mandatory vs voluntary continuing education

7. A baccalaureate degree in nursing as the entry level into practice for professional nurses

8. A master's degree in nursing as a requirement for practice in critical care units

9. Third-party payment for nurses

10. Political action in nursing to effect change in the quality of health care

11. Relicensing exams for nurses every 5 years in one's specialty area to assure competence

12. The media's portrayal of nurses and nursing

13. Refusal of treatment by patients who are not expected to die in the near future

14. Salaries of critical care nurses

Exercise 9–11

Values Issues/Conflicts/Dilemmas

Briefly describe a values issue, conflict, or dilemma you have experienced or are presently experiencing. Use the questions posed to help you clarify and resolve the conflict. You can do this strategy alone or use it as a means of encouraging members of your team to talk together.

1. *Who* is involved? *How* are they involved? *What* is involved? Make a *concise statement of the problem* you are experiencing.
2. *Identify the values* that are important to you in this issue. Which of your values are *in conflict* in this dilemma?
3. State your position on this issue based on your values.
4. Identify some *alternatives* for resolving this conflict and determine which ones are *consistent with your values.*
5. As accurately as possible, *predict the consequences* of any of the alternatives that you feel are reasonable ways to resolve this issue.
6. *Prioritize the alternatives that are acceptable* courses of action for you and develop a plan of action.
7. *Implement the plan* for resolving the conflict.
8. Carefully *evaluate the action* you've taken and the degree to which it has effectively resolved the problem. Ask yourself, "Did I do the 'right' thing?" "Were my actions ethical?"

(The steps presented here can be found in more depth in the decision-making model found in Uustal D: Values and Ethics in Nursing: From Theory to Practice. E Greenwich, RI, author, 1985)

Exercise 9–12

Identifying Values in Clinical Situations

After you or your colleagues have had experience in identifying, discussing, and prioritizing values, take the time to listen to each other about the *situations that cause conflict*. If you are doing this exercise alone, recall a few conflicting situations and identify the values in each.

If you are doing this exercise as a group, focus on identifying values that seem to influence your choices and behavior consistently and on resolving the conflict by being clearer on your values. This is an excellent strategy that can be incorporated in team conferences or postclinical discussions. As critical care nurses you constantly confront value conflicts in the clinical area. Conflicting situations and values can be identified more clearly through discussion than if the values are learned unconsciously in the clinical area and the conflicts in values never identified, discussed, clarified, and resolved.

Here are some clinical situations that have posed conflicts in values. They are excellent for discussions with your colleagues.

1. Conflicting loyalties in nursing: to whom is the nurse primarily accountable? To the doctor, the institution, the patient? Describe a situation in which these conflicting loyalties posed a conflict in values for you. Identify your values in the situation.

2. The nurse manager of your critical care unit is resistant to open discussion regarding the poor morale and lack of colleagueship. How can change be initiated and sustained? Identify, analyze, and prioritize your values in this situation.

3. You are working in a large teaching hospital. You feel that one physician constantly manipulates patients into treatments that they really do not want. He asks you to sign an informed consent form, but you do not know what has been shared with the patient. Identify and prioritize your values. How do your values influence your behavior?

Exercise 9–13

Balancing Choices Among Values

You know that values are conceptions of what is right, good, or pleasing. When we learn about them, they are usually taught one at a time, as if they exist in and of themselves. They are taught simplistically and as absolutes. For example, most of us were taught to "tell the truth" or "don't lie," or "don't steal," "don't cheat" and "keep your promise." But fewer of us were taught to prioritize the values we've learned when they come into conflict or when a choice between two values is necessary. What do you do when you've been taught to value truth telling and also to be sensitive and not hurt another's feelings? On one hand, truth telling is of value, and yet, in telling the truth a person's feelings may be hurt. On the other hand, in not telling the truth, the person's feelings may be spared (for how long and for what reasons?), but you've not upheld the value of truth telling. Conflicts in values such as these can be simple or complex. The *prioritization of your values in relation to your other values* can be a matter of confusion and controversy and can certainly stimulate introspection and lively discussions that lead to clarity in what values tend to be centrally motivating for you.

This strategy will encourage you to reflect on the *relative importance* of values *when compared one to another*. It will also help you to evaluate the importance and interrelationship of values that may conflict in different situations.

1. Choose the values from List I, II, III, or IV. Prioritize them in order of their importance to you. Number 1 means that value is most important and so on.

2. Talk with your colleagues and share how and why you prioritized your list.

Discuss the similarities and differences in your priorities and what contributes to your preferences.

3. Talk about whether people with the same value priorities can make different decisions and behave differently—or whether their decision and behavior will be the same.

Exercise 9–14

Balancing Choices Among Values

List I

patience
trust
curiosity
fairness
honesty
competence
dedication
lovingness
helpfulness
creativity
loyalty

List II

determination
kindness
caring
respectfulness
sharing
learning
responsibility
giving
understanding
friendship
discipline

List III

accountability
responsibility
autonomy
compassion
caring
honesty
empathy
flexibility
nonjudgmental attitude
acceptance
organization commitment

List IV

colleagueship
pride
competence
sanctity of life
patient's right to make choices
belief in yourself
individualized care
cost consciousness
patience
humor
creativity

If you want to explore further:

1. Discuss a situation that is typical and portrays conflict familiar to the partic-

ipants. Then ask them to prioritize the values on one of the lists in order of preference and *in relation to the conflict situation.*

2. Discuss the idea that some values emerge as consistently preferred and are therefore called central motivating values. Other values, by comparison, have a less significant impact on choices and behaviors and are typically chosen to influence behavior less frequently in relation to central values. These values are therefore called supporting values. *The importance of this exercise is in examining the relative importance of values in relation to each other.*

3. In a brainstorming session, have the group generate a list of values that are important to them (or do this on your own). Next, have each person prioritize these values and with a partner discuss the *meaning* of each of the values, their *relative importance* to one another, and how they *prioritize conflict* between/among these values.

4. Generate your own list of nursing values rather than using those identified above and proceed with the exercise.

Chapter 10

Legal Reflections on Ethics

Elizabeth A. Chaney

Ethics committees and *patient advocacy* are concepts that receive considerable attention in the nursing ethics literature and in nursing discussions of health care decision making and patient care dilemmas. The consensus seems to be that both ethics committees and patient advocacy are good activities that nurses ought to engage in, and that both are essential to closing the gap between what is technologically possible and what is humanely desirable. Often missing from the discourse is an appreciation for the way in which questions of law differ from questions of ethics, how the law's different concerns for dispute prevention and dispute resolution parallel the functions suggested for ethics committees, and how the court's concern for questions of law affect judicial attitudes about advocacy conduct.

Questions of Law

Ethics literature frequently conveys the opinion that courts are not the desirable arenas in which to resolve ethical and moral issues raised in today's critical care setting. It is difficult to quibble with the reasons cited. Litigation is an awesomely costly venture for all parties. The process is, for all, torturously slow. The outcome is uncertain. Publicity surrounding the court action is thought to evoke more extreme and rigid positions on all sides, as is the adversarial nature of court proceedings. The court, as a social institution, considers and may overrule the individual's wishes in the light of compelling and opposing social interests. The nature of subject matter jurisdiction necessarily limits the court to a review of legally relevant facts and does not facilitate an exchange of attitudinal and emotional information that might lead to a decision more inclusive of the parties' values and notion of morality. All these criticisms, however, may well be beside the point. Courts do not decide questions of ethics; courts decide questions of law. What is under judicial review is not ethical rights and duties, but legal rights and duties.

Perceiving that courts do not decide questions of ethics is sometimes made difficult because social values and ethics arguments are considered by legislators and by judges as they work through a process of forming what is regarded as law. Furthermore, lawyers and ethicists use a common language base for discussing rights and duties. Thus, when a judge determines that a patient's right to self-determination requires that his wish for treatment withdrawal be respected, the reader may think "Aha! That judge has decided an ethical question." In fact, the judge has decided a legal question of constitutional and long-standing common law origins. If the right to self-determination did not have a legal foundation, there would have been no legal decision.

Law is commonly described as a set of rules for social behavior that is enforced by external constraints such as threat of some sort of penalty or punishment. While such a description is valid as far as it goes, it does not go far enough to be useful in understanding how the law works.

Another way of conceiving the law is to hold that law concerns itself with preventing and resolving disputes: disagreements over what is to be done, over what may be done. The law seeks to bring peace to the actual or potential disputants in a manner reasonable to them, and to those who follow in their paths.[1]

In Anglo-American tradition, dispute prevention is the principal responsibility of legislative bodies. Thus, legislative lawmakers are absorbed in the continuous task of devising a system of policies and rules that will prevent dispute among society's members by making known what may and may not be done.

Courts, on the other hand, are concerned with resolving disputes that arise when the application or interpretation of existing policies and rules breaks down and there is disagreement as to what may or must be done.[2] Thus, a hospital, patient, or family seeks judicial intervention in the belief that a policy or a rule has been or might be violated, that the wrong rule has been or might be applied, or that the tension created by uncertainty about a rule's application or interpretation is unbearable. To make the matter one of dispute, the responding party necessarily has a different point of view as to the relevant law, relevant facts, or resulting legal rights and duties of the parties.

A petition for judicial review puts the court into the business of deciding what the parties are unable or unwilling to agree upon for themselves. What are the legally relevant facts? What is or ought to be the law? How does the law apply to these particular sets of facts? But judicial intervention also results in another crucially important and distinctive level of decision making. Having determined the relevant facts and law, and how the law applies, the court also decides what must be done by the parties so as to give expression to their resulting and respective legal rights and duties.[3]

It is at the point where the court decides what must be done that the distinction between deciding questions of law and questions of ethics becomes most apparent. Suppose that a court's legal determination of the patient's right to have treatment withdrawn is at odds with the health care provider's determination of its ethical/moral duty to continue treatment. Will the court force the health care provider to act contrary to a perceived ethical/moral duty? Although rogue decisions undoubtedly exist, the court is traditionally reluctant to extend its authority to matters of ethical and moral duty. Thus, the ethically/morally dissident health care provider who calls attention to the moral dilemma is more likely to be ordered to turn the patient's care over to a provider who can and will carry out the legal duty prescribed by the court. The rightness or wrongness of the provider's ethical/moral position is not judged.[4]

What of those decisions that order a patient to receive a treatment the patient wishes to refuse on religious or moral grounds? Again, such decisions do not involve a judging of the rightness or wrongness of the patient's religious/moral position. Whether the matter came before the court upon petition by the patient or the health care provider, the question to be resolved must be stated as a question of law, not of ethics or morality.

When a patient is ordered to accept treatment the legal question decided is often stated as follows: "Does an individual have the legal right to refuse medically indicated treatment that carries a strong probability of success when refusal of said treatment jeopardizes the well-being of others who are dependent on the individual for their economic and social support?" Or, the question may be phrased: "Does an individual's constitutional right to religious freedom extend to refusal of medically indicated treatment that carries a strong probability of success when refusal of said treatment jeopardizes the well-being of others who are dependent on the individual for their economic and social support?" What is placed in context, therefore, is not the question of one's ethical right to make such a decision, but one's legal right to do so.[5]

Although the decisions in such cases are often characterized as compelling the patient to accept the treatment, the court order typically authorizes the health care provider to override the patient's legal objections to treatment because the patient's legal right to refuse treatment is overcome by a superior legal duty to innocent third parties. Arguably, the patient is still free to leave the control of the health care provider who has been authorized to administer the treatment and, therefore, free to exercise his or her religious or moral belief.

The fact that ethicists, employing the language and process of ethical analysis, might arrive at a conclusion similar to the court does not alter the conclusion that courts decide questions of law, not questions of ethics.

Ethics Committees

Transformation of a conflict into a question of law suitable for judicial intervention is, in itself, abhorrent to a number of individuals. The physician has long shunned judicial intervention as an unnecessary and unwelcome intrusion into the privacy of the physician-patient relationship. More recently, though, nurses and other health care providers have been promoting the idea of setting up an intra-institutional, multidisciplinary ethics committee as an alternative to court review of critical care decisions. The ethics committee is conceived as an answer to the frustration that health care providers feel in the face of legislative inaction and the complexity associated with judicial intervention.

As noted in Chapter 3 of this text, the ethics of decision making in critical care has gained increasing attention as the gap has widened between what is humanly desirable and what is medically possible. Courts have responded to this widening gap by suggesting that some kind of intra-institutional review might facilitate fact-finding and decision making concerning the patient's prognosis.[6] There would be a panel, coined a "prognosis committee," comprised of physicians with expertise in assessing the particular disease or illness. The findings of the committee would serve as a backup to a physician's decision to recommend continued treatment or withdrawal of treatment.

Contrary to popular belief, impetus for establishing multidisciplinary ethics committees has not come from the courts, nor have the courts recognized legal authority for such a committee to decide questions of continuing or withdrawing medical treatment.[7]

Neither have legislators recognized a decisional role for such a committee. Even federal regulations concerning the treatment of neonates created an institutional review committee that served more a coordinating, red-flagging, and clearinghouse function than one of decision making.

The movement for a multidisciplinary approach to the ethics of health care decision making has emerged from the literature on health care and bioethics.[8] The idea certainly makes sense because so many disciplines are actively involved in the patient's care and have access to information that can affect the decision-making process. In fact, the idea makes so much sense that just about anyone who has ever struggled or thought of struggling with the questions and conflicts common to critical care decision making has at least one idea of what the ethics committee could do to make things better.

A nonexhaustive list, casually compiled from readings and conversation, would assign to ethics committees one or more of the following functions: education of staff, patients, families, the community at large; complaint review and mediation of conflicts between medical and nursing staff regarding code orders; complaint review and mediation of conflicts between nursing staff and administration regarding environmental requirements for ethical nursing practice; mediation of conflicts among patient, family, and physician regarding treatment decisions; consultation; prognosis review; forum for dialogue, debate, and reaching a consensus within the hospital and between and among staff, patients, and families; policy, protocol, and procedural guidelines development for medical and nursing practice with the terminally ill, the comatose, the questionably incapacitated, the newborn, the elderly, the family, or the surrogates and others; and case review concluded by recommendations or decisions concerning the ethically appropriate course of action or referral to outside agencies or institutions including protective services and courts.

The list incites several reactions in most managers who examine it. First, the list is terribly long and the tasks all appear time-consuming and therefore costly. Second, some of the functions are or should be managed by other groups within the hospital setting. The call for an ethics committee to mediate physician/nurse disputes or nurse/administration disputes, for example, indicates that weaknesses exist in the current organizational process. Third, the skills required to perform these functions are so varied that it would seem many ethics committees, or subcommittees, would be necessary. Coordination of so many functions would again take time and manpower.

Critical reactions such as these mean neither that ethics committees cannot exist in a hospital setting nor that managers are hostile to the idea. The reactions do suggest that each hospital needs to examine its own laundry list of reasons for establishing an ethics committee and should decide which of those reasons could only or best be served by an ethics committee and which could be served by a different group within the organization.

The list is especially intriguing to a lawyer because it seems that all the functions can be placed in one of two categories: dispute prevention or dispute resolution. If that is the case, then ethics committees are asked to perform both quasilegislative and quasijudicial functions. Quasijudicial functions, such as mediation and case review, are understandably attractive to those who want to keep decisions about what to do out of the courtroom. Where reconcilable differences do exist, as the result of misinformation or miscommunication, mediation can be an effective tool for heading off major confrontations in the courtroom.

However, not all differences are reconcilable and not everyone wants to "get to yes" through mediation. No authority exists to compel participation in mediation proceedings, and involuntary participation would not augur well for success. Undoubtedly the parties one would most want to engage in some kind of review process are those least likely to participate voluntarily.

Other problems can emerge. Efforts by hospitals to offer mediation services can open the hospital-based mediator to charges of conflict of interest, particularly today when certain kinds of treatment decisions may be more costly to the institution than others.

Mediation is a skill that is not acquired by membership on an ethics committee. Conceivably, dissatisfied participants in a mediation process could entertain a negligence claim against the mediator, alleging harm resulting from a failure to meet certain standards or mediation practice. Furthermore, information brought forth in mediation could become an object for discovery in a subsequent court action. The prospects of today's discussion becoming a part of tomorrow's court transcript often chill open communication. Thus, the advantages sought through mediation services need to be weighed against the burdens acquired, particularly if taken on by persons who lack technical preparation in mediation.

Case review is often viewed as an attractive mechanism for shedding light on chronic and acute decision-making problems in a setting. The review can take place prospectively or retrospectively. Retrospective reviews serve educational as well as policy assessment and evaluation functions. There is precedent for such committee activity in the quality assurance and peer review activities already existing in most hospitals. Unless the results of the retrospective reviews are used to affect staff privileges or opportunities within the setting, liability exposure seems minimal.

Prospective case review is a different matter entirely because the reviewers become participants in the case by virtue of their examination of the facts and their capacity to influence the outcome by issuing recommendations or decisions. If parties involved in a case agree to submit to the ethics committee's "jurisdiction" and to be bound by the committee's decision or recommendations, then the process used by the committee to gather information and arrive at its decisions must be prepared to withstand the scrutiny of even the formal judicial system.

What will the committee decide? Questions of law? Questions of ethics? Both? Will the opinions be written? How will minority opinions be expressed? How will appearances before the committee be compelled? Can decisions be rendered without appearances by all the parties in interest? Can any of the proceedings or committee deliberations be protected from discovery in subsequent litigation? To whom is the committee beholden? How is conflict of interest to be prevented or resolved?

What are the legal and ethical implications of a physician submitting his or her professional judgment to a decision by a committee or by nonphysicians? What are the legal and ethical implications of a nurse submitting his or her professional judgment to a decision by a committee comprised of non-nurses? If parties differ with the committee decision or recommendation, what rights of appeal are available? What are the implications to health care providers who disregard the decision or recommendation to follow the dictates of their own professional judgment? How do professionals reconcile their duties to report medical neglect with the role of impartial fact finder? Can a case review committee with decisional or recommending powers be all that different from a court of law? And, if not, what is the point of adding yet another costly, time-consuming layer of review?

On the other hand, the quasilegislative function is an urgently needed, more promising , and less hazardous activity for ethics committees. Dilemmas and conflicts often arise in the presence of misinformation about relevant ethical and legal principles, and in the absence of sufficiently descriptive policies, procedures, and guidelines within the institution. Clinicians in medicine, nursing, social work, and other related disciplines are familiar with using consultants for added problem-solving expertise and commonly view such resources as enhancing and valuable.

Hospitals have long been in the business of preparing educational programs, developing policies and procedures to guide staff in complex situations, providing consultation to staff, and conducting a variety of medical and nursing practice review functions to improve patient care. As hospitals mature in carrying on the quasilegislative activities through a multidisciplinary ethics committee, the product of such efforts shows promise in providing legislators with a data base from which to derive public policies on critical care decision making, which, at best, will bring peace of mind to health care providers and health care consumers alike—and, at the least, narrow the field of questions that require judicial intervention.

Quasilegislative functions pose fewer hazards because they do not engage the hospital and committee members directly in the conflict-ridden, emotionally charged process of choosing what to do in particular patient care dilemmas. It is important, however, to recall that policies and procedures set standards that can be introduced to establish the legal standard of care that should have been followed in a particular patient care situation. Thus, as in other circumstances, the policies and procedures need to be clinically rational, and, therefore, reasonably attainable.

Clinical nursing, clinical medicine, and clinical social work skills in negotiating safe passage through the mine fields of interpersonal relationships have a long and honorable history. If some of these skills seem to have broken down in the critical care arena, it may be for want of an adequate administrative framework to nourish and support staff. An ethics committee that successfully conducts staff and community education, develops policy/procedure guidelines, and provides consultation may be all that is needed to restore participants in the critical care drama to the equilibrium needed to work out reasonable solutions to the majority of dilemmas right at the bedside. And, is the bedside not the most effective place for insuring individualized decisions, taking into account the widest array of variables that come to bear on a given human life?

If education, comprehensive policy/procedural guidelines, consultation, and clinical skills together fail to resolve the indecision or conflict about what to do, perhaps judicial intervention is what is needed. Surely those health care providers and consumers in the jurisdiction controlled by the *Bartling*[9] and *Barber*[10] decisions have more certain legal parameters for critical care decision making than existed before the parties went to the time, expense, and discomfort of seeking judicial review.

Patient Advocacy

Nurses who encounter unsafe working conditions, patient abuse, invasive medical treatment against the patient's wishes, demands to assume medical functions without legal authority, and other situations that jeopardize the patient's dignity and safety are often stymied in their efforts to bring about a change in what they perceive as unethical or illegal practices by their employers or others. In frustration, such a nurse may decide that, on ethical and moral grounds, advocacy requires that he or she discontinue performing that part of any work responsibility that acquiesces to the objectional circumstance. When, in response to this announcement, the employer terminates the nurse's employment, does the nurse have recourse in law? Possibly. Success will turn largely on what it is the nurse is objecting to and what is relied upon to justify the nurse's conduct.

Courts have been unreceptive to arguments that rely on professional ethical standards to justify refusal to perform a job. Such standards are commonly viewed as self-serving, personal, and proprietary, especially if the standards result in a nonperformance of work that is associated with preserving life. Consequently, they are not recognized as legitimate expressions of "public policy" that support and protect the employee's actions.[11]

While the courts are willing to accept regulations and statutes as legitimate expressions of public policy, the language of the law must be specific in supporting and protecting the conduct selected to advocate for patient welfare. For example, licensing board regulations that address in global terms the nurse's responsibility for patient welfare or safety have not been found sufficiently specific as expressions of support for a nurse's refusal to accept what she or he believed were unsafe staffing levels. Again, the nurse's refusal to act would be viewed as based on personal belief and of no greater weight than the employer's personal belief that the conditions were sufficiently safe.

Would a different outcome result if the nurse were to point to a specific violation of state licensing requirements for staffing levels? While this might be a stronger argument, the employer might successfully argue that even if there were a violation, the nurse would not be committing an illegal act if she or he did work and might be placing the clients in greater jeopardy by refusing to work. The employer's argument might well call forth the state's "compelling interest" in preservation of life to take legal priority over the nurse's individual opinion that refusal to work was ethically justified.

In 1985 the California Board of Registered Nursing adopted regulations defining competency to include the following:

> [The nurse] acts as the client's advocate, as circumstances require, initiating action to improve health care, to change decisions or activities which are against the interests or wishes of the client, giving the client the opportunity to make informed decisions about health care before it is provided.[12]

While this regulation specifically supports a patient advocacy role, it is not clear that support is given for nurses to refuse, on grounds of personal or professional ethics, to perform their job responsibilities. Rather, the language seems to require that the nurse act affirmatively to "improve health care," "change decisions" when necessary, and act in terms of what the patient wants or what a reasonable person in the patient's situation would want.

One state, Illinois, has enacted a statute that prohibits an employer from "all forms of discrimination, disqualification, coercion, disability or imposition of liability" based on an employee's "conscientious refusal to . . . perform, assist, counsel, suggest, recommend, refer or participate in any way in any particular form of medical care contrary to his or her conscience."[13]

Nurses practicing under such a statute would appear to have considerable support in public policy to exercise broad discretion in refusing to participate in any situation that violated their personal ethical and moral standards. Such a statute offers splendid opportunity to test, in vivo, the courts' concern that chaos would result if individuals were able to decide whether to perform a task based on individual, personal beliefs.

Legal arguments that the employer wrongfully terminated employment in violation of a public policy are of course strengthened when the attorney can cite a specific statute that expressly prohibits termination for refusing to participate in the particular job circumstance. For example, forty-two states have enacted statutes that protect employees from termination for refusing to participate in performing abortions.[14]

Advocacy of course does not necessarily involve a refusal to perform one's job duties. What if the nurse chooses to advocate *for* a patient by continuing to provide treatment in the face of what she or he believes is an improper "do not resuscitate" or withdrawal of treatment order? Suppose the nurse is then terminated for acting in an insubordinate manner or for refusing to follow medical orders, and brings suit for wrongful termination based on a violation of public policy?

The outcome of the suit would be affected by numerous factors, not the least being whether the jurisdiction recognized a public policy basis for wrongful termination claim. Assuming technical problems were overcome, the nurse would seem to have support in the argument that the action had been in accord with the compelling state interest to preserve life. However, the nurse's position would be vastly enhanced if the action were also in accord with the patient's express wishes to continue living, if statutory or regulatory law imposed specific advocacy responsibilities on the nurse, and if hospital procedures for determining DNR or treatment withdrawal orders had been violated by the physician.

In some instances, the duty to advocate may require the nurse to speak out within the agency or to take the patient care problem to an outside agency for investigation and review. Does law offer support to such a nurse? A definite trend has developed in legislative law to offer some degree of protection to employees who report an employer's illegal activities to state agencies.[15] Furthermore, the California legislature, as one example, has created a rebuttable statutory presumption of retaliation if an employee is fired within 120 days of reporting a health facility violation to the state licensing agency.[16]

In the absence of strong legislative protection, however, the nurse must be prepared to offer substantial objective evidence that the conditions or circumstances warranted the action taken against the employer. Evidence suggesting that the nurse acted with malice could, for example, fatally taint the advocacy argument where the nurse was relying on common law principles.

Summary

The distinction between questions of law and questions of ethics is not merely one of words. How one perceives the court's role shapes not only our expectations about what courts decide, but also our expectations of what emerging ethics committees can and should accomplish and how the courts will respond to the nurse's assertion of rights and responsibilities in an advocacy role.

Notes

1. Llewellyn KN: The Bramblebush. New York, Oceana Publications, 1930
2. Ibid, pp 12–13
3. Judicial decisions are not advisory opinions or recommendations. Procedurally, the decision is effected by an "order of the court" that directs the parties to take specified action.

The power to decide what is to be done, and to compel the doing, is consciously tempered by restraint in determining what is proper subject matter for judicial intervention.

4. See Bartling v Superior Court, 163 Cal App 3d 186, 1984

5. Most nurses will recognize this fact pattern as it has appeared when an adult patient who has minor children and is a member of the Jehovah's Witnesses faith refuses to accept a blood transfusion that is medically determined to be necessary to preserve the adult's life.

6. See In re Quinlan, 355 A 2d 647, 1976; see also Matter of Welfare of Coyler, 669 p 2d 738, Wash, 1983

7. While the Quinlan court called for a multidisciplinary ethics committee to protect hospitals, physicians, and others, the court prescribed for the committee the task of reviewing the diagnosis and agreeing/disagreeing with the physician's conclusion that the patient had no reasonable possibility of emerging from a comatose state. This multidisciplinary model for medical decision making was rejected in Matter of Welfare of Coyler, 660 p 2d 738, Wash, 1983:

   > The Quinlan court recommended a hospital ethics committee, made up of physicians, social workers, attorneys, and theologians, to oversee the decisions. This type of a committee has been criticized, however, for its amorphous character, for its use of non-medical personnel to reach a medical decision, and for its bureaucratic intermeddling. . . . We agree that such an administrative body does not best serve the desired function. In actuality, what is needed is a prognosis board to confirm the attending physician's diagnosis. . . . Thus, we recommend that in future decisions of this nature, there should be unanimous concurrence from a prognosis board or committee. Such a committee should consist of no fewer than two physicians with qualifications relevant to the patient's condition, plus the attending physician.

8. Cranford R, Doudera AE: Institutional ethics committees and health care decision-making. Ann Arbor, Health Administration Press, 1984. See also President's Commission for the Study of Ethical Problems in Medicine and Biomedical and Behavioral Research: Deciding to Forego Life-Sustaining Treatment. Washington, DC, Government Printing Office, March 1983

9. Bartling, op cit. (Adult patient, or his surrogate, with underlying, progressive, irreversible fatal illness may refuse to accept life sustaining treatment.)

10. Barber v Superior Court, 147 Cal App 3d 1006, 1983

11. In Warthen v Toms River Hospital [488 A 2d 229, 118 BNALRRMK 3179 (NJ Sup Ct, 1985)], the court rejected a nurse's attempt to rely on the ANA Code for Nurses, observing that preservation of life is the most fundamental of public policies and that "it would be a virtual impossibility to administer a hospital if each nurse or member of the administrative staff refused to carry out his or her duties based upon a personal private belief concerning the right to live." In Pierce v Ortho Pharmaceutical Corporation [417 A 2d 505 (NJ 1980)], the Hippocratic Oath did not protect a physician from employment termination when he refused on ethical grounds to continue working on a project: "Chaos would result if a single doctor engaged in research were allowed to determine according to his or her individual conscience, whether a project should continue. . . . An employee at will who refused to work in answer to a call of conscience should recognize that other employees and their employer heed a different call."

12. 16 CAL ADM CODE Section 1443. 5, 1985

13. Illinois Stat, Ann, Ch, 111 1/2, Sections 5302–5313, West Supp, 1985

14. They include Alaska, Arizona, Arkansas, California, Colorado, Delaware, Florida, Georgia, Hawaii, Idaho, Illinois, Indiana, Iowa, Kansas, Kentucky, Louisiana, Maine, Mary-

land, Massachusetts, Michigan, Minnesota, Missouri, Montana, Nebraska, Nevada, New Jersey, New Mexico, New York, North Dakota, Ohio, Oregon, Pennsylvania, Rhode Island, South Carolina, South Dakota, Tennessee, Texas, Utah, Virginia, Washington, Wisconsin, and Wyoming.

15. For example, federal law prohibits any reprisal or personnel action against a federal employee for disclosing information that she or he believes provides evidence of a violation of law, rule, regulation, mismanagement, waste of funds, abuse of authority, or substantial and specific danger to public health or safety unless such disclosure is specifically prohibited by law or specifically required to be kept secret by executive order for national security or foreign affairs reasons. [5 USC Section 2302(b) (8) (a) (1980)] Some states have also enacted whistle-blowing statutes. MICH COMP LAWS ANN Section 15.362 (1980); 1983 CONN ACT 578; ME REV STAT ANN Title 26, Sections 831, 832; 1984 NX LAWS 660.

16. CAL HEALTH AND SAFETY CODE 1432(a), 1432(c) (1984).

Chapter 11

Piecing Together the Ethical Puzzle: Operationalizing Nursing's Ethics in Critical Care

Marsha D. M. Fowler

Whether plumb bob and trowel, parchment and quill, or *pH* and stethoscope, every discipline has tools necessary to its trade. Normative ethics is no different; it has ethical norms and processes or mechanisms for the resolution of ethical dilemmas. This chapter will examine the principles and values discussed in the preceding chapters in the light of nursing organizational policies and will then look at institutional mechanisms for coming to grips with moral issues in clinical practice.

Values and Principles in Practice

The principles and rules that the preceding chapters have discussed include the duties of respect for autonomy, nonmaleficence, beneficence, fidelity, veracity, and justice, as well as one's duties to one's self. The moral values that have been either implied or explored include responsibility, accountability (answerability), nonmalevolence, benevolence, faithfulness, dependability, honesty, integrity, justness, fairness, ''care-fullness,'' skill, knowledgeableness, competence, humaneness, compassion, authenticity, empathy, sensitivity, respectfulness, impartiality, courage, self-regard, other-regard, and autonomy. The nonmoral values identified (whether goods in, or ends of, nursing) include autonomy, justice, fairness, advocacy, health, care, comfort, human dignity, well-being, and respect for persons. All of these, and more, are the moral norms that nursing, as a profession, demands, strives for, and hopes to realize in the work-a-day world of clinical practice.

This is, admittedly, a rigorous expectation of the profession's members. It can also be an impossible expectation. It is impossible to live out these norms if the professional environment does not reward it, if the moral milieu discourages it, if the administrative climate impedes it, or the fiscal priorities of the institution prohibit it. How then can these norms be realized? There are a number of mechanisms that will aid in implementing sound ethical decision making, in fostering the moral values nursing wishes to cultivate, and in achieving the ends that nursing seeks. These mechanisms include professional policies and institutional procedures that are "enabling" factors within the community of moral discourse.

However, before discussing those factors, it is necessary to address two questions. The first is, "What is the ethical decision-making process?" and the second is, "Why should nursing or nursing organizations formulate policy, promulgate guidelines or position statements, or establish mechanisms or processes for ethical review of issues or cases?"

What Is the Decision-Making Process?

Decision making in ethics, as in nursing and medicine, is decision making under conditions of uncertainty. Unfortunately, in the face of hard moral decisions in clinical practice we cannot simply peer into that longed-for crystal ball to foretell consequences, or weigh principles on the balance scales of rightness, or even trust that, as with an erector set, we can attach part A to segment B at joint C and inevitably produce result D. Nursing and medicine face the same predicament in nonethical clinical decision making. How does one overcome some of these uncertainties? Usually by resort to a *process* of decision making.

A process is a stepwise method of analyzing and evaluating a situation, choosing an action and acting, then reevaluating. There is a caveat, however. In ethical decision making, even with a method for analysis and evaluation of a moral dilemma, ethical choices remain hard choices by nature because they make conflicting claims upon us, or present us with seemingly equally unsatisfactory alternatives. Thus, simply to come to the "right" answer ethically does not necessarily free us from the personal pain of a situation; it simply clarifies the moral appropriateness of an alternative, provides us with greater confidence, and frees us from vague but gnawing feelings of guilt, apprehension, or doubt. Nonetheless, a method for ethical decision making can provide us with a general structure for a thoughtful consideration of moral problems. In brief, reflection upon an ethical problem will generally entail the following steps:

Problem Identification: Identify, as clearly as possible, what you consider to be the ethical problem. It is possible that more than one ethical problem may exist. Are there competing ethical claims made upon you, that is, do you sense a conflict of duties? Is there a conflict of either personal or professional values? What are they? Is this your ethical conflict, or does it rightly belong to another?

Identify the Morally Relevant Facts: Not all facts of the situation are morally relevant. Examine the context of the dilemma. How did it occur? Could it have been avoided? Is it likely to arise again, avoidably or unavoidably? Who are the participants and decision makers in the situation? What are the viewpoints and vested interests of each actor (patient, professional, family, others)? Are there relevant nonmoral considerations, including medical, administrative, economic, political, legal, prudential, or aesthetic concerns?

Evaluate the Ethical Problem: Examine professional ethical norms as seen in the ethical literature of nursing, in the codes of ethics, or in the moral tradition of the profession. Do they speak to the situation and provide moral action guides? Consider also the broader ethical principles, such as justice and autonomy, which give rise to those professional norms and which have been discussed throughout this book. Do they provide adequate direction in this situation? Consider, too, the norms of moral value and nonmoral value that have been discussed. Do they assist in providing direction for action? Factor in those aspects of the situation that individualize it. Examine the situation in the light of the ethical principles, weighing and prioritizing them in accord with both professional and personal ethical demands.

Identify and Analyze Action Alternatives: What action alternatives are open to you? Are there new or creative alternatives that can be considered? What are the harms and goods that are likely to result from each alternative? Who will be harmed and who will be helped? Which actions will produce subsequent dilemmas? How would you ethically analyze each action alternative? Are there institutional procedures for addressing this particular type of dilemma? If so, how can they help?

Choose and Act: On the basis of your ethical evaluation of the dilemma and the options for action, choose a plan of action. Modify that plan of action if necessary to make it accord with legal or other values while remaining consistent with your moral norms. Then, act.

Evaluate and Modify Your Plan: What are the results of your action? How did you feel, at a moral level, about your action in this instance? If you were in this sort of situation again, are there new considerations or actions you might weigh? Could this sort of situation be avoided in the future? If so, how could you practice preventive ethics? How should you modify your plan of action now, in this situation?

It is not by accident that the steps of ethical analysis and evaluation in clinical practice vaguely resemble those of the nursing process. Though they have different content, both processes require a situational analysis and evaluation, and action (that is, application to practice), under conditions of uncertainty. Both are intended to provide a systematic and thoughtful approach to the resolution of dilemmas, whether nursing-diagnostic or ethical, bringing a supporting foundation of theory to bear upon those situations. The resolution of clinical dilemmas is, however, dependent on the existence of procedures and policies that support action, which brings us to our second important question.

Why Should Nursing Formulate Policies, Position Statements, and Guidelines?

Why should nursing or nursing organizations formulate policy, promulgate guidelines or position statements, or establish mechanisms or processes for ethical review of issues or cases? After all, medicine has published a variety of guidelines, hospitals are creating ethics committees, the President's Commission has published rather thoroughgoing reports, the American Hospital Association has a Patient's Bill of Rights, most institutions have institutional review boards, and consumers are increasingly aware of their rights and responsibilities with regard to health care.

Well, true enough. The moral picture is changing. Ethical precepts are no longer regarded as irrelevant or frivolous concerns in the face of medical, scientific, and technological innovation. Many groups, not to mention individual professionals and "consumers," (an unfortunate term), certainly attend to the moral realm with greater sophistication and regard. But the moral expressions of others, whether professions, institutions, or even patients, do not give voice to nursing's particular concerns.

A Voice for Nursing's Ethics

At an abstract level (a concrete example will follow), it has been maintained that different disciplines select or even isolate specific observable *phenomena of concern*, that is, specific events, occurrences, needs, conditions, manifestations, or relationships that the discipline wishes to investigate, control, or manipulate. For nursing, the phenomena of concern are actual or potential responses to health problems.[1] For critical care nursing, the phenomena of concern are human responses to actual or potential *life-threatening health problems*[2] (see Appendix A). The way in which the profession, discipline, or theorist interrelates the variety of phenomena of concern with the role and scope of the profession forms a *conceptual model*. A conceptual model gives a perspective on a profession, what it is and does, whom it serves, how it serves, and so on. But professions and disciplines are interested in concepts at an even more abstract level than "human responses" and conceptual models.

They are interested in what are called *metaparadigm concepts*, the root conceptual constructs that combine to form a larger *metaparadigm*, which is something of a profession's world view. Professions are uniquely identified by the metaparadigm concepts that form their metaparadigm. That being the case, it then follows that distinctively different professions will hold distinctively different perspectives on the world.[3] The difference in perspectives will necessarily produce differences in moral perspectives, even when there may be some areas of shared professional interest. Thus, one can expect to see some similarities, but a cumulatively different ethical emphasis, for different professions.

To make this less abstract, there is considerable agreement that nursing has four *metaparadigm concepts*: *person, environment or society, nursing, and health*.[4] Every nursing theory or conceptual model will, at some point, have to deal with each of these metaparadigm concepts, even if the model evades outright definition of the concepts. While the definitions of the concepts themselves are of considerable importance, the relationships between the concepts are of equal and sometimes greater significance. For instance, most models define health. Illness, however, is often left undefined, its definition to be found indirectly in the interaction between two or more of the metaparadigm concepts: some models, such as Nightingale's, locate illness in the interaction between person and environment; others place it in the linkage between person and health, as in Orem's model. Some models emphasize one concept over another; emphasis is placed on environment in some models, as in Roy; in others it is placed upon person, as in Johnson's model. Differences in metaparadigm concept definitions and concept relationships constitute the differences among nursing models. These are the differences between the models of Nightingale, Johnson, Roy, Levine, King, Rogers, and others. They all remain, however, *nursing* models specifically because of their participation in the nursing metaparadigm.

The metaparadigm concepts of medicine are different. Medicine is concerned to define the metaparadigm concepts of *person, environment or society, physician, and pathophysiology,* and the relationships between these concepts. Just as in nursing today, there have, of course, been a number of different medical models, some of which persist. At one time (in the late 1800s and early 1900s) alternative medical models competed with the allopathic model, which is the dominant form of Western medicine today. Still, some competing models do survive and include osteopathy, homeopathy, naturopathy, and chiropracty, though chiropracty has considerably narrowed its claims in recent decades. Despite differences in how health and disease and how the role of the physician and the patient/person are defined, each of these models is a medical model by virtue of its subscription to the medical metaparadigm. The phenomena of concern to medicine, though at some points shared with nursing, are not those of nursing. In addition, the values and obligations inherent in medicine's metaparadigm are not identical to those that nursing would express.

Because nursing is a distinctive profession, with a distinctive metaparadigm, metaparadigm concepts, and phenomena of concern, it will inevitably have a particular ethical expression—a *distinctive nursing ethics.*[5] Given that nursing is not a subvariety of medicine, it is proper then to discuss nursing's ethics separately from medicine's ethics.[6] It is both proper and necessary, also, to articulate nursing's moral values and concerns in separate documents, rather than to allow the positions of other professions or groups to be determinative of our own.

Nursing Organizational Policies

Though there are a number of specialty nursing organizations, two of the most relevant to the professional life of the critical care nurse are the American Association of Critical-Care Nurses (AACN) and the American Nurses' Association (ANA). Both organizations have clearly demonstrated an awareness of the moral nature of nursing and an interest in the moral dilemmas that confront nurses in practice. Even more, however, both organizations have come to an awareness of the absolute necessity of professional policy and position statements that support the moral norms of the profession, and set standards for professional behavior, decision making, priorities, and goals.

This is one of the major contributions that a professional organization can make toward assuring that its members can deliver high-quality nursing care. Professional organizations, as distinguished from clinical or practice organizations, serve to represent a profession or group to the public, to legislators, the judiciary, and others. While practice organizations are principally concerned with assisting the nurse at the bedside level, the "microlevel" (through continuing education, research, collaboration , and so forth), professional organizations focus their energies on broader issues—those at the "macrolevel." They form political action groups, set national standards for practice and education, promote the economic and general welfare of their members, and represent the profession (or a specialty group) at a national or international level. Some organizations attempt to serve both functions, but generally separate the focus as the organization grows; state and local groups will emphasize clinical concerns while the national body emphasizes what are called professional concerns. Both emphases are crucial to assuring high-quality nursing care; it is a serious error to neglect to participate in a professional organization, having mistaken the functions of the two sorts of organizations for one another.

The AACN, through its position statements, definition of critical care nursing, legislative influence, and other activities, serves as a professional voice for critical care nurses. However, it also demonstrates a clear practice focus through the National Teaching Institute, regional teaching institutes, clinically oriented publications, and local chapter meetings. Similarly, the ANA, though largely a professional organization, does attempt to meet a practice focus through such activities as special interest groups, publication of the *American Journal of Nursing*, and sponsored research.

In an examination of their position and policy statements, it is clear that both AACN and ANA are concerned to give voice to the moral concerns and values of the profession. The principles and values discussed in the preceding chapters are evident in a number of the documents of these organizations. In some instances, they demand attention like the beam of a search light; in other cases they glimmer and flicker like the flame of a candle.

These documents are crucial to the practice of the critical care nurse for they provide statements of the ethical foundation of the nurse's practice, set standards of ethical practice, and are documents to which the nurse can resort for support and direction. Knowledge and ethical understanding of these documents are, thus, essential to every critical care nurse; they are both the sword and the shield of ethical action in clinical nursing. Consequently, this chapter will examine various position statements for their support of each of the principles and values discussed in the previous chapters, and will conclude with an examination of processes and mechanisms that can be used to bring these positions to bear upon dilemmas in practice.

Principles, Values, and Position Statements—Autonomy, Advocacy, and Accountability

Respect for Persons

Respect for persons, as a principle that is broader than respect for autonomy, is clearly emphasized in the Code for Nurses. (See Appendix B.) The preamble of the Code states:

> When making clinical judgements, nurses base their decisions on consideration of consequences and of universal moral principles, both of which prescribe and justify nursing actions. The most fundamental of these principles is *respect for persons* [italics added].[7]

The Code mentions, elsewhere and repeatedly, the efforts and responsibilities of nurses to respect the worth and dignity of every patient. Likewise, though not specifically addressing the larger principle of respect for persons, the AACN position statements *Conceptual Model of Critical Care Nursing* (Appendix C), *Scope of Critical Care Nursing Practice* (Appendix D), and *Principles of Critical Care Nursing Practice* (Appendix E) all declare the responsibility of the nurse to respect the individuality, wholeness, uniqueness, integrity, dignity, and rights of all persons; these are part and parcel of what it means to respect persons.

But, respect for persons is a bit abstract and must be operationalized to make it more useful in the clinical setting. This is usually done through the doctrine of informed consent, which is intended to assure patients the right to exercise a measure of autonomy or self-determination.

Informed Consent

It is unfortunate that most of the nursing ethical literature links informed consent and self-determination to issues of nursing research. Informed consent in health care, the right of a patient to determine what will be done with her or his body, must be seen more broadly as a right to determine to accept, continue, reject, or partially reject nursing (or medical) intervention of any sort. The Code affirms this position when it states in provision one (section 1.1, "Respect for Human Dignity"):

> Clients have the moral right to determine what will be done with their own person; to be given accurate information, and all the information necessary for making informed judgements; to be assisted with weighing the benefits and burdens of options in their treatment; to accept, refuse, or terminate treatment without coercion.[8]

Thus, the informed consent process must not be limited to situations of nursing research, but must also be used in situations involving "ordinary" nursing intervention. This passage from the Code incorporates both the informedness and consent (as voluntariness) aspects of informed consent, heavily emphasizing the notion of self-determination in health care. The Code also mentions informed consent in the provision on nursing research (provision 7, section 7.2, "Protection of Rights of Human Participants in Research"), stating:

> Individual rights valued by society and by the nursing profession that have particular application in research include the right of adequately informed consent. . . . Inherent in these rights is respect for each individual's rights to exercise self-determination, to choose to participate or not, to have full information, and to terminate participation in research without penalty.[9]

The Code does not make any further specification of the particularities of informed consent. That information is found in two excellent and important documents, ANA's *Human Rights Guidelines for Nurses in Clinical and Other Research*, and AACN's Statement on *Ethics in Critical Care Research* (see Appendix F).

The *Human Rights Guidelines* declare "the need for human protection as a priority in ethical considerations in nursing": considerations of human rights are considered to be an ethical duty for nurses.[10] To exercise this moral duty, the *Guidelines* specify information that must be offered for the patient to be fully informed. This includes an explanation of the study, its procedures and purposes; a description of any attendant risks, discomfort, threats to privacy or dignity; and an explanation of the means by which anonymity and confidentiality will be safeguarded. In terms of voluntariness, the *Guidelines* simply assert that "the subject must give consent voluntarily and without being subject to overt or covert coercion or deception."[11] These guidelines are principally concerned with external influences on voluntariness, actions such as coercion, duress, undue influence, deception, or fraud. There is no extended discussion of those conditions that are permanent or temporary influences on voluntariness, conditions such as electrolyte imbalance, hypoxia and hypercapnia, psychological disequilibrium, or disease states. It is a generic document that covers the canvas with broad strokes, though with more detail than the Code, but does not deal extensively with specialty populations (such as the critical care or pediatric patient), particular situations (such as emergencies), or varieties of consent (such as waiver of informedness with valid consent). It does, however, provide both a backdrop for the necessity of informed consent in nursing research, and a discussion of one institutional mechanism (the institutional review board [IRB]) for ensuring that subject rights are protected in research. It is a more professionally than practice-focused document.

The AACN statement on ethics in nursing research has a different emphasis; it is a practice-oriented document that, when coupled with the ANA guidelines, provides both the broad strokes and the finer detail, a more complete picture, of informed consent. AACN's statement ratifies the contents of the ANA document, yet operationalizes it at the practice level, specifically for a critical care population of subjects, including *status populations* such as adolescents, children, mentally incompetent patients, and unconscious patients.[12] Status populations include those whose status precludes the legal capacity to consent (minors), those who cannot be fully informed (the very young, the cognitively impaired), those who cannot exercise self-determination (the comatose patient), and those whose situation is inherently coercive (students, some patients, those with severe pain or suffering, those who are affectively disturbed). Special precautions must be taken with status group members to assure that their rights are protected.

AACN's statement grounds the conduct of research involving human subjects in the ethical principles of autonomy, beneficence, and justice. Thus, it more explicitly though briefly discusses ethical principles and at points articulates what is implicit in the ANA guidelines.[13] Both the ANA and AACN papers provide excellent references for further investigation of the moral bases and requirements of informed consent, as a mechanism for assuring patient self-determination in nursing research. Together they serve as a powerful base for nursing implementation of the informed consent process in both patient care and nursing research.

Advocacy

Given its importance, and its current dominance as a model for nursing, the advocacy aspects of the nursing role receive rather modest, though forceful, attention in nursing's ethical documents. The Code openly declares the nurse to be an advocate for the client (section 3.1):

> The nurse's primary commitment is to the health, welfare, and safety of the client. As an *advocate for the client*, the nurse must be alert to and take appropriate action regarding any instances of incompetent, unethical, or illegal practice [italics added].[14]

This is a bold, profound, and ethically warranted assertion—and in need of further ethical research and exploration, after the fashion of Fry and others, to bring the concept to its moral and theoretical maturity.

Advocacy is, of course, related to nonmaleficence and beneficence, the protective (sometimes called "whistle-blowing") functions of the nurse. It is linked to what the ANA *Social Policy Statement* terms the "distinguishing characteristics of nursing . . . practices that are nurturant, generative, or protective in nature."[15] Advocacy is, in part, an exercise of *nurse autonomy*. Autonomy, or respect for autonomy, is not limited to patient autonomy; it is a universal principle and applies to the nurse as well.

The AACN position statements do not directly discuss the moral autonomy or the advocacy role of the nurse. The position statement *Collaborative Practice Model: The Organization of Human Resources in Critical Care Units* states that "nurses are autonomous when dealing with issues that affect nursing practice."[16] The intent of the statement is really to ensure that nurses can autonomously practice nursing, rather than an assertion of the duty of the nurse to exercise moral autonomy through advocacy.

Despite the lack of explicit development as a concept, however, both the ANA and AACN implicitly express a notion of nursing advocacy for patients through consistent expression of concern for the rights and values of the patient and the demand to respect the inherent worth and dignity of the patient. Thus, all three models of advocacy are emphatically affirmed, though not sorted out, in the statements of both groups. Both groups do go farther by demanding accountability and responsibility of the nurse, for without accountability and responsibility, advocacy is of no effect.

Accountability and Responsibility

Provision 4 of the Code for Nurses is devoted entirely to nurse accountability and responsibility. It reads, "The nurse assumes responsibility and accountability for individual nursing judgements and actions."[17] Accountability, as Fry notes, is understood as answerability and remains without substantive content in the nursing literature. It is yet another moral concept that requires additional ethical research to explore its place in nursing and the variety of models that might support its demands. Responsibility is always tied to accountability, but is not always given a definition that distinguishes it from accountability. Accountability can be narrowly defined and limited to "accounting for" one's actions (or inaction), that is, justification of one's behavior. Responsibility would then entail the assignment of moral blameworthiness or praiseworthiness. (It should be noted that a nurse could be morally blameworthy without being legally blameworthy. In his book *Punishment and Responsibility*, legal theorist H.L.A. Hart discusses varieties of responsibility and categorizes them as causal, role, liability, and capacity responsibility.)[18] Accountability or answerability, however, can be more broadly defined to incorporate the ideal of responsibility, collapsing responsibility into accountability as one aspect of it.

Virtually all of the AACN position statements mention accountability, dividing it along role-related lines. Nursing administrators are responsible and accountable for the development of practice-related guidelines, and for the effective functioning and evaluation of care of the unit (position statements on *Clarification of Resuscitation Status in Critical Care Setting* [Appendix G]; *Collaborative Practice Model: The Organization of Human Resources in Critical Care Units* [Appendix H]). AACN is responsible and accountable for "promoting professionalism and accountability of nurses caring for the critically ill" (Position statement on *AACN's Purpose, Long Range Goals, and Intermediate Strategies* [Appendix I]). The responsibility and accountability of the individual nurse extend to professional judgments, respect for persons, maintaining clinical competence, promotion and restoration of health, and alleviation of suffering (Appendices C, D, E). Both the ANA and AACN have heavily incorporated the concepts of accountability and responsibility in their documents as recognized duties, and consequently as standards for professional behavior. To be answerable, then, requires that the nurse "provide moral justification, in terms of standards or norms recognized by the profession" in the Code generally, and in position statements specifically (see Chapter 3).

Answerability and responsibility, as duties, emanate from the relationship of *trust* between the nurse and the patient (alluded to in the AACN position statements, Appendices C, D). What remains to be developed in the general nursing and critical care nursing ethical literature is a fuller exploration, at both the theoretical and concrete levels, of the *ethical nature* of the nurse-patient relationship. Only after this is done can we hope to more definitively develop the concept of answerability in nursing.

Nonmaleficence and Beneficence

While it is possible to divide a discussion of nonmaleficence and beneficence, for the convenience of exploring the principles individually, it is virtually impossible to do so when addressing their implementation in clinical practice. It is rare to find pure statements of nonmaleficence in the nursing ethical literature, except perhaps in the Nightingale Pledge, which states that the nurse "will not take or knowingly administer any harmful drug."[19] Virtually all other statements join nonmaleficence with beneficence. For the sake of simplicity, we will refer to these as statements of beneficence.

Beneficence is customarily couched in terms of "safeguarding the health and safety of the client," "protection of the public from misinformation and misrepresentation," and "promoting communal and national efforts to meet the needs of the public."[20] In a sense, it can be argued that every effort of the profession or the individual to establish or maintain standards of practice are efforts to "do good" for those who would require nursing services. To do so would be broadly to place all nursing activity, even collective bargaining (which is linked to retention of well-prepared nurses and quality of care), under the rubric of the principle of beneficence. While it is true that principles and their demands do overlap, conceiving of beneficence quite that broadly muddies the ethical waters. Beneficence is more appropriately limited to the fairly direct infliction of good or evil, leaving debates for or against activities affecting the economic and general welfare of the nurse to be argued on other moral grounds.

In contemporary nursing, beneficence has become so linked with respect for autonomy that, in some instances, beneficence *means* respect for autonomy. Anything a nurse does that negatively influences patient autonomy is then seen as the infliction of harm and morally impermissible. Discussions that so strongly align beneficence with respect for autonomy will inevitably focus on patient informedness and self-determination, respect for rights of the patient and family, and the implementation of the duties and observation of the values generally discussed under autonomy, advocacy, and accountability.

Though it is true that failure to show respect for persons does do them harm, there are problems with the collapse of beneficence into respect for autonomy. First, there are more ways to harm a patient than simply to fail to respect his or her autonomy. For instance, to deny access unjustly to critical care resources constitutes the infliction of harm (not to mention injustice) without violating the patient's autonomy. Second, discussions of respect for autonomy apply *by definition* to those patients who have the capacity to exercise their autonomy. In instances in which the patient cannot speak or decide on his or her own behalf, the question of autonomy does not arise. Doing good for these patients, or not inflicting harm on them, raises the issue of beneficence without a concurrent discussion of autonomy.

Considerations of the noninfliction of harm and doing good consequently fall out, not entirely neatly, into categories of beneficence and the autonomous patient, and beneficence and the nonautonomous patient. Further discussion projects the principle of beneficence to the macrolevel and examines nursing's duties to or within society.

Beneficence and the Autonomous Patient

In nursing it is very clear, today, that in planning and implementing a plan of care the patient's wishes should prevail. The limit to that autonomy is, of course, the proviso that others will not be harmed. As noted previously, the Code acknowledges a patient's right to accept, reject, or terminate treatment, or to refuse to participate or withdraw from participation in research. The human rights guidelines for nursing research for both the ANA and AACN strongly affirm this position.

Added support for nursing's position comes from the President's Commission document *Deciding to Forego Life-Sustaining Treatment*. The Commission maintains:

> Nothing in current law precludes ethically sound decision making. Neither criminal law nor civil law—if properly applied . . . forces patients to undergo procedures that will increase their suffering when they wish to avoid this by foregoing life-sustaining treatment.[21]

To force a patient to undergo treatment against his or her wishes, when no significant harm will accrue to others, constitutes both a violation of autonomy and the infliction of harm. In cases such as these, the autonomous *patient* determines what constitutes unwarranted suffering.

Clinically, it often seems more difficult, and less morally defensible, to withdraw treatment once begun. However, if the treatment does not benefit the patient, there is no logical or moral reason that compels us to continue it. The President's Commission notes this by saying:

> The distinction between failing to initiate and stopping therapy—that is, withholding and withdrawing treatment—is not itself of moral importance. A justification that is adequate for not commencing a treatment is also sufficient for ceasing it.[22]

Nursing generally has less difficulty with participation in the withdrawal of high-tech machinery than it does with the withdrawal of food and fluid. In recent years medicine has come to regard food and fluid, particularly when administered through "artificial means" as a treatment. This position has been supported, in many quarters, by ethical analyses that declare such feedings/fluid to be either extraordinary (non-obligatory) treatment or a burden to the patient. It is a stronger position to rest the argument on the obligatoriness or nonobligatoriness of continued feeding and fluid than to argue its artificiality, extraordinariness, or even burdensomeness. (Arguing from the point of obligatoriness requires an analysis of the situation and an ethical justification; burdensomeness, extraordinariness, and artificiality are conclusory concepts, not analytical tools.) Despite ethical and medical argumentation to the contrary, nurses often resist designating food or fluid as treatment and are hesitant to withdraw it.

For nurses, food and fluid are often regarded as comfort measures, though this has not yet been physiologically established through nursing research. Alternatively, nursing has regarded food and fluid as what is humanly due another (as rooted in the nurse-patient relationship), or as a comfort measure even when physically detrimental to comfort (and consequently as an aspect of the quality of life). For instance, infants whose gastrointestinal problems cannot be surgically repaired, and whose medical condition would generally result in an NPO order, nonetheless seem comforted by sucking small amounts of fluid. Or, consider the patient dying of renal failure who has been ordered NPO who receives comfort from eating food that will ultimately harm him.

In some instances there is ample moral justification for withholding or withdrawing food or fluid, even in the presence of serious emotional or psychological reluctance to do so. In other cases there is not. Nursing needs to explore the issue of food and fluid, especially the role-related differences in medical and nursing moral perspectives on its use or withdrawal.

Some clarification of the nurse's role in the withdrawal of life-sustaining treatment and the withdrawal of food and fluid is forthcoming. The ANA Committee on Ethics is in the initial phases of formulating position statements covering these two issues. While the two issues are really one, the committee felt that the withdrawal of food and fluid was of such particular concern and significance to nurses in practice that it deserves separate consideration.

The President's Commission's recommendations for decisions deciding to forego life-sustaining treatment highlight a concern for patient self-determination, the non-infliction of harm, and the necessity for adequate procedures and policies to support ethically right-making decisions. They are to:[23]

1. Respect patient choices even to forego life-sustaining treatment
2. Provide mechanisms and guidelines for decision making for patients who cannot decide
3. Presume in favor of sustaining life if in doubt
4. Provide respectful, responsive, supportive care when no further medical care is available or chosen
5. Encourage institutions to establish procedures for decision making, available to all patients

In terms of beneficence, the autonomous patient is well protected in the documents of the health professions, and by the recommendations of the President's Commission.

Beneficence and the Nonautonomous Patient

The nonautonomous patient is in a theoretically slightly more precarious position in the ethical literature, particularly with regard to nontherapeutic nursing research. The word *theoretically* is important here. Clinically the AACN and ANA guidelines provide a comprehensive, conservative, stringent, and well-articulated guideline for protection of human subjects in nursing research. However, beneficence and the *nonautonomous patient* is not given a great deal of attention in either the Code or the ANA or AACN guidelines. It can certainly be inferred, and must be, that respect for human dignity, wholeness, rights, and uniqueness extends to the nonautonomous patient. But the means for actually living out that respect is not well articulated.

The Code states that a "surrogate decision maker should be designated" for the patient who lacks the capacity to make decisions (but does not comment on who the surrogate is).[24] Both the Code and the AACN position statements, as well as the ANA *Social Policy Statement*, accord the family a role, if not responsibility, in health care planning and decision making. It can often be assumed and demonstrated that the family is in the best position to represent the values and rights of a nonautonomous patient, though this is not always the case. Nursing needs to give additional theoretical and practical consideration to articulating more clearly, in its ethical literature and position statements, (1) who the patient is—family and patient or patient alone, (2) who represents the nonautonomous person who is ill in matters of nursing concern, and (3) who represents the nonautonomous person in matters of nursing practice when there is no family, no fictive family, or when those closest to the patient appear to be making injudicious or inappropriate decisions for the patient (including but not limited to decisions regarding treatments that sustain life or enhance comfort).

Beneficence, Nontherapeutic Nursing Research, and the Nonautonomous Patient

Perhaps the place where nursing most urgently needs to turn its ethical attention regarding beneficence is to clarifying the issue of nontherapeutic research on the nonautonomous patient, particularly the comatose or nonresponsive patient. The Code states that the nurse must assure informed consent in nursing research and that patients may permissibly decline to participate in nursing research.[25] Both the AACN and ANA documents on nursing research give great weight to informed consent. The AACN paper states that the organization supports "conduct of research in a manner which assures that patients give informed consent for participation," while the ANA paper states that "the subject needs to be assured that his rights will not be violated without his voluntary and informed consent."[26,27] Thus, the autonomous patient has the right to decline to participate in nursing research, whether it is or is not of therapeutic benefit, and for reasons sufficient unto the patient alone.

Both the ANA and AACN documents are absolutely clear that an extra measure of protection is due to status individuals who become research subjects. The ANA guidelines state:

> Nurses must be increasingly vigilant in their concern for subjects and patients who by reason of their situation or illness are not able to protect themselves effectively from an externally imposed threat or injury. [This does not necessarily mean that they are nonautonomous.] They must also be sensitive to the possibility of exploitation of captive populations such as students, the poor, patients in institutions, or prisoners. . . . The choice of minors or groups with limited civil freedom as research subjects can be justified in most instances only if benefits will accrue in the future to them or to others in similar situations or classes. Strict standards governing the use of minors and other groups (including the unborn and the dead) lacking capacity to give informed consent are being established with increasing frequency by various governmental statutes and regulations.[28]

Both the AACN and ANA documents indicate that second-party consent can be accepted in lieu of patient consent: "If critically ill patients cannot consent to enter a research study, family members or significant others may be asked to give second party consent"; "to safeguard the basic human right of self-determination, consent to participate in research or unusual clinical activities must be obtained from the prospective subject or his legal representative."[29,30] So, all told, we have surrogate, family, significant others, or legal representatives giving consent for a nonautonomous patient.

The moral bind of nontherapeutic research is this:

Nursing demands informed consent from autonomous patients; nursing demands protection of human subjects in its research; nursing demands extra protection for status (including nonautonomous) individuals who participate in nursing research; nursing declares itself to be a patient advocacy profession, seeking the ends of the patient; nursing is based on a relationship of trust with the individual patient or patient family; nursing can justify research on the nonautonomous patient when benefit accrues to that patient and second-party consent has been secured; but, how can nursing justify nontherapeutic research on vulnerable populations, including the critically ill, for the collective good, in situations in which the autonomous patient would have the right to refuse to participate in nursing research?

Does the comatose, nonresponsive, or critically ill patient have fewer rights than the autonomous patient? Does he or she have an obligation to participate in nontherapeutic nursing research that will benefit that class of individuals? Does nursing have an obligation to refrain from doing research with these kinds of patients? Is the nonautonomous, nontherapeutic research subject simply a means to the nurse-researcher's own ends? Can it be held that benefit to others, without benefit to one's self, is sufficient moral justification for the inclusion of nonconsenting patients in nontherapeutic research? Is there any class of nursing research that nursing, because it is nursing, ought not to do?

The answers to these and collateral questions are not clear and must soon be attended to. What is clear is that nursing must continue to research its interventions in order to benefit current and future patients through expansion of a sound knowledge base. It is also clear that beneficence in nursing demands protection of patient rights and values, protection from undue risk of harm, protection from frivolous or ill-constructed research projects, and an additional measure of protection for vulnerable individuals. And, it is clear that nursing has formally established research standards that recognize its tradition and duties in a remarkably rigorous articulation of concern for human subjects as expressed in documents such as those promulgated by the ANA and AACN.

Fidelity and Veracity in Nursing

Early in this century, Wilber Wright, in a discussion of efforts at human flight, wrote in *Century Magazine*: "With the machine's moving forward, the air flying backward, the propellers turning sideways and nothing standing still, it seemed impossible to find a starting point from which to trace various simultaneous reactions."[31]

With the motion and commotion in nursing, ethics, medicine, technology, and health care financing, fidelity seems to have become difficult to trace among the "simultaneous reactions": fidelity is the lost imperative of nursing.

Fidelity can be discussed as a duty, as a moral value (virtue), or as a nonmoral value (a good or end). Early nursing ethics leaned heavily on an ethics of virtue, heavily linked to other virtues such as devotion, obedience, and faithfulness. The nurse was, by moral character, to be unquestionably (and unquestioningly) devoted. From earliest nursing in the United States, through the 1950s, the nurse "devoted [herself] to the welfare of those committed to [her] care."[32]

From about the 1960s forward, nursing ethics began to shift away from a virtue-based ethics to an ethics of obligation that shunned questions of virtue and regarded them as "private morality."[33] This shift was influenced by a number of social forces including the movement of nursing education into colleges and universities, the advance of medical science and technology, a prior cultural movement away from virtue-based concerns, and the increasing freedom accorded women in society.[34] In nursing the notion of fidelity was obscured in the shift. As a moral value fidelity does have a correlative duty to act fidelitously.

Discussions of fidelity subsequent to the shift have pretty much cast it simply as a duty to keep promises. It has taken a flavor of fidelity to promises, rather than fidelity to the patient. Though promise keeping is a major aspect of fidelity, it is not the whole of the principle. Fidelity truly includes the moral values of devotion, loyalty, faithfulness, dedication, and commitment—to the patient—as well as honesty, veracity, and integrity. As a principle fidelity most often appears in the ANA and AACN papers as promise keeping and truth telling, or implicitly in discussions of trust or of the nurse-patient relationship. The Code actually identifies fidelity as promise keeping and sees veracity as truth telling and as a separate principle.[35] Both are seen to derive from the basic principle of respect for persons.

Fidelity, like autonomy, is linked to the concept of advocacy. It speaks to the proper object of commitment of the nurse: "The nurse's primary commitment is to the health, welfare, and safety of the client. As an advocate for the client."[36] Statements of this principle generally do not use the language of fidelity; rather, they tend to be less direct:

> Nursing practice has been health-oriented for more than half a century, partly because of its focus on individuals as persons, and on the family as the necessary unit of service. . . . Health becomes the center of nursing attention, not as an end in itself, but as a means to life that is meaningful and manageable.[37]

It is implied that, in the end, it is the patient himself or herself who is the object of commitment of the nurse, and that commitment to patient health and welfare is only to recognize them as instrumental goods by which nursing commitment to the patient can help the patient achieve the end of meaningful and manageable life.

Veracity, as a moral duty, appears most often in relation to informed consent and the exercise of self-determination. The Code declares that "truth-telling and the process of reaching informed choice underlie the exercise of self-determination, which is basic to respect for persons."[38] The AACN Ethics in Critical Care Research (Appendix F) states, "Informed consent is knowing consent of a competent individual who is able to exercise free power of choice without undue inducement or any element of force, fraud, deceit, or any other form of coercion."[39]

Indeed, deceit, whether directly by lying or indirectly by omitting the truth, and all the shades of disclosure in between, is coercive. Violation of the principle of veracity is not limited to lying: it includes any attempt deliberately to deceive.

Some research, however, because of the nature of the study itself, requires that all the details of the study *not* be disclosed to the participant. The AACN guidelines on partial disclosure discuss when its use may be justified. Partial disclosure should be used when full disclosure and valid or reliable results are absolutely incompatible. It should never be used to secure participation from a subject who would have refused to participate if the facts of the study were known. When partial disclosure is used, the patient should be informed that the study is "blind" or that unspecified variables will be measured and should be offered the choice of participation under those conditions. The decision to propose a research project that utilizes partial disclosure should not be undertaken lightly or unilaterally. Researchers have the responsibility to make decisions in the light of day and to have them ratified by other professionals through mechanisms such as the IRB. The decision to withhold information from a subject is a grave one and should stand up to the moral scrutiny of one's peers, in true accountability.

While fidelity is a lost emphasis in nursing, veracity, which receives relatively little discussion in the nursing literature, is not. Veracity is so intrinsic to the nurse-patient relationship that it is a general presumption in a way that fidelity is not. Nursing, as a profession, has a long and honorable tradition of devotion to the patient, which encompasses truth telling, and many characteristics that are essential to a truly caring relationship—fidelity and veracity being among them.

Justice in Nursing

For many years now, nursing has been swimming upstream in its declaration that nursing, and health care generally, should be distributed on the basis of need. Nursing has not taken account of two factors: (1) need outstrips resources and (2) the current health care delivery system has a one-wheel drive.

Declarations that nursing services at the macroallocation level should be distributed on the basis of need are consistent with nursing's special concern for the vulnerable person—who has traditionally been called "the lame, the halt, and the blind," "the widow, the orphan, and the stranger in your land." It seems that nursing's approach to distributive justice has been, strongly, to define it in compensatory terms, superimposed on a concern for equal access to health care for all.

Provision 11 of the Code addresses the issue of the macroallocation of nursing/health care and directs the nurse toward collaboration with others at a local, state, national, and international level. It is an implicit recognition that distribution at the macrolevel is a political issue that requires nursing input.

Need, however, is greater than resources. When all needs cannot be met, nursing ethics enjoins the nurse to promote or foster *equal access,* or fairness in access, to nursing and health resources. Access to health care resources is and will continue to be the single most demanding ethical issue of our day. It is an area in which nursing needs to conduct research, to explore, and to become politically involved: this is the arena for nursing advocacy at the societal level.

Health care is medically driven. If a patient needs nursing but does not need medicine, nursing is difficult to obtain. There is, of course, no legal prohibition against the direct delivery of nursing services. The prohibition is more subtle: nurses generally cannot be reimbursed for nursing services not authorized by a physician. We are not "free" to deliver our services on the basis of need. Perhaps when society realizes that it is less costly to deliver needed nursing services without unneeded medical services, we will see the rise of independent nursing institutions that accept nursing or medical referral—and reimburse the nurse for services rendered.

The critical care nurse is in a particularly difficult position with regard to the macroallocation of nursing services. Critical care nursing, which differs from intensive nursing, is intrinsically tied to medicine when defined as "nursing which deals specifically with human responses to life-threatening problems." Life-threatening health situations invariably require medical aid as well as nursing care. Thus, critical care nurses cannot offer their services except in a context that also offers medical care. Consequently, to bring about a more just distribution of nursing, critical care nurses must work to assure a just societal distribution of critical care in general.

Though there are those who excel in the political arena, and who can work toward that goal, all the work should not be left to those few, or to the organization behind them. At the very least, the critical care nurse owes "the unknown patient" the support of the collective voice of nursing's professional organizations and associated political action. This is, in part, the emphasis of AACN's position statement *Process for Addressing Practice, Political, and Professional Issues* (see Appendix J). It is also a concern of ANA's *Social Policy Statement,* a critically important document. Nursing services must also be allocated at the microlevel. Nursing is very clear that the only just ground for discrimination between patients, in terms of the allocation of services, is *need.* In the light of the Code, it is morally impermissible for nurses to allow the patient's personal attributes, socioeconomic status, or the nature of the patient's health problems to be used as grounds for allocation. The interpretive statements of the 1985 revision of the Code go even farther, stating, "The need for health care is universal, transcending all national, ethnic, racial, religious, cultural, political, educational, economic, developmental, personality, role, and sexual differences. Nursing care is delivered without prejudicial behavior."[40] Patient attributes serve only as factors that influence the individualization of nursing care for the welfare, self-respect, and dignity of the patient.

As at the macroallocation level, when injustice exists, the nurse has a responsibility to act, whether directly or indirectly through the support of others. Within an institution, the critical care nurse is responsible to support procedures and policies that assure a just utilization and access of critical care nursing services. And, as at the macrolevel, collective action is often more forceful a voice than that of an individual nurse.

But, the allocation of patient care services is not the only concern of justice. It is clear from the AACN position statements that there must also be a concern for the just allocation of nursing education. Both the position statement *Entry into Professional Nursing Practice* and *Resolution Supporting the Continuation of BSN Programs* address this issue. Many nurses who graduated before or around the time of the 1965 ANA position paper on entry into practice (declaring the BSN as entry level into professional practice) could have been left in a less than just position, had not articulation programs and grandfathering been espoused. This was the case because few BSN articulation programs were available, and those nurses, mostly diploma-prepared nurses, were left to repeat virtually their entire basic nursing education to obtain a degree. Should nursing eventually decide that the MSN is the appropriate entry level into professional practice (and some hold that position—and beyond), a somewhat similar problem would obtain for those who possess a BSN only.

Nursing, in justice, needs to assure that a sufficient number and distribution of articulation programs are available to those who wish to continue their professional education. At the same time, the profession needs to continue to work toward achieving a BSN-prepared professional work force as a minimum entry level to assure high quality nursing care to all in need of nursing.

Issues in justice, in the distribution of burdens and benefits in society, are far reaching. They include the allocation of nursing resources to the patient, the allocation of nursing resources to nurses, and the allocation of social goods (such as wages and salaries) to the nurse. It is under the principle of justice that nurses argue for just compensation for nursing services provided. This presents a rather stronger moral argument than the argument that nurses should be justly paid so that well-prepared nurses can be recruited and retained, that patient care may continue to be "high quality." (This is an argument distally related to beneficence.) While that may be true, and a point worth arguing, it is also worth arguing that the nurse is justly due social benefits, including social esteem, apart from any benefit that may accrue to patients. The 1976 Code grounds its argument for the economic and general welfare of the nurse in the welfare of the patient. Traditionally, nursing has been loathe to argue for its own welfare as a good in itself, rather than as an instrumental good. Provision 9 of the Code states that "the nurse participates in the profession's efforts to establish and maintain conditions of employment conducive to high-quality nursing care." The interpretive statements of the Code of 1976 (the provisions themselves did not change in the 1985 revision) linked the provision directly to the economic and general welfare of the nurse. A justice argument works better here than does a beneficence argument.

The revised interpretive statements, rightly, broaden the intent of the provision to include control of practice, professional autonomy, and standards of practice. While nurses stand to gain, personally, from such conditions, they are principally patient focused. That is, when arguing for work conditions as economic and general welfare, we nurses are really concerned about justice as it relates to the nurse. When, on the other hand, nurses argue for work conditions vis-à-vis quality patient care, they are principally concerned for beneficence.

Nursing has always hesitated, even today, to appear "self-serving," by demanding a more equitable pay scale. There is, however, a point at which a claim to justice, though self-serving, is legitimately so. Nurses have not always remembered that they themselves are worthy of the same regard that they demand be accorded the patient.

Duties to Self

Integrity

The Code does acknowledge, directly and indirectly, that the nurse has duties to self. Section 1.3 of the interpretive statements falls under the ethical category of integrity and pertains to refusal to participate in interventions to which the nurse has moral objections.

> If ethically opposed to interventions in a particular case because of the procedures to be used, the nurse is [morally] justified in refusing to participate. Such refusal should be made known in advance and in time for other appropriate arrangements to be made for the client's nursing care. If the nurse becomes involved in such a case and the client's life is in jeopardy, the nurse is obliged to provide for the client's safety, to avoid abandonment, and to withdraw only when assured alternative sources of nursing care are available.[41]

The nurse does have a duty to self to refuse to participate in interventions that would violate that nurse's moral integrity. The grounds for refusal are *moral* ones, and are not matters of personal preference, prejudice, convenience, or arbitrariness. As a part of duty to self, however, the nurse must understand that refusal on moral grounds does not necessarily have any legal standing; neither does it always protect the nurse from termination of employment. In some cases of conscientious objection, there may be a penalty for ethically right-making behavior, if the issue is pursued and pressed. Such decisions should be made with full informedness and free consent on the part of the nurse. The fact that moral objections to participation in a procedure have, sometimes, led to termination points up the fact that institutional mechanisms for voicing moral concerns (without fear of reprisal) have not always been available. Close working relationships, a unified nursing staff, and a community of moral discourse at the unit level can go a long way to avert "disasters" for individual nurses, even in the absence of institutional processes. One would hope that the tenor of the unit would be such that nurses (and physicians) could swap patients among themselves for the moral well-being of their peers.

If the client's life is in jeopardy, life takes priority over moral scruples until such time as assignments can be changed. For the sake of all concerned, moral prohibitions against participation in categories of procedures should be made known in advance, at the time of employment. The employer should have the opportunity to decline to hire a nurse who will not participate in procedures routinely done by the institution. The usual types of interventions for which nurses need to examine their values and ethics customarily include surgical procedures such as abortion, transsexual surgery, experimental surgeries (primate-to-human heart transplant, artificial heart), and radical surgeries (hemicorporectomy), which may be done routinely in some specialty or teaching hospitals. The situations differ from one of objecting to a single intervention with a particular patient, such as a "learner's biopsy" of the liver on a terminally ill glioblastoma patient. Here, the issue is primarily one of patient advocacy rather than the nurse's moral integrity.

The AACN document on ethics in research contains a section (question 14) on the nurse's ethical stance on research.

> Nurses are not morally obligated to cooperate in experimental procedures about which they have ethical concerns. Indeed, they may have an ethical obligation [to themselves as well as to the patient] to refuse to participate in such activities and to bring their concerns to the attention of others who can assist the patient and review the appropriateness of the research activity.[42]

The statement is very savvy with regard to refusal to participate. It goes on to state, wisely, that

> Personal consequences exist for both reporting and not reporting perceived ethical injustices. Individuals perceived as interfering with another's project may be ostracized, harassed, or even fired. However, the personal consequences of not reporting conduct which violates one's ethical principles may be unacceptable to the nurse and to the profession.[43]

Personal consequences, the violation of one's moral integrity, are serious. It is not unreasonable to maintain that more than one nurse has summarily left the profession, not because of working conditions or pay, but because of a political or practical inability to preserve her or his moral integrity in a specific clinical setting. Recognition of uniqueness, *wholeness*, dignity, and rights is not limited to a concern for the patient.

Professional–Personal Moral Integration

Early nursing engaged in close scrutiny of the moral purity and character of the probationer, trainee, and graduate, and it included everything from dress and bowel habits of the nurse to [her] relationships with patients and with all males. Fortunately, nursing has moved away from this. Unfortunately, it overshot its mark. So concerned has nursing been to shun the more repressive aspects of its past that it now regards private moral behavior as a virtually separate domain, unrelated to professional moral behavior. There is a level at which this is appropriate, and nursing has no right to fiddle with a nurse's private life.

However, given the virtues as habits of character, it is rather difficult to conceive of a nurse who could be dastardly privately and saintly professionally. Individuals are not fractionated and compartmentalized like isoenzymes or immunoglobulins. Persons, even those who lead troubled or difficult lives, are at some levels invariably whole, or integrated, or at the very least partially consistent. Moral values are so fundamental an aspect of human character that personal and professional morality, even if undernourished or not fully integrated, are never wholly separate.

The 1968 version of the Code is the first version to omit a clause about the private ethics of the nurse. Concern for the personal morality of the nurse remains a lost note for about a decade, when we again begin to hear the overture to a recognition of the importance of moral integration. The AACN position statement *Principles of Critical Care Nursing Practice* states, "The American Association of Critical-Care Nurses recognizes that its members are often faced with difficult and sensitive situations involving nurse-patient relationships. These Principles of Practice define, promote, and uphold the highest standards of *personal* conduct among members [italics added]."[44] This is a clear recognition that the nurse's personal and professional conduct are, at the moral level, inseparable.

Self-Judgment

Virtually all nursing documents that deal with standards of practice mention the nurse's responsibility to remain competent. This is true of the Code, and of the AACN position papers that specify, to some extent, areas of competence related to differing roles. In these documents, competence is directly linked to an increase in a nurse's knowledge; enhancement of clinical analysis and problem solving; professional preparation; adherence to standards of the profession (including moral standards); and continued learning.

Though the Code (section 5.2) recognizes peer evaluation as a "hallmark of professionalism and a method by which the profession is held accountable to society," it is, first and foremost, a personal professional responsibility.[45] Indeed, the nurse has a personal professional responsibility for self-judgment and is additionally accountable to the profession through peer review.

Values and Critical Care Nursing

Just as personal integrity is a moral value, an end, and an obligation in nursing, so is the integrity of the profession, but it is neither the single nor the highest end of the profession. Nursing affirms a plurality of nonmoral values that include health, healing, scientific care, patient comfort, well-being, welfare, dignity, safety, patient-as-end, high-quality nursing care, effective care, advocacy, and respect.

Nonmoral values are important to nursing because they are the goods and ends—and ultimate ends—that the profession seeks. Nonmoral values are important to the individual nurse because (1) they are the goods and ends the nurse seeks, (2) they influence moral decision making, and (3) they may or may not be congruent or compatible with the values of the profession. Just as the nurse has a responsibility to self-judge clinical competence, there is also a responsibility to self-judge or self-examine one's values and value system. (The exercises at the end of Chapter 9 are designed to assist in doing this.)

Self-examination must not stop there. Values clarification, as clarification, is descriptive and a part of self-discovery. That self-examination must extend to an examination of the normative values of the profession, and an evaluation of the compatibility of one's own and the profession's values.

The nurse or prospective nurse who cannot affirm a respect for persons, irrespective of the personal attributes of the patient, or who cannot support an advocacy role, or who cannot generally place patient autonomy over imposing good on the patient cannot hope to be "a nurse" in the moral sense. While personal values and those of the profession are never identical or co-extensive, they must be compatible. If not, nursing will never "feel right" to the person, will make moral demands that cannot be met, and will produce an intolerable moral dissonance.

Those who would be nurses would profit from an examination of the essential documents of the profession. The *Code for Nurses with Interpretive Statements* and *Nursing: A Social Policy Statement* are a starting point. Both make an open declaration of the values of the profession and are a fruitful source of values information in exploring nursing either as a potential lifework or as a member of its community.

Nursing is caring. It is an affirmation of life and health, of human dignity and worth. It is an inherently moral endeavor that demands a great deal of its members and gives back in terms of an honored and honorable tradition and the relationships that are formed.

Law and Ethics

Relationships in nursing have moral, legal, political, and economic import. Though ethics has been our principal concern, ethics is not wholly untouched by the long arm of the law; they do interact, customarily but not always, with reconcilable differences.

On the whole, ethicists make poor ad hoc lawyers, and lawyers make awful ad hoc ethicists. Unfortunately, this point is only sometimes recognized. In a discussion of the legal side of medical ethics at the far edges of life, a judge encountered an ethicist and the following exchange took place:

B.A.G. (a sometime lawyer): As a lawyer I feel uncomfortable with these ethical problems.
A.R.J. (a philosopher): As a lawyer you should.[46]

Practically, and prudentially, the ethicist or clinician making an ethical judgment needs to be aware of what the law might say concerning practice issues. Nonetheless, there needs to be a recognition that ethical decisions are not legal decisions and vice versa.

The confusion between law and ethics, or perhaps the conflation of law and ethics, often occurs because, as Chaney notes, "lawyers and ethicists use a common language base for discussing rights and duties" (see Chapter 10). Lawyers define rights as "an area of liberty to act without interference." Goldberg has stated, "To a lawyer a right is that which one may do without incurring legally enforceable liability, or that which one may legally require another to do for him or refrain from doing for him. The legal right may or may not be ethical."[47]

Definitionally, this is profoundly different from the ethical understanding of a right. In ethics rights are "a complex web of relationships and duties between individuals defining what they morally should or should not do."[48] A moral right may or may not be legally actionable. To let a baby drown in a puddle of water is not legally actionable (unless perhaps if you yourself put the baby there). Such an action is unquestionably morally reprehensible and morally actionable, insofar as moral suasion has "teeth" in any given setting.

Law and ethics have an intricate relationship that has been explored from many vantage points over the centuries. (The Hart-Devlin debate over the legislation of morality is one example.) It is not within the scope of this book to explore that relationship in any depth. It is important, however, to acknowledge that while law influences ethical decision making, ethics *can* influence legal decision making. In the Saikewicz decision, it is noted, "Medical ethics which influence a doctor's decision as to how to deal with the terminally ill patient are not . . . controlling, [but] they ought to be considered for the insights they give us."[49]

Even where the law does not interact with ethics at the bedside, at the microlevel, it does profoundly influence ethics at the macrolevel. It is through the law that reimbursement policies are controlled, that "rationing" takes place, that access to health care is ultimately facilitated or impeded. The Code recognizes the importance of law and the political nature of living out the profession's ethics. Provision 11 speaks to the nurse's responsibility to work for the welfare and safety of all people—as incorporated in the goals and commitments of nursing—"by active participation in decision making and institutional and political arenas."[50] These arenas are reached through the appropriate use of institutional and political mechanisms.

Processes and Mechanisms for Moral Action in Critical Care Nursing

Just as nursing ethics requires policies and position statements to articulate its concerns in professional practice, policies and position statements require mechanisms and processes for their implementation in practice. These include the institutional ethics committees, as well as ethics education of professionals and the laity.

Institutional Ethics Committees (IECs)

IECs, mentioned in virtually every chapter of this book, are interdisciplinary groups that, though still in the stage of clinical trials, have received widespread support. As a concept, they have been endorsed by the American Medical Association, the

American Nurses' Association, and the President's Commission. The ANA has published a document entitled "Guidelines for Nurse's Participation and Leadership in Institutional Ethical Review Processes" (1985).

In brief, with the recognition that clinical decisions often contain a moral component that cannot be collapsed into a question of medical or nursing fact, ethics committees have been established to help clarify and illuminate moral dilemmas in clinical practice. They are an advisory—and not a decision-making—body, designed to assist with moral decisions as necessary in patient practice.

To that end, they engage in several functions, including education, preparation of general guidelines for handling categories of moral dilemmas, family or staff counseling in decision making, conduct of ethics research, clarification of the moral dimensions of a case, and arbitration of moral disagreement (with attendant pitfalls as noted by Chaney in Chapter 10). The most used functions tend to be those of education, consultation, and guideline preparation.

Not all ethics committees have the resources (or need) to carry out all of the possible functions of an IEC. Some rightly limit the scope of their activity. Institutions that do not have the necessary resources can form an inter-institutional ethics committee to share the burdens and resources that the activities of the committee create. Ethics committees can function both well and appropriately by establishing consistent institutional ethics policies through guidelines, by being "immediately" responsive to the need of the clinician or the patient, by helping to resolve nonlegal ethical questions, by referring legal nonethical questions, and by raising the level of staff (and self) ethics consciousness and knowledge.[51]

While it is true that the courts do not decide questions of ethics, it is also true that some ethics questions end up in the court. This is not a failure of either law or ethics: it simply points up the fact that there has not always been an adequate forum for the exploration of the moral dilemmas that are encountered in daily practice. The IEC gives us such a forum for the serious exploration of ethical questions and the resources, or access to the resources, that shed light on those questions.

Institutional Review Boards (IRBs)

IRBs were originally designed to say aye or nay to research projects that proposed to use human or animal subjects within any institution that received federal dollars. Because this includes hospitals (through Medicare), most hospitals have had to form an IRB, though the process for review (or exemption from review) varies somewhat from institution to institution. (Some places exclude research on the institution's nurses or other personnel from the review process.)

IRBs are designed to protect the rights and welfare of human subjects by peer review of research proposals, before the start of data collection. Because they deal with questions of rights, they do encounter questions of ethics in the review process. They are not an ethics committee, and as they may not have a committee member conversant with ethics, IRBs deal with ethical questions in research with varying levels of sophistication. With the growth in numbers of IECs, IRBs now have an excellent consultative-advisory resource for addressing ethical questions in research. In addition, ethics guidelines for research are now available as organizational publications and as sections (however brief) in a few textbooks on the research process. The IRB, because it is peer-review based, is a group to which researchers are accountable and which is itself accountable for the human rights conduct of research within an institution.

Nursing Ethics Councils

The newspapers are rife with articles that, often sensationalistically, bring ethical dilemmas in health care to the public attention. Some cases (Baby Fae, artificial hearts, conjoined twins, Bouvia, Herbert, Brophy) receive ongoing, blow-by-blow attention from the media and so keep these dilemmas in our awareness. And certainly, these cases and less dramatic ones are the stuff of ethics committee deliberations.

However, some categories of dilemmas do not tend to be addressed by IECs, ones that nurses confront in their daily practice. While committees grapple with the ins-and-outs of a case, it is the nurse at the bedside, giving care, who by law must institute CPR on the patient if she should "code," in situations in which the nurse perceives CPR to be morally wrong-making. And what about when acuity levels of the patient load are ignored to squeeze in another admission—or the charge nurse who must help decide on the allocation of beds *and* the accompanying nursing resources? There are many dilemmas in nursing practice that simply do not make it to the IEC agenda.

The creation of a nursing ethics council is one way to address these sorts of nursing issues. Nursing ethics councils *do not* function as a parallel IEC. Rather, they are a group of nurses, interested in ethics, who convene to examine and explore *nursing-specific* issues and questions not addressed by the IEC.

Nursing ethics councils have several possible functions:

1. Education of council members and nursing staff in ethics generally, and historical perspectives on the nursing profession and its ethics specifically
2. Provision of a forum for open discussion of nursing-based questions and issues
3. Service as a resource group within the institution
4. Development or distribution of nursing ethics educational or resource materials for staff
5. Review of ethics materials (including films and study guides) that might be useful tools in nursing education
6. Institution of interhospital communication among nurses to enhance local ethics resources in nursing
7. Provision of a forum for investigation of the moral tradition of nursing, the nursing philosophy of the institution, and the impact of its perspectives on nursing, health, and clinical practice

Nurses confront ethical dilemmas daily in their clinical practice, but without the concepts or language to articulate their concerns are left with an indefinable moral dis-ease. Nursing ethics councils can serve the nurse through ethics education, exploration and, and discussion in such a way as to prevent some dilemmas from arising, and by preparing nurses to discuss others that consistently resurface. One way to do this is to have the ethics council participate in establishing and conducting unit-based ethics rounds.

Preventive Ethics: Unit-Based Ethics Rounds

Unit-based ethics rounds, conducted or sponsored by the IEC or the nursing ethics council, can be either interdisciplinary or nursing based, depending on the nature and climate of the unit. Optimally, they are eventually co-sponsored and interdisciplinary. Initially, however, in the educational phases these rounds may be best conducted in a unidisciplinary fashion until the nursing staff becomes well enough acquainted with ethics content to feel comfortable with ethics analytical skills. Ethics rounds are conducted as are any other rounds—the participants focus on cases, in an organized fashion, with an "attending ethicist" or facilitator. In ethics rounds, the clinical aspects of the case are the backdrop for a discussion of potential issues or questions that might arise and action alternatives that might be considered.

The skill of the facilitator is an important ingredient. That person must have a sound basis in ethics, professional nursing, and patient care, as well as reasonably adept group skills. Ethics rounds are intended to be "preventive ethics" as well as clinical education, with those purposes made clear. Poorly facilitated rounds can deteriorate into case review of a less than constructive nature. Well-conducted ethics rounds can help to avert some morally difficult situations, help to clarify others, and result in a nursing staff that is more confident and articulate in the expression of its ethical values, obligations, and concerns.

Nursing Grand Rounds and Conferences

Both grand rounds and conferences, as vehicles of education, have their strengths and weaknesses. If well put together and executed, both can effectively *sensitize* nurses to ethical issues or situations. But neither one, even when well done, provides more than a modest introduction to the full spectrum of professional nursing ethics. Ethics rounds and conferences can be gripping and useful as a starting point for the initiation of ethics councils or unit-based participation in ethics education. By its very nature, ethics education requires prolonged exposure, discussion, and application that can only be enhanced or perhaps revitalized by conferences.

Processes and Mechanisms

The mechanisms previously discussed are not uniformly available and are useful for differing purposes. Given these mechanisms, how, from the bedside, is the nurse to initiate moral discourse and the change or resolution of moral dilemmas? There are two fundamental processes.

The Code for Nurses discusses the traditional process, which is still the only available process in a number of hospitals. If the nurse encounters a "questionable practice," the nurse is to call that practice to the attention of the perpetrator, specifying the "possible detrimental effects upon the client's welfare," and to a responsible administrator if it is a problem of the system itself.[52] The nurse should also report to the "appropriate authority within the institution, agency, or larger system."[53]

The Code further states: "There should be an established process for the reporting and handling of incompetent, unethical or illegal practice within the employment setting so that reporting can go through official channels without causing fear of reprisal."[54] It is important to underscore the necessity of using official channels where they are available, both to minimize the potential for reprisal and to foster moral discourse; "lone ranger ethics" bodes ill for the individual nurse, for hope of moral discourse, and ultimately for the effectiveness of patient advocacy.

Essentially, the nurse works up the institutional ladder of communication, through verbal reports supported by factual documentation in memoranda of concern. When the rungs of the ladder are refractory to moral concern, and the situation persists without attempts at amelioration, the nurse is warranted in reporting to other appropriate authorities "such as practice committees of the pertinent professional organizations or the legally constituted bodies concerned with licensing."[55] Accurate, factual reporting and documentation in writing are essential every step of the way. State nurses' associations and professional organizations can often provide support and counseling as to documentation, as well as avenues to pursue for recourse. In instances of ethical concerns regarding a research project, the nurse is obliged to bring the observations to the attention of the principal investigator, then to the nursing administration or the peer review board if warranted.[56]

This process, though traditional and available to all, is cumbersome at best. With the institution of IECs a second and more responsive and efficient process is established. When moral dilemmas develop in a hospital that has a functioning IEC, the nurse must first approach the party involved and attempt to rectify the situation in that fashion, pointing out the effects on the patient and guidelines covering such situations (as available). If met with resistance or unresponsiveness, the nurse can formally report those concerns to the appropriate supervisor and to the chairperson or representative of the IEC. It must be remembered, however, that the IEC functions in an advisory capacity and that there are difficulties associated with their participation in arbitration, particularly with reluctant participants. It is more effective and prudent to approach an IEC on a prospective or preventive basis, to anticipate and forestall dilemmas whenever possible, and to foster an environment of open, free moral discourse.

Nursing Ethics Beyond the Bedside

Processes within an institution are meant to serve those involved with specific cases. Larger issues require working through one's professional or specialty organization, or both. In some cases, commendably, the organizations themselves collaborate on issues of concern to both groups. (See the AACN *Principles of Critical Care Nursing Practice* [item 6] and the AACN *Definition of Critical Care Nursing*: both draw upon prior ANA work.)

The AACN policy statement *Processes for Addressing Practice, Political and Professional Issues* (see Appendix J) goes beyond the bedside and presents a process for addressing macrolevel concerns, including ethical ones. Like the Code (provision 11), it recognizes both the organization's political responsibility and the power of the collective voice to speak nursing's values and goals into the public arena, through political action committees, generation of standards, and other means. The expression of nursing advocacy is first at the bedside and then beyond, using all the institutional and political mechanisms and processes necessary to assure that the integrity of the nursing profession is maintained and that high-quality nursing care can be delivered to those in need of nursing.

It is not by happenstance that the first object of the ANA articles of incorporation was to "establish and maintain a code of ethics." Nor is it by chance that nursing organizations are developing ethics guidelines for research on human subjects. Neither is it simply a curiosity that nursing has literally hundreds of journal articles that grapple with ethical issues and concerns from the inception of the profession in this nation.

Nursing Is . . .

Nursing is, of course, a profession. It is also the diagnosis and treatment of human responses to actual or potential health problems. But it is also much more than that. It is a worthy, courageous, and honorable tradition that embodies a profound regard for humanity and a concern to express that regard through nurturing, generative, and protective care to all in need. It is, at its very core, in its essence, an ethical expression of human concern for one another.

Notes

1. ANA: Nursing: A Social Policy Statement, p 9. Kansas City, MO, ANA, 1985
2. AACN: Position Statement. AACN's Definition of Critical Care Nursing. Newport Beach, CA, AACN, 1984
3. Kuhn TS: The Structure of Scientific Revolutions, 2nd ed, pp 10–65. Chicago, University of Chicago Press, 1962
4. Flaskerud JH, Halloran EJ: Areas of agreement in nursing theory development. Advances in Nursing Science 3(1):1–7, 1980
5. Fowler MDM: The moral identity of nursing: Toward a distinctive nursing ethics. Prepublication manuscript, 1983
6. Fowler MDM: Nursing's Ethics, 1893 to the Present. In preparation
7. ANA: Code for Nurses, p i. Kansas City, MO, ANA, 1985
8. Ibid, p 2
9. Ibid, p 12

10. ANA: Human Rights Guidelines for Nurses in Clinical and Other Research, p 2. Kansas City, MO, ANA, 1985
11. Ibid, p 12
12. AACN: AACN's Statement on Ethics in Critical Care Research, p 7. Newport Beach, CA, AACN, 1985
13. Ibid, p 4
14. ANA, Code, op cit, p 6
15. ANA: Nursing: A Social Policy Statement, p 18. Kansas City, MO, ANA, 1985
16. AACN: Collaborative Practice Model: The Organization of Human Resources in Critical Care Units. Newport Beach, CA, AACN, October 1982
17. ANA, Code, op cit, pp 7–8
18. Hart HLA: Punishment and Responsibility. New York, Oxford University Press, 1968
19. Gretter L: The Florence Nightingale Pledge, 1893
20. ANA, Code, op cit, pp 6, 15, 16
21. President's Commission for the Study of Ethical Problems in Medicine and Biomedical and Behavioral Research: Deciding to Forego Life-Sustaining Treatment. Washington, DC, Government Printing Office, March 1983
22. Ibid, p 89
23. Ibid, pp 44–170
24. ANA, Code, op cit, p 2
25. Ibid, p 12
26. AACN, Statement on Ethics, op cit, p 1
27. ANA, Human Rights, op cit, p 3
28. Ibid, pp 6–7
29. AACN, Statement on Ethics, op cit, p 3
30. ANA, Human Rights, op cit, p 12
31. Wright O: Exhibit quotation (San Diego Aerospace Museum). Century Magazine
32. Gretter, op cit
33. Fowler, op cit (see n 6)
34. Ibid
35. ANA, Code, op cit, p i
36. Ibid, p 6
37. ANA, Social Policy Statement, op cit, pp 5–6
38. ANA, Code, op cit, p 2
39. AACN, Statement on Ethics, op cit, p 5
40. ANA, Code, op cit, p 3
41. Ibid, p 4
42. AACN, Statement on Ethics, op cit, p 14
43. Ibid
44. AACN: Principles of Critical Care Nursing Practice. Newport Beach, CA, AACN, 1981
45. ANA, Code, op cit, p 9
46. Goldberg A: The legal side of medical ethics. In Syllabus of the California Conference on Applied Clinical Geriatrics, vol 1, p 125. Davis, University of California at Davis, 1986
47. Ibid
48. Ibid

49. Ibid, p 134

50. ANA, Code, op cit, p 16

51. Fowler M: Institutional ethics committees: Response to a primal scream. Heart Lung 15:101–102, 1986

52. ANA, Code, op cit, p 6

53. Ibid

54. Ibid

55. Ibid, p 7

56. AACN, Statement on Ethics, op cit, p 14

Postscript
Information Resources on Ethics in Critical Care Nursing

Joyce A. Crump

As many recent publications attest, there are gray areas where dilemmas of life and death are involved. The nurse, as a member of a multidisciplinary team, is involved in joint decision making, but the nurse's unique contribution is in the giving of care, with respect to the quality of life, to those for whom cure may or may not be possible.[1] As nurses become more involved in the debate on ethical problems, they need to be informed in ethics to discuss issues from a reasoned, knowledgeable perspective rather than as an emotional response. A description of library sources and a discussion of how to use them will facilitate securing ethics information for application to clinical practice.

Library Resources

Monographs

Reference books provide brief answers to questions about definitions, addresses, statistics, drug data, and so forth. Monographs on specific subjects, such as on ethics for nurses, provide an overview of the topic and comprehensive coverage with chapters devoted to subordinate aspects.

In a small medical library, where the National Library of Medicine (NLM) classification scheme is posted, it will be relatively easy to find the general subject area—for example, nursing is in the WY section, then the particular nursing subject is found by scanning the shelves. All monographs are arranged alphanumerically.

To find what the library has by a particular author, or on a particular subject, or if a needed title is in the collection, it will be necessary to consult the library's catalog. Medical libraries use subject headings designated by the NLM. These are similar to the "MeSH" (medical subject headings) used in *Index Medicus*.[2]

University libraries use the Library of Congress (LC) Classification System, an alphanumeric system; public and school libraries use the Dewey Decimal System. Both systems use subject headings in their cataloging derived from the LC List of Subject Headings. Thus, the same monograph can be given one of three different classification numbers, depending on the type of library. To illustrate, consider the book *Ethical Dilemmas and Nursing Practice* by Davis and Aroskar.[3]

Classification System	Classification Number	Subject Headings
NLM	WY85 D261e	1. Ethics, nursing
LC	T85 D33	1. Nursing ethics 2. Medical ethics
Dewey	174.2	1. Nursing ethics 2. Medical ethics

In addition to shelf scanning, and use of the library's catalog, another method of selecting monographs is through bibliographies that identify the key texts on medical or nursing subjects. An excellent example is "Selected List of Nursing Books and Journals" by Alfred N. Brandon and Dorothy R. Hill, which appears biennially in *Nursing Outlook*, the March/April issue in even years.[4] Brandon and Hill also issue a bibliography known popularly as "the Brandon list," which contains sections of recommended texts (nursing, ethics, among 53 subject areas), and a list of core journals.[5] It is published in the April issue of *Bulletin of the Medical Library Association* in odd-numbered years. Many publishers issue reprints of these lists and distribute them at professional meetings where vendors have display booths.

Once several texts on the same subject have been located, is there any quick method of comparison? Scanning the tables of contents gives one an idea of the scope of the text. Examination of the index will reveal whether specific aspects of the subject are covered and how many pages are devoted to them. Of course, readability must be considered, and the authors' qualifications taken into account.

Periodicals

Periodicals offer timeliness. Most articles in them cover topics of current interest. Accounts of scientific research are reported first in journals for official documentation.

Periodicals also may feature "review" articles. These survey the history of a subject, summarize and appraise previously published research, and describe the subject's "state of the art." They are a good starting point for anyone beginning an in-depth study of a subject because they mention key authors and "landmark" papers.

Periodicals of particular interest to critical care nurses include *Critical Care Quarterly (CCQ); Journal of Emergency Nursing (JEN); Heart & Lung: The Journal of*

Critical Care; Journal of Obstetric, Gynecologic and Neonatal Nursing (JOGN); Emergency Medicine; and *Journal of Trauma.* All of these include occasional articles on ethical concerns. Journals that devote more space to critical care nursing ethics are *Dimensions of Critical Care Nursing (DCCN); Critical Care Nurse; Focus on Critical Care;* and *Critical Care Medicine.*

Lay periodicals deal with medical issues of concern to the general public. News stories, editorials, features, and columns all identify timely topics such as AIDS, Baby Doe, heart transplants, withholding or withdrawing life support, and so forth. They often provide background information not usually supplied in the medical or nursing literature. Important news magazines include *Time, Newsweek, U.S. News and World Report;* major daily newspapers include the *New York Times, Christian Science Monitor, Wall Street Journal, Washington Post,* and other journalistically responsible periodicals. Apart from locating desired journal titles in their alphabetical location in the library, in bibliographies, or in indexes given at the end of each journal's volume (usually at the end of the December issue—sometimes also in June), access to articles on specific topics is accomplished through the use of indexes. It is important to select the index most likely to deal with the topic, and to consider that more than one index may be needed.

Indexes

1. *Cumulative Index to Nursing and Allied Health Literature.*[6] Commonly referred to as CINAHL ("sin-all"), this index covers all nursing literature published in the English language. It indexes approximately 300 nursing and allied health (respiratory therapy, physical therapy, food management, etc.) journals. There are five bimonthly paperback issues per year (through October) followed by an annual cumulation. CINAHL also includes lists of book reviews, pamphlets, and audiovisual materials.

   CINAHL has an author and a subject section in each index. The subject heading and cross reference thesaurus is in the "yellow pages" in the back of each annual volume. Articles are cited only under first authors. Secondary authors have "see" references to first authors.

   A list of all publications indexed is included in the introductory part of each issue of CINAHL. Addresses of publishers are listed in the annual volume under the alphabetical list of abbreviated journal titles. Examples of subject headings in CINAHL are:

   Critical Care Nursing
   Critical Care Nursing—Education, Continuing
   Critical Care Nursing—Legislation & Jurisprudence, U.S.
   Critical Care Nursing—Organizations
   Critical Care Nursing—Psychosocial Factors

Under the last heading above, the following citation appeared in the January/

February 1986 issue of CINAHL: the role of critical care nurses in the ethical decision-making process. (Kemp VH) *DCCN* 1985 Nov–Dec; 4(6):354–9 (10 ref).

Other subject headings illustrate hierarchical format (from the general to the more specific):

Ethics
Ethics, Nursing
Ethics, Nursing—Education

2. *Index Medicus* is the world's major index to medical periodical literature. It covers English and foreign language medical and health-related journals and proceedings of congresses and symposia. It is published monthly and is cumulated annually. Access is by author or by subject. Citations are given only under the first author of each article; secondary authors are listed with "see" references to the first author. Subject access is by the subject headings listed in *Medical Subject Headings*, commonly called "MeSH," a separate section mailed each January. The following guidelines with examples will help you locate subjects in MeSH:

- Use the most specific form of the term first.

    Erythromycin is used; therefore, it is not necessary to look under Antibiotics for articles on erythromycin.

- Consider variants.

    Direct form: cerebral aneurysm
    Inverted form: anemia, hemolytic; ethics, nursing
    Synonyms (or near-synonyms): vertigo *is* used, *not* dizziness
    Noun form: liver, kidney, brain, heart
    Adjectival form: hepatic, renal, encephalic, cardiac
    Function: thinking *is* used, *not* brain, for this aspect
    Techniques: angiography, plasmapheresis
    Broader vs narrower terms: breast diseases vs breast neoplasms

- Use the organ, substance, or disease, *not* the technological term or an age group.

    Radiography of the pancreas: use pancreas
    Rickets in infants: use rickets

- Scan terms above and below the term you are considering. There may be a better term nearby.

    Life support care
    Life support systems

- Consider cross references.

    See: directs you from the term *not* used to the term that *is* used.
    X: refers to terms *not* used, which are "see references" to the term you are considering. These X terms save you from looking for them in vain as headings in *Index Medicus*.

XR: refers to related terms that *are* used. One of these may be better for you.

XU: refers to terms *not* used, but that are under a more general heading that *is* used.

- If there are no cross references and you cannot locate the subject heading best suited to your needs, use a dictionary or encyclopedia to obtain synonyms or variant forms, then try again.
- Once you have found the correct subject heading, use the *Cumulated Index Medicus* for the previous year to get a quick overview of what was indexed on your topic during the past year. Then use the monthly issues of *Index Medicus* for leads to the most recent articles.

Index Medicus has three other important parts. (1) The *Bibliography of Medical Reviews* cites under MeSH headings articles that are reviews. They include many references that are given in parentheses: e.g., (72 refs). In many cases a review article is enough to satisfy a user's ordinary requirement for information on a given topic. (2) *Literature Searches* are bibliographies prepared by NLM on subjects considered to be of wide interest. They are available free of charge from NLM, or your library may have copies. AIDS is a topic for which several editions of NLM literature searches have been issued. (3) In the January issue of *Index Medicus*, the *List of Journals Indexed* provides the full titles of the journals indexed, and a list of abbreviated journal titles, with the full titles of the journals directly under each abbreviation. The online version of *Index Medicus, MEDLINE,* and its back files, cover 1966 to the present. The new series of *Index Medicus* began with volume 1 in 1960, but preceding series, with varying titles, index medical literature since 1879.

3. *International Nursing Index*[7] is a quarterly publication, with each succeeding issue cumulating the previous quarterly issue. The fourth quarterly issue is therefore an annual cumulation. *INI* indexes over 200 nursing journals, including those in foreign languages. It also includes nursing articles that appear in any of the non-nursing journals indexed in *Index Medicus*. It has an author and a subject index and uses MeSH headings. Online access is via *MEDLINE* and its back files because all the citations in INI are included in *MEDLINE*.

4. *Hospital Literature Index*[8] is a quarterly publication indexing English language journal articles relating to all aspects of hospital administration, management, and health care delivery. Included are support services not directly involved in patient care, such as environmental services, accounting, and community relations. *HLI* is a primary source for articles on supervision, personnel and staffing, and such timely topics as DRGs. *HLI* uses MeSH headings for subject access and also has an author index. The online version of *HLI* is called the Health Planning and Administration File of the MEDLARS databases.

5. *Nonmedical Indexes*. Three indexes not usually found in medical libraries that are heavily used in most large public libraries are *Reader's Guide to Periodical Literature*,[9] *Magazine Index*,[10] and *National Newspaper Index*.[11] These provide

access to the writings of persons outside the health care field and to the lay perspective on issues of concern to nurses and others. All three are available online, but a brief discussion here will cover the standard versions. The first is a printed index, and the other two are computer output microfilm strips.

- *National Newspaper Index* cites articles in five of the nation's leading newspapers: *The New York Times, The Wall Street Journal, The Christian Science Monitor, The Los Angeles Times,* and *The Washington Post.* The tape, at any given time, covers a three-year period, current to the previous month. Subject headings have clarification where necessary:

  > Life Support Systems (Critical Care)
  > Life Support Systems (Space Environment)

  Cross references are copious: for example, in July 1986, under Medical Ethics, there were 18 "see also," 20 subheadings, and 94 citations. The subheadings, with the number of cited articles, were: Medical Ethics: Analyses (33). Cases (20), Conferences and Congresses (2), Economic Aspects (2), Evaluation (1), Interpretation and Construction (1), Investigations (3), Law & Legislation (3), Management (3), Moral & Religious Aspects (1), Philosophy (1), Political Aspects (3), Psychological Aspects (1), Public Opinion (4), Research (1), Rules & Regulations (5), Seminars & Workshops, etc. (1), Social Aspects (5), Standards (3), Study & Teaching (1). This detailed array illustrates the depth of indexing provided to these key newspapers.

- *Magazine Index* covers 400 titles over a four-year span and is updated monthly. In July 1986, magazine articles from April 1982 through June 1986 were indexed. Under Medical Ethics there were 21 "see also," 19 subheadings, and a total of 74 citations. Under the subheading "Analysis," there were 22 citations spread among 17 titles. A look at these diverse titles reveals the range of public interest in the subject: Medical Ethics—Analyses (22): *Newsweek* (1), *National Catholic Reporter* (2), *Christian Century* (1), *TIME* (1), *Nation* (1), *MacLeans* (1), *America* (4), *New Republic* (1), *USA Today* (1), *Technology Review* (1), *Science News* (1), *New York Times Magazine* (1), *Saturday Night* (1), *Present Tense* (1), *U.S. News & World Report* (1), *People* (1).

  Ten of the subheadings under Medical Ethics were similar to those used by *National Newspaper Index.* The nine different subheads included Medical Ethics: Addresses, Essays, Lectures; Catholic Church; Forecasts; History; Innovations; International Aspects; Personal Narratives; South Africa; Surveys.

- *Reader's Guide to Periodical Literature.* This "granddaddy" of the popular indexes began in 1900. It now indexes 185 general interest periodicals, and is issued semimonthly, with annual cumulations covering March through the following February. It provides author and subject access. The annual volume for March 1984—February 1985, under Medical Ethics, had 14 "see also" references and 12 citations for the one-year period covered. *Reader's Guide* is time consuming to use because each semimonthly and annual issue must be examined separately. Bear in mind that using these indexes on your own before you request any online searches provides a realistic overview of "what's out there," and under what terms it is being indexed.

Vertical File

The vertical file maintained in most libraries is an often overlooked resource. Articles on subjects of potential interest to library users have been preselected for their pertinence. Most of the files are "weeded" regularly to keep the contents of the file current, except in those cases where landmark articles are important to retain. Finding a previous report prepared on the same subject for which you need to write a report provides a springboard for new ideas, while at the same time it reveals aspects that might be overlooked today.

The vertical file usually uses the same subject headings as the monograph catalog, with added entries for ephemeral areas.

Online Databases

Most health science libraries in hospitals and medical centers are now equipped with terminals or computers that provide access online to information in medical, nursing, and allied health databases, as well as to subjects covered by the complete range of the Dewey Decimal System. Not all journals cited in databases will be available in-house. They may have to be requested through interlibrary loan or obtained directly at another library.

1. *Medical Literature Analysis and Retrieval System* (MEDLARS) is the online system of the National Library of Medicine's indexes, the most famous of which is MEDLINE. The database from which the printed *Index Medicus* is derived, MEDLINE contains over 7 million citations to articles in over 3000 of the world's medical journals. Other MEDLARS databases include the Health Planning and Administration File; Bioethicsline; Histline (History of Medicine online); Cancerline; Cancerproj; Clinprot; PDQ; AVline (audiovisuals online); SDIline (selective dissemination of information online); among others.

2. *Nursing and Allied Health,* the online version of *Cumulative Index to Nursing and Allied Health Literature* (CINAHL) has been available since 1984. Its print counterpart is published bimonthly and cumulates into annual volumes.

3. *Nonmedical Databases.* By special arrangement with commercial database vendors, such as DIALOG and BRS, medical librarians are able to access databases that are bibliographic (providing references to literature) or factual (numerical, tabular, or textual information). DIALOG alone offers over 250 databases. Popular among these are ERIC[12] (Educational Resources Information Center); Magazine Index (popular magazines); National Newspaper Index; Psychinfo[13] (Psychological Abstracts); Scisearch[14] (Science Citation Index); Biosis[15] (Biological Abstracts); and Social Scisearch[16] (Social Science Citation Index).

Manual Versus Online Searching

1. *Topics Requiring Only One Subject Heading.* Manual searching is warranted here. The searcher is able to locate articles quickly by looking under the heading that applies. The desired citations can be either photocopied or jotted down. Retrieval is faster if the complete citation is recorded: author, title, journal name, date, volume/issue, and pagination for each article. Online searching will provide a printed list for the requester. The cost of a search needs to be considered.

2. *Topics Requiring More Than One Subject Heading.* In manual searching, the searcher must look under each appropriate heading. Key articles should be indexed under each. This is a tedious, time-consuming activity. Retrieval is only as good as the titles of the articles can reveal. Some titles are very specific, but there are many that are so ambiguous that they are frustrating. There is no way to know, without seeing the article itself, what weight either subject has. For example, suppose one wanted articles on morphine for the relief of pain in terminal cancer patients. It would be necessary to look under Morphine or under Morphine—Therapeutic Use and under Pain—Drug Therapy. A given article could be emphasizing morphine, or it could be just one of several pain killers. Conversely, the use of morphine for cancer patients may only be mentioned briefly, and other uses (burn victims, etc.) could predominate. The great strength of online searching is the ability the searcher has to coordinate two or more concepts to retrieve a set of articles.

3. *Topics That Have No Appropriate Subject Headings.* During manual searching, it is almost impossible to locate articles by using new terminology for access in printed indexes, unless by chance the words of the concept appear when titles are scanned under established headings. Examples of this problem, which NLM made into MeSH headings quickly after the terms proliferated in the literature, are Toxic Shock Syndrome; Diagnostic Related Groups; and AIDS, for which the MeSH is Acquired Immunodeficiency Syndrome. Before these headings were established, it was perplexing to determine which MeSH terms applied.

   Online systems enable searching for "text words" in titles and abstracts. Thus pertinent articles that use the precise words required can be retrieved.

4. *Advantages of Manual Searching.*
   - *Convenience.* Most of the time, a library user can browse in printed indexes, locate appropriate subject headings, and find articles on the subject in question. There is no need to request, wait for, or pay for online searching.
   - *Extended Coverage.* Printed indexes usually cover more extensive time periods than their online counterparts, which were developed more recently and tend to cover shorter time spans.

5. *Advantages of Online Searching.*
   - *Speed.* Online searching can be done in minutes, even when many aspects of the subject are searched.

- *Timeliness.* Online databases usually provide access to current literature before their printed counterparts are published.
- *Coordination of Terms.* Boolean operators—and, or, and not—are used to combine subject headings and/or text words to tailor searches.
- *Depth.* Online searches can utilize more terms to retrieve citations than their printed counterparts. Some subject headings not used in printed indexes exist in online databases; text word searching offers virtually unlimited access; and other online capabilities expand the retrieval. For example, in MEDLINE a hierarchical term can be "exploded" to retrieve not only citations under the primary term, but also those from subordinate terms. If the term *Interpersonal Relations* is exploded, citations from the following subordinate terms will also be located: Interprofessional Relations; Professional-Family Relations; Professional-Patient Relations (with its subordinate terms, Dentist-Patient Relations; Nurse-Patient Relations; or Physician-Patient Relations).
- *Cross-Database Access.* Searches can be run in one database, "saved," and then run in other databases. This saves online time, which is charged by the minute.
- *Remote Access.* One can search databases that have no print counterparts, or that may have print versions, but that the library does not own. Through online searching, "the sky's the limit" when access to the world's periodical literature is desired.

Some Online Ethics Searches

1. *Bioethics.*[17] This database is one of the MEDLARS group. It can be searched using MeSH, keywords (KW) from the Bioethics thesaurus, or free-term searching using the text word (TW) capability. Unlike the other databases of the NLM sponsored set, *Bioethics* indexes a variety of document types, including analytics (chapters in monographs), audiovisuals, bills, court decisions, laws, journal and newspaper articles, monographs, and unpublished documents. Sources selected for indexing represent literature of medicine, nursing, biological science, philosophy, religion, law, behavioral science, and popular media. A look at two searches, one specific and the other general, will illustrate the range of retrieval.

   - *Specific.* The numbers in parentheses on the right show the number of citations in the database.

     (KW) allowing to die (2518)
     (KW) prolongation of life (641)
     (KW) nursing ethics (214)
     searching nursing ethics with either one of the above topics (31)

   Of the preceding 31 citations, the document types were as follows: monographs (10), journal articles (11), bibliographies (pamphlet-size, 3), court case (1), dissertation (1), analytics (3), newspaper articles (2).

- *General.* Retrieval was much less than expected when broad concepts were combined:

    (TW) critical: and care: (135)
    (KW) intensive care units (160)
    (TW) ICU: or CCU: (9)

Nursing ethics and any of the above topics (5)

The five references resulting here were analytics (2), videocassettes (1), newspaper article (1), journal article (1). All the citations retrieved in these searches were pertinent.

The following two examples show the range of information.

2. *National Newspaper Index on DIALOG*

    s critical()care (23)

    s Nurs? (1192)

    the above topics searched together (0)

    s ethic? or guideline? or policy? or policies? (123089)

    (critical()care) and (ethic? or guideline? or policy?) (11)

All 11 articles seemed excellent when judged by the headlines that serve as titles of the citations. Nine articles were in the *New York Times* and two in the *Washington Post.*

3. *MEDLINE.* The search below with asterisked terms was intended with those subjects as main points of the articles.

    *life support care or *life support systems (22)
    ethics, nursing (341)
    both of the above subjects searched together (12)

All but two of the preceding twelve articles were in nursing journals. Those two were in *Critical Care Medicine* and in *Law Medicine and Health Care.*

Conclusion

In this paper, the typical print and online resources available in most hospital and health care institution libraries have been described and discussed. Suggestions for their use have been indicated.

In a pithy article on ethical issues involved in the nursing care of the elderly, Gunter states, "Knowledge without ethics or ethics without sufficient or appropriate knowledge establishes a context fraught with dangers for patient care."[18] It is to be hoped that nurses wanting to increase their understanding of the ethical issues surrounding caring for the critically ill will seek to obtain such knowledge. The resources are not far from them. Four bibliographies are appended:

1. Monographs
2. Journal articles (see note)

3. Guidelines for ethical decision making and action
4. Bibliographies (list of sources) of ethics in health, medicine, and nursing.

Bibliography

Monographs

Abrams N, Buckner MD: Medical Ethics: A Clinical Textbook and Reference for the Health Care Professions. Cambridge, MIT Press, 1983

American Hospital Association, Special Committee on Biomedical Ethics: Values in Conflict: Resolving Ethical Issues in Hospital Care. Chicago, AHA, 1985

Beauchamp TL, Childress JF: Principles of Biomedical Ethics, 2nd ed. New York, Oxford University Press, 1983

Benjamin M, Curtis J: Ethics in Nursing. New York, Oxford University Press, 1981

Campbell AV: Moral Dilemmas in Medicine: A Coursebook in Ethics for Doctors and Nurses, 3rd ed. New York, Churchill Livingstone, 1984

Creighton H: Law Every Nurse Should Know, 5th ed. Philadelphia, WB Saunders, 1986

Curtin LL, Flaherty MJ: Nursing Ethics: Theories and Pragmatics. Bowie, MD, Brady Communications Co, 1982

Doudera AE, Peters JD: Legal and Ethical Aspects of Treating Critically and Terminally Ill Patients. Ann Arbor, AUPHA Press, 1982

Fenner, KM: Ethics and Law in Nursing: Professional Prospectives. New York, Van Nostrand Reinhold, 1980

Fromer MJ: Ethical Issues in Health Care. St Louis, CV Mosby, 1981

Jameton A: Nursing Practice: The Ethical Issues. Englewood Cliffs, Prentice-Hall, 1984

Jonsen AR, Siegler M, Winslade WJ: Clinical Ethics: A Practical Approach to Ethical Decisions in Clinical Medicine, 2nd ed. New York, Macmillan, 1986

Kastenbaum RJ: Death, Society, and Human Experience, 3rd ed. St Louis, CV Mosby, 1986

Mappes TA, Zembaty JS: Biomedical Ethics, 2nd ed. New York, McGraw-Hill, 1986

Muyskens JL: Moral Problems in Nursing: A Philosophical Investigation. Totowa, NJ, Rowman & Littlefield, 1982

Purtillo R, Cassell CK: Ethical Dimensions in the Health Professions. Philadelphia, WB Saunders, 1981

Ramsey P: Patient as Person: Explorations in Medical Ethics. New Haven, Yale University Press, 1970

Rosoff AJ: Informed Consent: A Guide for Health Care Providers. Rockville, MD, Aspen Systems, 1981

Shannon TA: Twelve Problems in Health Care Ethics. Lewiston, NY, E Mellen Press, 1984

Tate BL: Nurse's Dilemma—Ethical Considerations in Nursing Practice. Geneva, International Council of Nurses, 1977

Thompson IE, Melia KM, Boyd, KM: Nursing Ethics. New York, Churchill Livingstone, 1983

Thompson JB, Thompson HO: Ethics in Nursing. New York, Macmillan, 1981

Veatch RM: A Theory of Medical Ethics. New York, Basic Books, 1981

Winslade WJ, Ross JW: Choosing Life or Death: A Guide for Patients, Families, and Professionals. New York, Free Press, 1986

Journal Articles

For journal articles, the reader is referred to the most current bibliographies, or the indexes described above, many of which are updated monthly or bimonthly. Cumulative annual bibliographies and indexes are also extremely useful. (The editors have deleted list of articles.)

Guidelines—Bioethics

American Academy of Pediatrics Infant Bioethics Task Force and Consultants: Guidelines for infant bioethics committees. Pediatrics 74:306–310, 1984

American Nurses' Association: Code for Nurses with Interpretive Statements. Kansas City, MO, ANA, 1985

Committee on Biomedical Ethics of the Los Angeles County Medical Association; Los Angeles County Bar Association: Principles and Guidelines Concerning the Foregoing of Life-Sustaining Treatment for Adult Patients. Adopted by the Board of Trustees of the Los Angeles County Bar Association on December 11, 1985, and by the Council of the Los Angeles County Medical Association on January 6, 1986

Duff RS: Guidelines for deciding care of critically ill or dying patients. Pediatrics 64:17–23, 1979

Guidelines for the determination of death. Report of the Medical Consultants on the Diagnosis of Death to the President's Commission for the Study of Ethical Problems in Medicine and Biomedical Behavioral Research. JAMA 246:2184–2186, 1984

Halligan M, Hamel RP: Ethics committee develops supportive care guidelines. Health Prog 66:26–30, 60, 1985

Natural Death Act: Section 7185–7195 of Chapter 3.9 California Health and Safety Code. (The nation's first "natural death act," enacted in 1976.)

Sherman SR, Dickey N, Burkhart JH, Chisholm WS, Epps CH: Bioethical Opinions of the Judicial Council of the American Medical Association. Chicago, AMA, 1984

Bibliographies

American College of Physicians: Ethics manual. Part II. Research, other ethical issues. Recommended reading. (Ad Hoc Committee on Medical Ethics.) Ann Intern Med 101:263–274, 1984

American Nurses' Association: Committee on Ethics. Ethics References for Nurses. Kansas City, MO, ANA, 1982

Brandon AN, Hill DR: Selected list of books and journals for the small medical library. Bull Med Libr Assoc 73:176–205, 1985

Brandon AN, Hill DR: Selected list of nursing books and journals. Nurs Outlook 34:74–82, 1986

Cassel CK, Meier DE, Traines ML: Selected bibliography of recent articles in ethics and geriatrics. J Am Geriatr Soc 34:399–409, 1986

Foulke GE, Albertson T, Fisher CJ: Critical care medicine: An annotated bibliography of recent literature. Am J Emerg Med 3:266–274, 1985

Goldstein DM: Bioethics: A Guide for Information Sources. Detroit, Gale, 1982

Hastings Center: The Hastings Center's Bibliography of Ethics, Biomedicine, and Professional Responsibility. Frederick, MD, University Publications of America, 1984

Jonsen AR, Cassel C, Lo B, Perkins HS: The ethics of medicine: An annotated bibliography of recent literature. Ann Intern Med 92:136–141, 1980

Lewis CS Jr: A library for internists: Recommended by the American College of Physicians. Ann Intern Med 102:423–437, 1985

Loepprich JC, Smith JL: Keeping up with nursing information resources: Building your personal library. Imprint 3:50–57, 1984

Pence T: Ethics in Nursing—an Annotated Bibliography, 2nd ed. New York, National League for Nursing, 1986 (NLN 20-9189)

Shmavonian N: Human Values in Medicine and Health Care: Audiovisual Resources. Valley Forge, PA, United Ministries in Education, 1983

Simpson MA: Dying, Death and Grief: A Critically Annotated Bibliography and Source Book of Thanatology and Terminal Care. New York, Plenum Press, 1979

Sollito S, Veatch R: Bibliography of Society, Ethics and the Life Sciences. Hastings-on-Hudson, NY, Institute of Society, Ethics and the Life Sciences, 1974; 1975 rev by Fenner D; 1976–77 rev by Taylor NK

Taylor NK: Bibliography of Society, Ethics and the Life Sciences. Hastings-on-Hudson, NY, Institute of Society, Ethics and the Life Sciences, 1977 (Full bibliography by Sollito S, Veatch R)

Walters L: Bibliography of Bioethics, vols 1–6. Detroit, Gale, 1975–80; vols 7–9, New York, Free Press, 1981–83; vols 10–11, Washington, DC, Georgetown University, Kennedy Institute of Ethics, 1984–85

Notes

1. Thomson WW: Nursing. In Duncan AS, Dunstan GR, Welbourn RB: Dictionary of Medical Ethics, 2nd ed, pp 311–312. New York, Crossroad, 1981
2. Index Medicus: Bethesda, MD, National Library of Medicine. 1960–(ns, v 1). (Online version, MEDLINE, 1966–)
3. Davis AJ, Aroskar MA: Ethical Dilemmas in Nursing Practice, 2nd ed. Norwalk: Appleton-Century-Crofts, 1983
4. Brandon AN, Hill DR: Selected list of nursing books and journals. Nurs Outlook 34:74–82, 1986
5. Brandon AN, Hill DR: Selected list of books and journals for the small medical library. Bull Med Libr Assoc 73:176–205, 1985
6. Cumulative Index to Nursing and Allied Health Literature: Glendale, CA, Glendale Adventist Medical Center, vol 1, 1956–. (Online, 1983)
7. International Nursing Index: New York, Am J Nurs. In cooperation with the National Library of Medicine, 1966–
8. Hospital Literature Index: Chicago, American Hospital Association. In cooperation with the National Library of Medicine, vol 11, 1955–. (Formerly called Hospital Periodical Literature Index, vols 1–10, 1946–54)
9. Readers Guide to Periodical Literature: New York, HW Wilson Co, vol 1, 1900–. (Online database, 1983–)
10. Magazine Index: Belmont, CA, Information Access Co, 1977–. (Online covers 1959–70; 1973–)
11. National Newspaper Index: Belmont, CA, Information Access Co, 1979–. (Online 1979–)
12. ERIC: Washington, DC, Educational Resources Information Center, 1966–. (Online, 1966–)

13. Psychinfo (Online database of Psychological Abstracts): Washington, DC, American Psychological Association, 1967–

14. SCISEARCH: Philadelphia, Institute for Scientific Information (Online database of Science Citation Abstracts), 1974

15. BIOSIS: Philadelphia, BioSciences Information Service (Online database of Biological Abstracts), 1969–

16. SOCIAL SCISEARCH: Philadelphia, Institute for Scientific Information (Online database of Social Science Citation Index), 1972–

17. BIOETHICS: Georgetown, Kennedy Institute of Ethics, in cooperation with the National Library of Medicine, 1973– . (Book form is Bibliography of Bioethics, vol 1, 1973– .) *See* p XX, Walters L, cited on preceding page

18. Gunter LM: Ethical considerations for nursing care of older patients in the acute care setting. Nurs Clin North Am 18: 411–421, 1983

Appendices

Appendix A

AACN Position Statement
AACN'S Definition of Critical Care Nursing

In *Nursing, A Social Policy Statement*, the American Nurses' Association defines nursing as "the diagnosis and treatment of human responses to actual or potential health problems." Critical care nursing is that specialty within nursing which deals specifically with human responses to life-threatening problems.

(Adopted by AACN Board of Directors, February 1984)

Appendix B

Code for Nurses with Interpretive Statements

Preamble

A code of ethics makes explicit the primary goals and values of the profession. When individuals become nurses, they make a moral commitment to uphold the values and special moral obligations expressed in their code. The Code for Nurses is based on a belief about the nature of individuals, nursing, health, and society. Nursing encompasses the protection, promotion, and restoration of health; the prevention of illness; and the alleviation of suffering in the care of clients, including individuals, families, groups, and communities. In the context of these functions, nursing is defined as the diagnosis and treatment of human responses to actual or potential health problems.

Since clients themselves are the primary decision makers in matters concerning their own health, treatment, and well-being, the goal of nursing actions is to support and enhance the client's responsibility and self-determination to the greatest extent possible. In this context, health is not necessarily an end in itself, but rather a means to a life that is meaningful from the client's perspective.

When making clinical judgments, nurses base their decisions on consideration of consequences and of universal moral principles, both of which prescribe and justify nursing actions. The most fundamental of these principles is respect for persons. Other principles stemming from this basic principle are autonomy (self-determination), beneficence (doing good), nonmaleficence (avoiding harm), veracity (truth-telling), confidentiality (respecting privileged information), fidelity (keeping promises), and justice (treating people fairly).

In brief, then, the statements of the code and their interpretation provide guidance for conduct and relationships in carrying out nursing responsibilities consistent with the ethical obligations of the profession and with high quality in nursing care.

Introduction

A code of ethics indicates a profession's acceptance of the responsibility and trust with which it has been invested by society. Under the terms of the implicit contract between society and the nursing profession, society grants the profession considerable autonomy and authority to function in the conduct of its affairs. The development of a code of ethics is an essential activity of a profession and provides one means for the exercise of professional self-regulation.

Upon entering the profession, each nurse inherits a measure of both the responsibility and the trust that have accrued to nursing over the years, as well as the corresponding obligation to adhere to the profession's code of conduct and relationships for ethical practice. The Code for Nurses with Interpretive Statements is thus more a collective expression of nursing conscience and philosophy than a set of external rules imposed upon an individual practitioner of nursing. Personal and professional integrity can be assured only if an individual is committed to the profession's code of conduct.

A code of ethical conduct offers general principles to guide and evaluate nursing actions. It does not assure the virtues required for professional practice within the character of each nurse. In particular situations, the justification of behavior as ethical must satisfy not only the individual nurse acting as a moral agent but also the standards for professional peer review.

The Code for Nurses was adopted by the American Nurses' Association in 1950 and has been revised periodically. It serves to inform both the nurse and society of the profession's expectations and requirements in ethical matters. The code and the interpretive statements together provide a framework within which nurses can make ethical decisions and discharge their responsibilities to the public, to other members of the health care team, and to the profession.

Although a particular situation by its nature may determine the use of specific moral principles, the basic philosophical values, directives, and suggestions provided here are widely applicable to situations encountered in clinical practice. The Code for Nurses is not open to negotiation in employment settings, nor is it permissible for individuals or groups of nurses to adapt or change the language of this code.

The requirements of the code may often exceed those of the law. Violations of the law may subject the nurse to civil or criminal liability. The state nurses' associations, in fulfilling the profession's duty to society, may discipline their members for violations of the code. Loss of the respect and confidence of society and of one's colleagues is a serious sanction resulting from violation of the code. In addition, every nurse has a personal obligation to uphold and adhere to the code and to ensure that nursing colleagues do likewise.

Guidance and assistance in applying the code to local situations may be obtained from the American Nurses' Association and the constituent state nurses' associations.

Code for Nurses

1. The nurse provides services with respect for human dignity and the uniqueness of the client, unrestricted by considerations of social or economic status, personal attributes, or the nature of health problems.
2. The nurse safeguards the client's right to privacy by judiciously protecting information of a confidential nature.
3. The nurse acts to safeguard the client and the public when health care and safety are affected by the incompetent, unethical, or illegal practice of any person.
4. The nurse assumes responsibility and accountability for individual nursing judgments and actions.
5. The nurse maintains competence in nursing.
6. The nurse exercises informed judgment and uses individual competence and qualifications as criteria in seeking consultation, accepting responsibilities, and delegating nursing activities to others.
7. The nurse participates in activities that contribute to the ongoing development of the profession's body of knowledge.
8. The nurse participates in the profession's efforts to implement and improve standards of nursing.
9. The nurse participates in the profession's efforts to establish and maintain conditions of employment conducive to high quality nursing care.
10. The nurse participates in the profession's effort to protect the public from misinformation and misrepresentation and to maintain the integrity of nursing.
11. The nurse collaborates with members of the health professions and other citizens

in promoting community and national efforts to meet the health needs of the public.

(Used with permission)

Appendix C

AACN Position Statement
Conceptual Model of Critical Care Nursing

Have you ever tried to draw a picture of critical care nursing? As you can imagine, trying to encompass all the aspects of critical care nursing in a brief picture is a challenging task. Our brief picture has been drawn utilizing a framework of the *Standards for Nursing Care of the Critically Ill* (AACN, 1980), the Scope of Critical Care Nursing Practice, and the Principles of Critical Care Nursing Practice. The Principles of Critical Care Nursing Practice are those characteristics of personal conduct that all critical care nurses use in approaching quality patient care.

These elements have been combined and are graphically represented (over) in a "Conceptual Model for Critical Care Nursing Practice." Briefly, this approach describes some beliefs about critical care nursing.

The model reflects the goal of critical care nursing practice as quality care. Quality care is achieved by the interactional elements of the nursing process. The nursing process encompassing assessment, planning, intervention, and evaluation is used in providing care to the critically ill. The framework for quality care is formed by the three components which serve as the structure within which critical care nursing is practiced, utilizing the nursing process. The *Standards for Nursing Care of the Critically Ill* provides the foundation of the model. Standards are the criteria essential to provide quality care.

The Scope of Critical Care Nursing Practice delineates the environment of critical care. The critical care nurse, the critically ill patient, and the physical facilities are defined.

The Principles of Critical Care Nursing Practice identify personal perspectives in delivering care which respects the dignity, worth, and rights of all. The conduct and character of the critical care nurse, in approaching quality care, form this element of the model.

All elements of the framework are essential for achieving quality care; without any one component, the balance is lost and quality care cannot be attained.

Principles of Critical Care Nursing Practice

The American Association of Critical-Care Nurses recognizes that its members are often faced with difficult and sensitive situations involving nurse-patient relationships. These Principles of Practice define, promote, and uphold the highest standards of personal conduct among members. A primary responsibility of the critical care

Conceptual Model of Critical Care Nursing

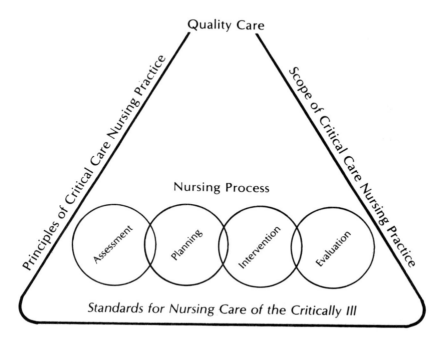

Quality Care

Principles of Critical Care Nursing Practice

Scope of Critical Care Nursing Practice

Nursing Process

Assessment

Planning

Intervention

Evaluation

Standards for Nursing Care of the Critically Ill

nurse is promotion and restoration of health, as well as alleviation of suffering for persons and families facing critical illness. Entrusted with this responsibility, the critical care nurse is accountable for respecting the individuality, wholeness, integrity, dignity, and rights of all humans.

1. The critical care nurse maintains the established standards of critical care nursing practice.
2. The critical care nurse continually updates knowledge necessary for competence.
3. The critical care nurse, as an integral part of the multidisciplinary health care team, coordinates care delivered to patients and supports families within the critical care environment.
4. The critical care nurse recognizes the stresses involved in the critical care environment, and creates a compassionate and humanistic climate by providing support to patients, families, and colleagues. The critical care nurse must also identify psychological and physiological limitations when providing care.
5. The critical care nurse respects the rights of patients, families, and colleagues in the promotion or prolongation of life by individualizing each patient situation.
6. The critical care nurse identifies the values of patients, families, colleagues, and

self, and incorporates those beliefs and attitudes into situations of ethical dilemmas.

7. The critical care nurse adheres to the Code of Ethics of the American Nurses' Association

(Code for Nurses with Interpretive Statements, 1976). [Now 1985 version.]

Appendix D

AACN Position Statement
Scope of Critical Care Nursing Practice

Critical care nursing practice is a dynamic process the scope of which is defined in terms of the critically ill patient, the critical care nurse, and the environment in which critical care nursing is delivered; all three components are essential elements for the practice of critical care nursing.

The Critically Ill Patient

The critically ill patient is characterized by the presence of real or potential life-threatening health problems and by the requirement for continuous observation and intervention to prevent complications and restore health. The concept of the critically ill patient includes the patient's family and/or significant others.

The Critical Care Nurse

The critical care nurse is a registered professional nurse committed to ensuring that all critically ill patients receive optimal care. This nurse's practice is based on the following:

a. individual professional accountability.
b. thorough knowledge of the interrelatedness of body systems and the dynamic nature of the life process.
c. recognition and appreciation of the individual's wholeness, uniqueness, and significant social and environmental relationships.
d. appreciation of the collaborative role of all members of the health care team.

To continually refine the practice, the critical care nurse participates in ongoing educational activities. In addition to basic preparation, the critical care nurse acquires an advanced knowledge of psychosocial, physiological, and therapeutic components specific to the care of the critically ill. Clinical competency and the ability to effectively interact with patients, families and other members of the health care team are developed. Additionally, an awareness of the responsibility for a therapeutic environment is cultivated.

The critical care nurse utilizes the nursing process as a framework for practice. In caring for the critically ill, the nurse will collect data, identify and determine the priority of the patient's problems/needs, formulate an appropriate plan of nursing care, implement the plan of nursing care according to the priority of the identified problems/needs, and evaluate the process and outcome of nursing care.

The Critical Care Environment

A critical care unit is any geographically designated area which is designed to facilitate the care of the critically ill patient by critical care nurses. It is an area where safety, organizational, and ethical standards are maintained for patient welfare. Although critical care nursing usually occurs in a critical care unit, it can occur in any setting that meets the environmental and nursing standards, such as an area which has a psychologically supportive environment for the patients and significant others, adequately functioning equipment and supplies, readily available emergency equipment, facilities to meet staff needs, and ready access to support departments.

This Scope of Critical Care Nursing Practice statement provides a definition and framework for nursing care of the critically ill. For critical care nursing practice to occur, all three components must be present: the critically ill patient, the critical care nurse and a therapeutic critical care environment. The *Standards for Nursing Care of the Critically Ill* (AACN, 1980) are viewed as an extension of the Scope of Critical Care Nursing Practice and offer more specific guidance to nurses delivering care to critically ill patients.

Appendix E

AACN Position Statement
Principles of Critical Care Nursing Practice

The American Association of Critical-Care Nurses recognizes that its members are often faced with difficult and sensitive situations involving nurse-patient relationships. These Principles of Practice define, promote, and uphold the highest standards of personal conduct among members. A primary responsibility of the critical care nurse is promotion and restoration of health, as well as alleviation of suffering for persons and families facing critical illness. Entrusted with responsibility, the critical care nurse is accountable for respecting the individuality, wholeness, integrity, dignity, and rights of all humans.

1. The critical care nurse maintains the established standards of critical care nursing practice.

2. The critical care nurse continually updates knowledge necessary for competence.

3. The critical care nurse, as an integral part of the multidisciplinary health care

team, coordinates care delivered to patients and supports families with the critical care environment.

4. The critical care nurse recognizes the stresses involved in the critical care environment, and creates a compassionate and humanistic climate by providing support to patients, families, and colleagues. The critical care nurse must also identify psychological and physiological limitations when providing care.

5. The critical care nurse respects the rights of patients, families, and colleagues in the promotion or prolongation of life by individualizing each patient situation.

6. The critical care nurse identifies the values of patients, families, colleagues, and self, and incorporates those beliefs and attitudes into situations of ethical dilemmas.

7. The critical care nurse adheres to the *Code of Ethics* of the American Nurses' Association.

(American Nurses' Association, *Code for Nurses with Interpretive Statements, 1976.*)[now 1985]

Appendix F

AACN Position Statement
Ethics in Critical Care Research

The purpose of the American Association of Critical-Care Nurses (AACN) is to promote the health and welfare of mankind by advancing the science and art of critical care nursing. Goals identified by AACN include those of encouraging scientific investigation in critical care and promoting professionalism and accountability of nurses caring for the critically ill.

WHEREAS, research is essential for developing knowledge to benefit critically ill patients, and

WHEREAS, ethical principles of autonomy, beneficence, and justice should underlie the conduct of research in critical care units, and

WHEREAS, informed consent and peer review are two mechanisms to ensure that ethical principles are observed, and

WHEREAS, any research conducted in critical care units directly or indirectly affects the practice of critical care nursing, and

WHEREAS, nurses have an obligation to protect patients from unnecessary harm and unethical practices,

BE IT HEREBY RESOLVED THAT, the American Association of Critical-Care Nurses therefore supports conduct of research in a manner that assures that patients give informed consent for study participation, and conduct of research in a manner that assures that patients' rights continue to be safeguarded during conduct of the study.

To facilitate these goals, the American Association of Critical-Care Nurses advocates that:

1. Health care institutions establish formal multidisciplinary peer review boards to ensure that ethical principles that underlie the conduct of research are followed when research is conducted.

2. At least one professional nurse with equal voting rights be a regular member of all multidisciplinary peer review boards, including Institutional Review Boards (IRB).

3. Nursing administrations establish procedures that ensure communication between the investigator and nurses involved in conducting the study so that adequate information regarding the research and its risks and possible benefits are understood by critical care nurses who

   a) function in the caregiver role for critically ill patients involved in research studies,

   b) assist the researcher with data collection,

   c) are directly responsible for unit management, or

   d) are asked to answer questions of patient participants regarding study participation.

4. Nursing administrations establish mechanisms for addressing nursing concerns about critical care research.

Critically ill patients are in a position to benefit greatly from the results of research. Critically ill patients also constitute a potentially vulnerable population due to physiological, psychological, pharmacological, and environmental influences. It is, therefore, important to ensure that ethical principles underlie the conduct of any research involving the critically ill. Informed consent and peer review of research are two essential mechanisms for ensuring that basic ethical principles are observed when research involves human subjects.

Fifteen Questions and Answers on Ethical Issues in Critical Care Research

1. *What is the difference between research and practice?*

   Although practice and research often occur together and influence one another, differences exist in the purpose and focus of these two activities. In 1979 the National Commission for the Protection of Human Subjects of Biomedical and Behavioral Research (also called the Belmont Commission) defined ethical principles for the protection of human subjects of research. This commission distinguished between practice and research as follows:

   Practice consists of interventions designed solely to enhance the well-being of an individual, and that have a reasonable expectation of success. The purpose of practice is to provide diagnosis, preventive treatment, or therapy to particular patients.

Research consists of activities designed to test a hypothesis, permit conclusions to be drawn, and thereby to develop or contribute to general knowledge. Research is typically described in a formal protocol which identifies an objective and a set of procedures to measure how variables are related to that objective.

When critical care nurses participate in research activities, they have ethical responsibilities related to the conduct of research as well as to patient care.

2. *Why are critically ill patients "at risk" in research projects?*
Captive populations are at risk in research studies because of their dependency on a system. Critically ill patients compose a captive population and thus are placed at risk in a critical care setting.

The autonomy of critically ill patients may also be altered due to physiological, psychological, pharmacological, and environmental influences. Any of these influences may alter decision-making abilities.

Underlying disease processes may diminish a patient's mental clarity. Physical discomforts resulting from disease or medical/nursing interventions may affect a patient's autonomous judgment about whether to enter or continue to participate in a research study. Sensory alteration, degree of consciousness, or unstable hemodynamic states may influence autonomy.

Psychological stress may compromise ability to make clear decisions. Anxiety, depression, denial, or withdrawal may result from experiences with life-threatening illness. Communication barriers induced by medical instrumentation or pharmacological agents may increase the stress experienced. Pharmacological agents may also alter a critically ill patient's autonomous decision-making ability. Barbiturates, sedatives, and narcotics are examples of drugs that may sedate the patient and thus compromise mental abilities.

The foreign environment of the critical care unit may induce further stress. Strange equipment, excess noise and illumination, change in sleeping patterns, disruptive unit routines, or lack of contact with family members may create a feeling of helplessness. These stressors may make it more difficult for the patient to weigh the risks and benefits of research participation. As a result, capacity for self-determination may be wholly or partially lost, and critically ill patients may submit passively to research studies.

If critically ill patients cannot consent to enter a research study, family members or significant others may be asked to give second party consent. Physical exhaustion, psychological stress, or mounting hospitalization costs may affect the ability of family members or significant others to appropriately weigh the risks and benefits of the study.

Although critically ill patients constitute an "at risk" population, they should not be prevented from entering research trials simply because they are seriously ill. However, safeguards should be used to ensure protection of their rights and welfare. These safeguards include informed consent, peer review, and communication between the investigator and nursing staff.

3. *What are the basic ethical principles that should underlie the conduct of research involving human subjects?*

There are three ethical principles important to research: autonomy, beneficence, and justice. Autonomy is the fundamental ethical principle in first party consent (consent given by the individual). Beneficence is the fundamental ethical principle in second party consent (an individual acting in the best interest of the research subject). Justice is a fundamental principle in both first and second party consent.

First party consent is based on the principle of autonomy. This principle establishes a person's right to make a free and informed choice about whether to participate, not participate, or withdraw from a research study. Autonomy is based on the fundamental principle of respect for persons. There is no requirement that individuals be prevented from participating in a research study that involves risk. They must, however, be told about any potential risk(s) and be allowed to decide freely whether or not to enter the study.

If autonomy is diminished (the person is unconscious, mentally incompetent, or a small child), a person then has the right to additional safeguards. These safeguards involve securing the consent of the next of kin or guardian.

Second party consent is based on the principle of beneficence. This principle establishes a person's right to protection from harm. Guaranteeing this principle involves first giving a fair assessment of known risks and benefits and then monitoring the person's response during the study (if consent is given).

The principle of justice is involved in both first and second party consent. This principle establishes that research subjects be selected from a variety of groups and not solely from those likely to be vulnerable to coercion (persons with severe mental or physical illness or persons who are educationally or economically disadvantaged).

4. *What mechanisms facilitate the conduct of research according to ethical principles?*

Informed consent and peer review of research are two essential mechanisms for ensuring that basic ethical principles are observed when research involves human subjects.

Informed consent is the knowing consent of a competent individual who is able to exercise free power of choice without undue inducement or any element of force, fraud, deceit, or any other form of coercion. Informed consent can also be given by an individual's legal representative if the individual is not competent to personally give consent.

Federal regulations mandate that human subjects have the following rights when participating in a research study:

a) To be informed of the nature and purpose of the experiment.

b) To be given an explanation of the procedures to be followed in the experiment, and any drug or device to be utilized.

c) To be given a description of any attendant discomforts and risks reasonably to be expected from the experiment.

d) To be given an explanation of any benefits to the subject reasonably to be expected from the experiment, if applicable.

e) To be given a disclosure of any appropriate alternative procedures, drugs, or devices that might be advantageous to the subject, and their relative risks and benefits.

f) To be informed of the avenues of treatment, if any, available to the subject after the experiment if complications should arise.

g) To be given an opportunity to ask any questions concerning the experiment or the procedure involved.

h) To be instructed that consent to participate in the experiment may be withdrawn at any time, and the subject may discontinue participation in the experiment without prejudice.

i) To be given a copy of any signed and dated written consent form used in relation to the experiment.

j) To be given the opportunity to decide to consent or not to consent to an experiment without the intervention of any element of force, fraud, deceit, duress, coercion, or undue influence on the subject's decision.

Participation of patients in research is based on trust that their rights will be respected when the research design is developed, when data are collected, and when findings of the research are shared with others.

The informed consent process, therefore, requires that the potential research subject a) be informed, b) be competent, c) have adequate information to make an enlightened decision, and d) be allowed to decide freely whether to enter a research trial. To the extent that any of these four necessary elements is jeopardized, the validity of the informed consent may be questioned.

The goals of peer review are to ascertain that the essential components of informed consent have been addressed, and to protect human subjects from undue research risks and from invasion of privacy. The scientific merits of a study are considered and weighed against foreseeable risks.

Peer review of research should determine that 1) risks to subjects are minimized, 2) risks to subjects are reasonable in relation to anticipated benefits, 3) selection of subjects is equitable, 4) informed consent will be sought from each prospective subject or the subject's legally authorized representative, 5) informed consent will be appropriately documented, 6) the data collection process will be monitored to ensure the safety of subjects, and 7) adequate provisions are included to protect the privacy of subjects and to maintain the confidentiality of data.

5. *Why obtain informed consent?*

Informed consent should be obtained for ethical and legal reasons. The American Nurses' Association Human Rights Guidelines for Nurses in Clinical and Other Research states that it is the ethical responsibility of the professional nurse to determine that the potential human subject is informed about the nature of the research. AACN's *Standards for Nursing Care of the Critically Ill* also emphasizes this responsibility. Informed consent is a legal requirement when federal funding is involved. The federal government has mandated specific guidelines to be followed for achieving informed consent for federally funded research projects. Some states have also enacted laws to protect the rights of human subjects. Both investigators and caregivers involved in research studies are bound by these regulations. State laws apply to all researchers in a state, not just those who receive federal funding.

Informed consent and peer review also provide personal liability protection. A written consent provides protection should a lawsuit be instituted. When a patient signs a consent, there is written documentation that the patient was apprised of possible risks and benefits before entering the study.

6. *Who can obtain informed consent?*

Responsibility for obtaining informed consent ultimately rests with the principal investigator. The principal investigator may personally obtain consent or delegate this responsibility to another member of the research team. Such delegation is acceptable if the person who obtains the consent understands the study, is able to sufficiently answer a patient's questions, and is cognizant of the elements of informed consent. It is the ethical obligation of all individuals involved in the study to assure that informed consent has actually been obtained.

7. *Who can give consent?*

Competent adults. Informed consent can be given by autonomous individuals who are able to make decisions about their own care.

Adolescents between 13 years and legal age. Adolescents 13 years to legal age (defined by each state) should sign a regular adult consent form, also countersigned by a parent. Liberated minors may give consent in some states.

Children. It is generally recognized that, by the age of seven, most children are capable of some reflective judgement and moral reasoning. Federal guidelines suggest that children aged seven through twelve years of age be given a simplified version of the consent form and be asked to assent (agree to participate in the research) along with their parents. Under federal guidelines, assent of the child is not a necessary condition for proceeding with the research if the child's understanding is limited so that he or she cannot reasonably be consulted, or if the research holds a prospect of direct benefit important to the health or well-being of the child.

Ideally, informed consent should be obtained from both parents of children under the age of seven. If there is disagreement between the child's parents about study entry, the child should not be included as a research subject.

Mentally incompetent or unconscious patients. When a patient is unable to understand a research project due to disease, illness, or injury, such a project should not be undertaken unless there is more direct benefit than there is risk. Second party or proxy consent can be given by others when subjects cannot give adequate consent on their own behalf. Individuals who can give second party consent include 1) spouse or legal guardian, 2) parent, 3) adult children, 4) adult grandchildren, 5) brothers and sisters, 6) nephews and nieces, and 7) grandparents. If there is disagreement among relatives, state regulations should be consulted regarding priority of next of kin.

8. *When is incomplete disclosure justified?*
   Incomplete disclosure presents a special problem. When this approach is used, the potential subject is not informed of all aspects of the research because revealment would lessen the validity and reliability of the research findings. Incomplete disclosure may be used in double-blind randomized studies or compliance studies. In double-blind randomized studies, subjects are informed that they will be randomly placed (by chance) in one of several groups. In compliance research the specific purpose of the research or some of the features of the research may not be disclosed until the research is concluded. The rationale for incorporating secrecy into the procedure should be explained in the study proposal and the peer review board should concur that incomplete disclosure is appropriate. When incomplete disclosure is used, peer review boards may require that the investigator inform patients about the purpose of the study after its completion.

9. *When is a consent not required?*
   Ethical principles require that either written or oral consent be obtained from patients. When oral consent is requested, patients should be given the same information orally as would be conveyed in a written consent. They should also be given an opportunity to ask questions of the researcher.
   Peer review boards may approve certain research studies without requiring consent. Under federal guidelines (Code of Federal Regulations), written consent is not required when the only research activities in which human subjects will participate fall in one of the following categories:

   a) Research conducted in established or commonly accepted educational settings, involving normal educational practices, such as (i) research on regular and special education instructional strategies, or (ii) research on the effectiveness of or the comparison of instructional techniques, curricula, or classroom management methods.

   b) Research involving the use of educational tests (cognitive, diagnostic, aptitude, achievement), if information taken from these sources is recorded in such a manner that subjects cannot be identified, directly or through identifiers linked to the subjects.

c) Research involving survey or interview procedures, except where all of the following conditions exist: (i) responses are recorded in such a manner that the human subjects can be identified, directly or through identifiers linked to the subjects, (ii) the subject's responses, if they become known outside the research, could reasonably place the subject at risk of criminal or civil liability or be damaging to the subject's financial standing or employability, and (iii) the research deals with sensitive aspects of the subject's own behavior such as illegal conduct, drug use, sexual behavior, or use of alcohol. All research involving survey or interview procedures is exempt, without exception, when the respondents are elected or appointed public officials or candidates for public office.

d) Research involving the observation (including observation by participants) of public behavior, except where all of the following conditions exist: (i) observations are recorded in such a manner that the human subjects can be identified, directly or through identifiers linked to the subjects, (ii) the observations recorded about the individual, if they became known outside the research, could reasonably place the subject at risk of criminal or civil liability or be damaging to the subject's financial standing or employability, (iii) the research deals with sensitive aspects of the subject's own behavior, such as illegal conduct, drug use, sexual behavior, or use of alcohol.

e) Research involving the collection or study of existing data, documents, records, pathological specimens, or diagnostic specimens, if these sources are publicly available or if the information is recorded by the investigator in such a manner that the subject cannot be identified, directly or through identifiers linked to the subject.

In addition, peer review boards may approve a consent procedure which does not include, or which alters, some or all of the elements of informed consent if

a) the research entails no more than minimal risk and involves no procedures that require written consent outside of the context of a research project;

b) the waiver or alteration will not adversely affect the rights and welfare of the subjects;

c) the consent form would be the only record identifying the subject, and potential harm could result from any breach of confidentiality; or

d) the research could not be carried out without the waiver, and subjects will receive additional information after participation.
(See Question #8, When is incomplete disclosure justified?)

In critical care research, some or all of the elements of informed consent may not be required when a research trial is designed to validate present care practices (i.e., compare two currently used suctioning techniques; compare two methods of recording pulmonary artery pressures). These procedures are part of routine patient care, would be carried out whether or not the research trial were being conducted, and are therefore considered to be of minimal risk to the patient. In compliance research, the consent may not be required to explicitly describe the study's purpose if revealing the purpose would bias the subject's replies. In research involving issues which could place the subject at risk of criminal or civil liability, requirement for written consent also may be waived. As noted previously, federal guidelines do not require review of all research. Peer review boards may elect to consider only research which must be reviewed under federal guidelines. Peer review boards may also elect to be more restrictive and require review of research protocols that are exempt by federal guidelines. Still others may require all proposals to be submitted but only review proposals as required by federal guidelines. Also, personal liability issues may prompt the individual investigator to decide to obtain written consent even though it is not a requirement.

10. *What is an institutional review board (IRB)?*

An IRB is a type of peer review board. This specific type of review is required by Congress when institutions perform research supported by federal funds. Congress has mandated that such institutions must establish an institutional review board (IRB). Specific requirements have been legislated for IRB membership, approval criteria, documentation, and record-keeping procedures.

Federal guidelines require that an IRB be composed of a minimum of five members, at least one of whom is a lay member not associated with the institution. Institutional review boards include members chosen from health care professionals directly or indirectly involved in research studies. Many include a lawyer, a member of the clergy, and an ethicist. AACN advocates that at least one professional nurse with equal voting rights be a regular member of all IRBs.

Before approving a research study, the IRB is required to determine that 1) risks to subjects are minimized, 2) risks are reasonable in relation to anticipated benefits, 3) selection of subjects is equitable, 4) informed consent will be sought from each subject, 5) consent will be documented, 6) privacy guaranteed, and 7) appropriate additional safeguards included for subjects with diminished autonomy. The scientific merits of a proposal are weighed against all foreseeable risks. The IRB will then decide to approve, disapprove, or reconsider after suggested changes are made.

11. *What review is appropriate if your institution does not have an IRB?*

Research supported by federal funds or conducted within an institution receiving any federal funding is required to undergo IRB review. No funding will be awarded unless the principal investigator documents that the study received IRB review and approval. There is, however, no legal requirement that research which is not supported by federal funds or not conducted within an institution receiving federal funds be reviewed by an IRB or research review committee except as required by individual institutional policy. Consequently, nurses may be asked to participate as data collectors in studies that have not undergone research review. Nurses may also conduct research without such a review if the institution or agency has no review requirement and federal funding is not involved.

While there is no legal requirement that all research receive peer or IRB review, such review is an ethical responsibility. Many institutions have established peer research review committees modeled after federal IRB guidelines.

If no review committee is established in the institution in which research is being undertaken, the principal investigator should follow the established institutional policies and procedures to obtain approval. Other options for the investigator include review in an institution with an established IRB or peer review.

Guidelines for setting up an IRB can be obtained from the Office for Protection from Research Risks, Department of Health and Human Services, National Institutes of Health. Additional information sheets can be obtained from the Food and Drug Administration, Office of Health Affairs, HFY-20, 5600 Fishers Lane, Rockville, MD 20857.

12. *What are the responsibilities of the principal investigator (PI)?*

Before initiating a research endeavor, the principal investigator (PI) is responsible for being familiar with ethical principles, designing the study with consideration of human subjects' rights, obtaining peer review and establishing a mechanism for securing informed consent. While the study is being conducted, the PI is responsible for establishing and maintaining communication with all persons involved in the study and for answering questions or concerns during the data collection period.

It is the researchers' obligation to share information regarding the purpose, methodology, risks, and benefits of the study with those caring for patient participants in a research study. The researcher must provide sufficient information that nurses functioning in the caregiver role can make appropriate decisions to notify the PI if the patient's condition changes, and continued study participation appears to place the patient at additional risk. As an example, a patient participating in a suctioning study may require different ventilator settings before the trial is completed. As a result, data collection may need to be rescheduled for another time or day.

The PI is responsible for reporting all untoward reactions or protocol changes to the peer review board and caregivers. If information is obtained during the study which may affect the patient's continued participation in the study, the PI should share this information with the patient.

After the research study is completed, it is the responsibility of the PI to submit a final report to the peer review board and, if requested, to the caregivers. Health professionals who assist with research as data collectors or research subjects should be acknowledged by the PI.

13. *What are some mechanisms to ensure optimal patient care while patients participate in a research study?*

    A nurse's primary ethical obligation is to patients, as opposed to any other professional relationship, when there is a conflict of interests.

    The professional nurse should be a patient advocate who demands, attains, and provides the highest quality of health care for patients and families. In the role of patient advocate, the nurse must judge between the requirements of the study and the changing needs of the patient.

    Nurses are at the patient's bedside 24 hours a day and are responsible for continually assessing and evaluating patient response to the treatment being provided. On the basis of this assessment and evaluation, the nurse must decide whether to continue the present data collection plan or to suggest to the principal investigator that changes may be indicated. Occasionally, changes in patient condition may necessitate temporary or permanent removal from the study. In making this decision, and acting on it, the nurse may experience conflict between the obligations to the patient and expectations of the research team.

    It is important to remember that primary responsibility for appropriate conduct of the research rests with the principal investigator. Nurses in the patient-advocate role are not responsible for policing the researchers but are responsible for assuring that patients' rights are respected.

14. *What should a critical care nurse consider before taking an ethical stance regarding a research study?*

    A thorough assessment of a situation is essential before taking an ethical stance. The nurse should

    a) identify the questionable practice or activity.

    b) consider how personal values influence perception of their situation.

    c) identify the risks and benefits to all parties involved.

    d) verify the facts with someone familiar with the research process.

    e) determine the amount of harm that may come from not communicating the ethical concern.

    f) bring the observations to the attention of the PI if it can be established that ethical principles, laws, rules, or regulations have been violated. Clarification of the research protocol may be needed.

    g) take the information to the nursing administration and/or peer review board if further clarification is needed after talking to the PI.

    h) utilize state and national nurses' associations to find resources to assist in resolving the ethical dilemma if unsatisfied with the results sought within the institution.

Nurses should be aware that their ethical beliefs color their perceptions of an ethical dilemma. Nurses are not morally obligated to cooperate in experimental procedures about which they have ethical concerns. Indeed, they may have an ethical obligation to refuse to participate in such activities and to bring their concerns to the attention of others who can assist the patient and review the appropriateness of the research activity.

Personal consequences may exist for both reporting and not reporting perceived ethical injustices. Individuals perceived as interfering with another's project may be ostracized, harassed, or even fired. However, the personal consequences of not reporting conduct which violates one's ethical principles may be unacceptable to the nurse and to the profession.

15. *What obligations do nursing administrators have in addressing nursing concerns about critical care research?*

Nursing administrators should exhibit leadership in developing a multidisciplinary peer review research board if none is established. Nursing administration should support the inclusion of at least one professional nurse, with equal voting rights, as a regular member of this review board and on established IRBs.

Nursing administrators should establish procedures that ensure communication between the investigator and nurses involved in critical care research and review mechanisms to ensure that these procedures are followed.

Nursing administrators should define a process for review of ethical stances of nurses concerning critical care research. An assessment of the stance should include defining the ethical stance clearly and verifying the accuracy of the situation with others. Determining the ethical principles involved in the stance along with the actual and/or potential effects on clinical nursing practice are essential. Violations of ethical principles should be reported to the chairperson of the peer review research board.

Nursing administrators have the ethical obligation to support a nurse who reports a reasonable ethical stance on questionable research practices or activities. The nurse should be assisted in analyzing potential resolutions for the dilemma. Appropriate referral to multidisciplinary peer review research boards and/or to state or local nursing organization ethics committees should be made if the dilemma cannot be resolved within the institution.

To lessen the potential for ethical conflicts in critical care research, nursing administration should inform nurses, before employment, of research roles they may be expected to perform.

By all of the above means, it is anticipated that conflicts between the nurse's obligations to the patient and the expectations of the research team will be lessened or resolved.

References

AACN: Bylaws, Article II, Purpose and Goals, 1983
AACN: Standards for Nursing Care of the Critically Ill. Reston, VA, Reston Publishing, 1981
ANA: Commission on Nursing Research. Human Rights Guidelines for Nurses in Clinical and Other Research. Kansas City, MO, ANA, 1975

Barkes P: Bioethics and informed consent in American health care delivery. J Adv Nurs 4:23–38, 1979

Cassileth BR, Zupkis RV, Sutton-Smith K, Marsh V: Informed consent—why are its goals imperfectly realized? N Engl J Med 302:896–900, 1980

Davis A, Aroskar M: Informed consent. In Davis A, Aroskar M: Ethical Dilemmas and Nursing Practice. Norwalk, CT, Appleton-Century-Crofts, 1983

Hannah GT, Christian WP, Clark HB: Preservation of Client Rights: A Handbook for Practitioners Providing Therapeutic Educational and Rehabilitative Services. New York, Free Press, 1981

Loanzon P, Weissman C, Askanazi J: Clinical research and nursing in the intensive care unit. Heart Lung 12:480–484, 1983

Miller P: A guide to informed consent. Dimensions of Critical Care Nursing 1:304–306, 1982

Office for Protection from Research Risks (OPRR). The Belmont Report. The National Commission for the Protection of Human Subjects of Biomedical and Behavioral Research. Dept of Health, Education, and Welfare. April 18, 1979

OPRR Reports. Protection of Human Subjects. Code of Federal Regulations 45 CFR 46, Dept of Health and Human Services, March 8, 1983

US Dept of Health and Human Services. A Suggested Self-Evaluation Guide: Human Subject Protection Institutional Review Boards. Office of Health Affairs, FDA, Rockville, MD, 20857, April 1984

US Dept of Health, Education, and Welfare, General Administration. Protection of Human Subjects. Federal Register 39:18914–18920, 1974

US Dept of Health, Education, and Welfare, National Institutes of Health. Protection of Human Subjects Policies and Procedures. Federal Register 38:31738–31749, 1973

US National Commission for the Protection of Human Subjects of Biomedical and Behavioral Research. Research Involving Children; Report and Recommendations. Washington, DC, Government Printing Office, 1977

University of California, Los Angeles, Office of Human Use Protection. Rights of Human Subjects in Medical Experiments. January 1979

Appendix G

AACN Position Statement
Clarification of Resuscitation Status in Critical Care Settings

Critical care nurses practice in an environment where life and death are becoming less clearly defined. As 24-hour bedside practitioners, critical care nurses need clear medical treatment goals to facilitate decision making. Frequently there are no written resuscitation orders or those written may be ambiguous. As a result, nurses are often confronted by a lack of or confusing directions in resuscitation efforts when time is of the essence.

Therefore, guidelines must be written denoting levels of resuscitation efforts for each patient within the critical care setting.[1]

Therefore, development and uniform implementation of the guidelines must be a collaborative effort between medicine and nursing (AACN, 1981). Nursing administrators of critical care units are responsible and accountable for responding to the critical care nurses' need to develop such guidelines when guidelines do not already exist.

Thus, guidelines must include, but are not limited to the following components:

- A system and process for classification of patient resuscitation status—a mechanism for documentation and review of resuscitation status and the process used to arrive at this decision
- A mechanism for assurance of patient and family rights
- Use of clearly defined terminology, and thus, the critical care nurse will:
  assure quality of patient care regardless of resuscitation status
  review daily with the physician the current resuscitation status of the patient
  reflect the resuscitation status in the patient's plan of care.

Note

1. Guidelines must reflect legal statutes applicable in each state.

References

AACN: Standards for Nursing Care of the Critically Ill, p 37. Reston, VA: Reston Publishing Company, 1981

Pontoppidan H: Optimal care for the hopelessly ill patient. N Engl J Med 295(7):362–364, 1976

Powner DJ, Grenvik A: Triage in patient care; from expected recovery to brain death. Heart Lung 8(6):1103–1108, 1979

Selected Readings

Aroskar M et al: The nurse and orders not to resuscitate. Hastings Cent Rep 7(4):27–28, 1977

Canhizzo CJ: "No code blue"—Should the order be entered in writing on the patient's permanent medical records? Hospital Forum 19(1):46, 1977

Gillick M: The ethics of cardiopulmonary resuscitation: Another look. Ethics in Science and Medicine 7(3–4):161–169, 1980

Greenlaw J: Orders not to resuscitate: Dilemma for acute care as well as long term facilities. Law, Medicine & Health Care 10(1):29–31, 1982

Huffman BR: No code? Slow code? Show code? Am J Nurs 82:133–135, 1982

LeBlang TR: Does your hospital have a policy for no-code orders? Legal Aspects of Medical Practice 9(3):4–5, 9(4):5—8, 1981

Miya PA: Do not resuscitate: When nurse's duties conflict with patient's rights. Dimensions of Critical Care Nursing 3(5):293–298, 1984

President's Commission for the Study of Ethical Problems in Medicine and Bioethical and Behavioral Research. Making Health Care Decisions: A Report on the Ethical and Legal Implications of Informed Consent in the Patient-Practitioner Relationship. Washington, DC, Government Printing Office, October 1982

Slemenda MB: Brain death determination and management in children. Crit Care Nurse (May–June):63–66, 1983

(Adopted by the AACN Board of Directors, February 1985)

Appendix H

AACN Position Statement
Collaborative Practice Model: The Organization of Human Resources in Critical Care Units

Collaboration has been identified as a pivotal component in the delivery of quality health care. The Joint Commission on Accreditation of Hospitals acknowledges the importance of collaboration in critical care units by requiring that the activities of such units be guided by a multidisciplinary approach that includes both nursing and medical input.[1] The National Commission on Nursing also urges collaboration by proposing as an immediate goal that trustees and health care administrators "promote and support complementary practice between nurses and physicians" and that they "examine organizational structure to ensure that nurse administrators are part of the policy-making bodies of the institution and have authority to collaborate on an equal footing with the medical leaders in the institution."[2] This should clearly extend to the unit level where care is delivered.

Recognizing that the impetus for true collaboration must originate with health care professionals themselves, the Board of Directors of the American Association of Critical-Care Nurses and the Council of the Society of Critical Care Medicine commissioned a task force of experienced critical care practitioners, managers, and educators to identify principles by which critical care units could successfully function through collaboration. Because different unit environments and hospital structures exist, no model is likely to be universally applicable. However, regardless of these differences, certain principles must be incorporated into the unit structure in order to assure optimal functioning of the unit.

Principles

1. Responsibility and accountability for effective functioning of a critical care unit must be vested in physician and nurse directors who are on an equal decision-making level.

2. These directors must be appropriately prepared and educated. In addition to competence in patient management, they need knowledge and experience in the following areas: management principles, resources management, and skills in interpersonal relationships (including conflict resolution).

3. The organizational structure of a critical care unit must ensure that physicians are autonomous when dealing with issues that affect medical practice.

4. The organizational structure of a critical care unit must ensure that nurses are autonomous when dealing with issues that affect nursing practice.

5. Some aspects of patient care require interdependence between physicians and nurses. These aspects must be identified and addressed jointly.

6. Every critically ill person requires medical and nursing care. The services of ad-

ditional disciplines may also be required in specific situations. In order to provide a holistic approach, the care delivered by other health team members must be coordinated by the physician and nurse directors.

7. Unit support services must be organized to enable the directors to optimally carry out their primary responsibilities in the practice of their respective disciplines (i.e., patient care).

8. The directors are accountable for the evaluation of the quality and efficiency of care and the financial provision of that care. They must develop a unit-specific system for the evaluation of care on a timely basis.

9. The directors are responsible for creating and maintaining an environment in which individuals have opportunities to realize their potentials.

10. Close collaboration between the directors is essential for successful management. This collaboration can be enhanced by daily rounds, weekly meetings, and other means that will ensure continuous, open communication.

Notes

1. Joint Commission on Accreditation of Hospitals: Accreditation Manual for Hospitals, p 182. Chicago, JCAH, 1982

2. National Commission on Nursing: Initial Report and Preliminary Recommendations, p 62. Chicago, JCAH, 1981

(Adopted by AACN Board of Directors and SCCM Council, October 1982)

Appendix I

AACN Position Statement
AACN's Purpose, Long-Range Goals, and Intermediate Strategies

Purpose

To promote the health and welfare of those experiencing critical illness by advancing the science and art of critical care nursing.

Long-Range Goals

1) To promote delivery of care in accordance with standards of nursing care of the critically ill.

2) To promote education of critical care nurses in accordance with standards for education and practice.

3) To provide educational opportunities for nurses caring for the critically ill.

4) To promote professionalism and accountability of nurses caring for the critically ill.

5) To facilitate effective communication among critical care nurses.

6) To encourage scientific investigation in critical care.

7) To maintain effective communication between critical care nursing and its publics regarding issues that have an impact on critical care nursing.

Intermediate Strategies

I. *To facilitate the ability of AACN members to practice within the framework of
professional nursing.*

Competence in practice is the goal toward which critical care nursing strives.
It is our greatest asset in these times when quality care in a cost-effective manner
is the key to survival.

Practicing within the framework of professional nursing encompasses a variety of aspects, including

- Implementing the nursing process.
- Incorporating into practice AACN's Definition of Critical Care Nursing:
    In *Nursing: A Social Policy Statement*, the American Nurses' Association
    defines nursing as "the diagnosis and treatment of human responses to
    actual or potential health problems." Critical care nursing is that specialty
    within nursing that deals specifically with human responses to life-threat-
    ening problems.
- Identifying nursing phenomena.
- Enhancing clinical analysis and problem-solving skills.
- Addressing issues related to critical care nursing practice, i.e., analyzing an
    issue and determining a course of action.
- Identifying and acknowledging the impact of critical care nursing on patient
    outcomes.

II. *To provide information to nursing and its publics in an effort to demonstrate the
value of professional critical care nursing practice through data collection, analysis, and dissemination.*

As an organization, AACN has the resources to acquire and disseminate information related to the important impact of critical care nursing practice on patients. AACN can provide information to critical care nurses and others about that
impact on health care. It is in the interest of our organization of critical care
nurses and our profession to provide that informational support to critical care
nurses and others.

In an era of cost control, the value of adequate numbers of nurses to care for
patients, appropriately prepared nurses to care for patients, and professional
nurses versus other health care professionals performing patient care may be
overlooked. How does the individual manager or staff nurse respond to threats
against professional nursing practice in critical care? Specific data consistently
provide the most persuasive argument. Most individuals do not have access to or

the resources for and the interest in acquiring and disseminating data to support critical care nursing practice.

III. *To influence the environment in which critical care nursing is practiced through facilitating member activities, developing leadership skills and providing management tools, and targeting general association activities.*

AACN has demonstrated an increasing commitment to influence the environment in which critical care is practiced. We have issued position statements, such as "Use of Technical Personnel in Critical Care Settings" and "Collaborative Practice Model"; we have established the ANA legislative liaison and provided input to legislators regarding issues related to critical care, among many other actions. While AACN should continue activities at the national level, we recognize that our members are an untapped source with great potential for influencing the environment. AACN needs to invest resources in developing leadership and management skills in our members and facilitating their involvement in influencing the environment. We need to teach our members how to use the data that AACN will disseminate (see Strategy II) to assure high-quality patient care. The overall impact will be an exponential increase in influence compared with national AACN activities alone.

(Adopted by the AACN Board of Directors, 1984)

Appendix J

AACN Position Statement
Process for Addressing Practice, Political, and Professional Issues

Controversial legislative and judicial issues in health care have the potential for major impact on critical care nursing. From time to time, these issues are brought to the attention of the AACN president and Board of Directors from a variety of sources, including chapters, individual members, other nursing organizations, and the consumer public. These individuals and groups frequently request information concerning the Association's official position on the particular issue.

As the world's largest specialty nursing organization, AACN's position statements represent an important responsibility for the president, board members, and the Association itself. When requests for AACN position statements began to increase, the Public Affairs and Clinical Practice Committees developed a policy and process for addressing practice, political, and professional issues. The accompanying diagram outlines the process approved by the board of directors in 1983.

The process is as follows: AACN's president will be informed of all issues brought to the association for action, and will screen each one in order to appropriately delegate responsibility for determining relevance and priority. For example, what impli-

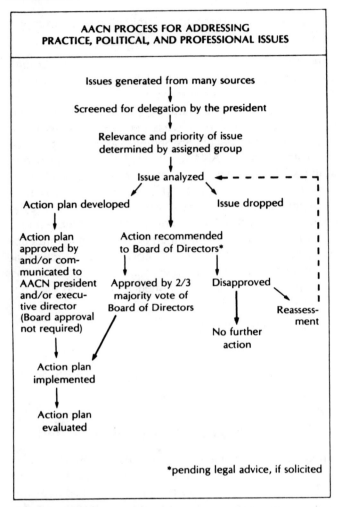

**AACN PROCESS FOR ADDRESSING
PRACTICE, POLITICAL, AND PROFESSIONAL ISSUES**

Issues generated from many sources

Screened for delegation by the president

Relevance and priority of issue
determined by assigned group

Issue analyzed

Action plan developed

Issue dropped

Action plan approved by and/or communicated to AACN president and/or executive director (Board approval not required)

Action recommended to Board of Directors*

Approved by 2/3 majority vote of Board of Directors

Disapproved

Reassessment

No further action

Action plan implemented

Action plan evaluated

*pending legal advice, if solicited

cations does the issue have for critical care nursing practice or for nursing in general? What are the potential effects of the recommended action or of no action?

When faced with controversial issues, developing a position statement is only one of several alternatives available to the AACN Board of Directors. The Board may approve the action, disapprove it and request reassessment, or disapprove it and take no further action.

Bibliography

Abrams N: A contrary view of the nurse as patient advocate. Nurs Forum 17:258–267, 1978

Abrams N, Buckner MD: Medical Ethics: A Clinical Textbook and Reference for the Health Care Professions. Cambridge, MIT Press, 1983

Allport G, Vernon P, Lindzey G: A Study of Values. Boston, Houghton Mifflin, 1960

American Academy of Pediatrics Infant Bioethics Task Force and Consultants: Guidelines for infant bioethics committees. Pediatrics 74:306–310, 1984

American Association of Critical-Care Nurses: Position Statement. Scope of Critical Care Nursing Practice. Newport Beach, CA, AACN, 1980

AACN: Position Statement. Principles of Critical Care Nursing Practice. Newport Beach CA, AACN, 1981

AACN: Position Statement. Use of Technical Personnel in Critical Care Settings. Newport Beach, CA, AACN, 1983

AACN: Position Statement. Definition of Critical Care Nursing. Newport Beach, CA, AACN, 1984

AACN: Historical Archives. Disk 100: AACN HIST. Newport Beach, CA, AACN, 1985

AACN: AACN's Statement on Ethics in Critical Care Nursing Research, Newport Beach, CA, AACN, 1986

American College of Physicians Ethics Manual. Part II. Research, other ethical issues. Recommended reading. (Ad Hoc Committee on Medical Ethics.) Ann Intern Med 101:263–274, 1984

American Medical Association: Proceedings, New Orleans, May 1869. Medical News 20:339–351, 1969

American Nurses' Association: Guidelines for Implementing the Code for Nurses. Kansas City, MO, ANA, 1980

ANA: Committee on Ethics. Ethics References for Nurses. Kansas City, MO, ANA, 1982

ANA: Statement on Nurses' Participation in Capital Punishment. Kansas City, MO, ANA, 1983

ANA: Code for Nurses with Interpretive Statements. Kansas City, MO, ANA, 1985

Anonymous: A Lady: The Young Lady's Friend (improved stereotype ed). Boston, American Stationers' Company, 1837

Aquinas T: Summa Theologiae, Batten RJ (trans). Vol 34, Charity, (par 2a2ae, quest 25, pt 4). New York, Blackfriars and McGraw-Hill, 1975

Aristotle: Nichomachean Ethics. Ostwald M (trans): Indianapolis, Bobbs-Merrill, 1962

Aristotle: Nichomachean Ethics, bk V, chap 11, 1138a–1720. Indianapolis, Library of Liberal Arts, 1962

Ashley JA: Nurses in American history, nurses and early feminism. Am J Nurs 75:1465, 1975

Baier B: The Moral Point of View: A Rational Basis of Ethics. Ithaca, Cornell University Press, 1958

Bandura A, Walters R: Social Learning and Personality Development. New York, Holt, Rinehart & Winston, 1963

Bartling v Superior Court, 147 Cal App 3d 1006, 1983

Bartling v Superior Court, 163 Cal App 3d 186, 1984

Beauchamp TL, Childress JF: Principles of Biomedical Ethics. New York, Oxford University Press, 1979

Beauchamp TL, Childress JF: Principles of Biomedical Ethics, 2nd ed. New York, Oxford University Press, 1983

Benjamin M, Curtis J: Ethics in Nursing. New York, Oxford University Press, 1981

Benjamin M, Curtis J: Virtue and the practice of nursing. In Shelp EE: Virtue and Medicine, pp 275–288. Dordrecht, D Reidel, 1985.

Bentham J: The principles and morals of legislation. In Melden AI: Ethical Theories: A Book of Readings, 2nd ed. Englewood Cliffs, Prentice-Hall, 1967

Birnbaum ML: High tech/low touch. Crit Care Med 12:1006, 1984

Bowie N: Role as a moral concept in health care. J Med Philos 7:57–63, 1982

Brandon AN, Hill DR: Selected list of books and journals for the small medical library. Bull Med Libr Assoc 73:176–205, 1985

Brandon AN, Hill DR: Selected list of nursing books and journals. Nurs Outlook 34:74–82, 1986

Bruce DA: The Pathophysiology of Increased Intracranial Pressure. Upjohn, Current Concepts, 1978

Burch GE: Changing concepts in cardiovascular therapy—a quarter century perspective. Am Heart J 93:413, 1977

Cadmus RR: Special care for the critical case. Hospitals 28:65, 1954

Cadmus RR: Intensive care reaches silver anniversary. Hospitals 54:98, 1980

Campbell AV: Moral Dilemmas in Medicine: A Coursebook in Ethics for Doctors and Nurses, 3rd ed. New York, Churchill Livingstone, 1984

Canadian Nurses' Association: CNA Code of Ethics: An Ethical Basis for Nursing in Canada. Ottawa, CNA, 1980

Cassel CK, Meier DE, Traines ML: Selected bibliography of recent articles in ethics and geriatrics. J Am Geriatr Soc 34:399–409, 1986

Chassin MR: Costs and outcomes of medical intensive care. MED Care 20:165, 1982

Christine M: Integrity in interprofessional relationships. In Agich GJ (ed): Responsibility in Health Care, pp 163–184. Dordrecht, D Reidel, 1982

Churchill L: The professionalization of ethics: Some implications for accountability in medicine. Soundings 60:40–53, 1977

Ciske KL: Accountability: The essence of primary nursing. Am J Nurs 79:891–894, 1979

Clark C: Classroom Skills for Nurse Educators. New York, Springer-Verlag, 1978

Committee on Biomedical Ethics of the Los Angeles County Medical Association and Los Angeles County Bar Association: Principles and Guidelines Concerning the Foregoing of Life-Sustaining Treatment for Adult Patients. Adopted by the Board of Trustees of the Los Angeles County Bar Association on December 11, 1985, and by the Council of the Los Angeles County Medical Association on January 6, 1986

Cone TE: History of the Care and Feeding of the Premature Infant. Boston, Little, Brown & Co, 1985

Cranford R, Doudera AE: Institutional Ethics Committees and Health Care Decision-Making. Ann Arbor, Health Administration Press, 1984

Creighton H: Law Every Nurse Should Know, 5th ed. Philadelphia, WB Saunders, 1986

Cullen DJ, Ferrara LC, Briggs BA, Walker PF, Gilbert J: Survival, hospitalization charges and follow-up results in critically ill patients. N Engl J Med 294:982, 1976

Curtin LL, Flaherty MJ: Nursing Ethics: Theories and Pragmatics. Bowie, MD, Brady Communications Co, 1982

Dalis G, Strasser B: Teaching Strategies for Values Awareness and Decision Making for Nurses. St Louis, CV Mosby, 1977

Davis A: Ethical and legal issues in a technological age. In Hockey L: Recent Advances in Nursing: Current Issues in Nursing. Edinburgh, Churchill Livingstone, in press

Davis A, Aroskar M: Ethical Dilemmas and Nursing Practice, 2nd ed. East Norwalk, CT, Appleton-Century-Crofts, 1983

Day HW: History of coronary care units. Am J Cardiol 30:405, 1972

Dennison C: Nursing service in the emergency room. Am J Nurs 42:777, 1975

Dock LL: The duty of this society in public work. In Proceedings of the Tenth Annual Convention of the American Society of Superintendents of Training Schools, Pittsburgh, Oct 7–9, 1903. Baltimore, JH Furst Co, 1904

Donagan A: The Theory of Morality. Chicago, University of Chicago Press, 1977

Donahue MP: Nursing—The Finest Art, an Illustrated History. St Louis, CV Mosby, 1985

Doudera AE, Peters JD: Legal and Ethical Aspects of Treating Critically and Terminally Ill Patients. Ann Arbor, AUPHA Press, 1982

Downie RS: Roles and Values: An Introduction to Social Ethics. London, Methuen London Ltd, 1971

Dreves KD: Nurses in American history—Vassar training camp for nurses. Am J Nurs 75:2000, 1975

Drews E, Lipson L: Values and Humanity. New York, St Martin's Press, 1971

Duff RS: Guidelines for deciding care of critically ill or dying patients. Pediatrics 64:17–23, 1979

Duff RS: Counseling families and deciding care of severely defective children: A way of coping with medical Vietnam. Pediatrics 67:317, 1981

Duska R, Whelan M: Moral Development: A Guide to Piaget and Kohlberg. New York, Paulist Press, 1975

Eisenberg PD: Duties to oneself: A new defense sketched. Review of Metaphysics 20:602–634, 1967

English HB, English A: A Comprehensive Dictionary of Psychological and Psychoanalytic Terms. New York, Longman, Green, 1958

Erikson E: Childhood and Society. New York, WW Norton, 1950

Ewing AC: Ethics. London, English Universities Press, 1953

Fagin C, Diers D: Nursing as a metaphor. N Engl J Med 309:116, 1983

Fenner KM: Ethics and Law in Nursing: Professional Prospectives. New York, Van Nostrand Reinhold, 1980

Fleury M: The Healing Bond. Englewood Cliffs, Prentice-Hall, 1984

Ford JA, Trygstad-Durland LN, Nelms BC: Applied Decision Making for Nurses. St Louis, CV Mosby, 1979

Foulke GE, Albertson T, Fisher CJ: Critical care medicine: An annotated bibliography of recent literature. American Journal of Emergency Medicine 3:266–274, 1985

Fowler MD: Doctoring or nursing under the influence. Heart Lung 15:205–207, 1986

Fowler MD: Ethics without virtue. Heart Lung 15:528–530, 1986

Fowler MD: The institutional ethics committee: Response to a primal scream. Heart Lung 15:101–102, 1986

Fowler MD: The role of the clinical ethicist. Heart Lung 15:318–319, 1986

Frankena W: Ethics, 2nd ed. Englewood Cliffs, Prentice-Hall, 1973

French J, Kahn R: A programmatic approach to studying the industrial environment and mental health. Journal of Social Issues 18:1–47, 1962

Fromer MJ: Professional accountability. In Fromer MJ: Ethical Issues in Health Care. St Louis, CV Mosby, 1981

Fry ST: Accountability in research: The relationship of scientific and humanistic values. Advances in Nursing Science 4:1–13, 1981

Fry ST: Ethics in community health nursing practice. In Lancaster J, Stanhope M (eds): Community Health Nursing: Process and Practice, pp 77–96. St Louis, CV Mosby, 1984

Gadow S: Existential advocacy: Philosophical foundation of nursing. In Spicker SF, Gadow S (eds): Nursing: Images and Ideals, pp 79–101. New York, Springer-Verlag, 1980

Geekie DA: Professional accountability and evaluation. Can Med Assoc J 20:346, 1973

Gewirth A: Reason and Morality. Chicago, University of Chicago Press, 1978

Gilligan C: In a Different Voice. Cambridge, Harvard University Press, 1982

Goldsborough J: Involvement. Am J Nurs 69:66, 1969

Goldstein DM: Bioethics: A Guide for Information Sources. Detroit, Gale, 1982

Greenfield HT: Accountability in Health Facilities. New York, Praeger, 1975

Guidelines for the determination of death. Report of the Medical Consultants on the Diagnosis of Death to the President's Commission for the Study of Ethical Problems in Medicine and Biomedical and Behavioral Research. JAMA 246:2184–2186, 1984

Halligan M, Hamel RP: Ethics committee develops supportive care guidelines. Health Prog 66:26–30, 60, 1985

Hastings Center: The Hastings Center's Bibliography of Ethics, Biomedicine, and Professional Responsibility. Frederick, MD, University Publications of America, 1984

Hennessy T (ed): Values and Moral Development. New York, Paulist Press, 1976

Hilberman M: The evolution of intensive care units. Crit Care Med 3:159, 1975

Hill TE: Servility and self-respect. The Monist 57:87–104, 1973

Hilliard AL: The Forms of Value: The Extension of a Hedonistic Axiology. New York, Columbia University Press, 1950

Hume D: An Enquiry Concerning the Principles of Morals. In Selby-Bigge LA: Enquiries, 2nd ed, pp 322–323 (268). Oxford, Oxford University Press, 1902

Illinois Stat, Ann, Ch, 111 1/2, Sections 5302–5313, West Supp, 1985

In re Quinlan, 355 A 2d 647, 1976; Matter of Welfare of Coyler, 669 p. 2d 738, Wash, 1983

International Council of Nurses: Code for Nurses (1973). In Jameton A: Nursing Practice: The Ethical Issues, p 300. Englewood Cliffs, Prentice-Hall, 1984

Jameton A: Nursing Practice: The Ethical Issues. Englewood Cliffs, Prentice-Hall, 1984

Joint Commission for the Accreditation of Hospitals: Rights and Responsibilities of Patients. AMA/86: Accreditation Manual for Hospitals. Chicago, JCAH, 1985

Jones H: Treating oneself wrongly. Journal of Value Inquiry 17:169–177, 1983

Jones WT: The Classical Mind: A History of Western Philosophy, 2nd ed. New York, Harcourt Brace Jovanovich, 1969

Jonsen AR, Cassel C, Lo B, Perkins HS: The ethics of medicine: An annotated bibliography of recent literature. Ann Intern Med 92:136–141, 1980

Jonsen AR, Siegler M, Winslade WJ: Clinical Ethics: A Practical Approach to Ethical Decisions in Clinical Medicine, 2nd ed. New York, Macmillan, 1986

Kant I: Lectures on Ethics. Infield L (trans): New York, Harper & Row, 1963

Kant I: The Doctrine of Virtue: Part II of the Metaphysics of Morals (1785). Gregor MJ (trans): Philadelphia, University of Pennsylvania Press, 1964

Kant I: Groundwork of the Metaphysics of Morals (1785). Paton HJ (trans): New York, Harper & Row, 1964

Kastenbaum RJ: Death, Society, and Human Experience, 3rd ed. St Louis, CV Mosby, 1986

Kluckhohn C: Values and value-orientations in the theory of action: An exploration in definition and classification. In Parsons T, Shils E (eds): Toward a General Theory of Action. New York, Harper & Row, 1951

Kluckhohn C, Strodtbeck F: Variations in Value Orientation. Evanston IL, Row, Peterson, 1961

Knaus WA, Draper EA, Wagner DP: The use of intensive care: New research initiatives and their implications for national health policy. Milbank Mem Fund Q 61:561, 1983

Knaus WA, Wagner DP, Draper EA, Lawrence DE, Zimmerman JE: The range of intensive care services today. JAMA 246:2711, 1981

Kohlberg L: The development of children's orientations toward a moral order, vol 1. Sequences in the development of moral thought. Vita Humana 6:11–33, 1963

Kohlberg L: Essays on Moral Development, vol 1. The Philosophy of Moral Development. San Francisco, Harper & Row, 1981

Kohlberg L: Essays on Moral Development, vol 2. The Psychology of Moral Development: Moral States and the Life Cycle. San Francisco, Harper & Row, 1981

Kohlberg L: Essays on Moral Development, vol 3. Education and Moral Development: Moral Stages and the Life Cycle. San Francisco, Harper & Row, 1981

Kohnke ME: The nurse as advocate. Am J Nurs 80:2038–2040, 1980

Kramer M, Schmalenberg C: Path to Biculturalism. Wakefield, MA, Contemporary Publishing, 1977

Lassen HCA: Preliminary report in the 1952 epidemic of poliomyelitis in Copenhagen. Lancet 1:37, 1953

Lave JR, Knaus WA: The Economics of intensive care units. In Bensch K, Abramson NS, Grenvik A, Meisel A (eds): Medicolegal Aspects of Critical Care. Rockville, MD, Aspen Systems, 1986

Lebacqz K: The virtuous patient. In Shelp E (ed): Virtue and Medicine, pp 275–288. Dordrecht, D Reidel, 1985

Leininger M: Transcultural Nursing: Concepts, Theories and Practices. New York, John Wiley & Sons, 1978

Leininger M: Caring: The essence and central focus of nursing. The Phenomenon of Caring: Part V. American Nurses' Foundation, Nursing Research Report, vol 12 (1), pp 2–14

Levine M: Nursing ethics and the ethical nurse. Am J Nurs 8:845–849, 1978

Lewis CS: A library for internists: Recommended by the American College of Physicians. Ann Intern Med 102:423–437, 1985

Llewellyn KN: The Bramblebush. New York, Oceana Publications, 1930

Locke J: Essays on the law of nature. In Raphael D: British Moralists 1650–1800, vol 1. Oxford, Oxford University Press, 1969

Lovejoy A: Terminal and adjectival values. Journal of Philosophy 47:593–608, 1950

Lyons AS, Petrucelli RT: Medicine—An Illustrated History. New York, Abrams, 1978

MacIntyre A: After Virtue: A Study in Moral Theory. Notre Dame, University of Notre Dame Press, 1981

Mappes TA, Zembaty JS: Biomedical Ethics, 2nd ed. New York, McGraw-Hill, 1986

Maslow A: Motivation and Personality. New York, Harper & Row, 1954

Maslow A: New Knowledge in Human Values. New York, Harper & Row, 1959

Maslow A: Psychological data and human values. In Maslow AH (ed): Towards a Psychology of Being. New York, Van Nostrand, 1968

Maslow A: The Farther Reaches of Human Nature. New York, Penguin Books, 1976

Massachusetts Nurses' Association: Ethics for Patient Protection: Guidelines for Nurses. Boston, MNA, 1986

Mayerhoff V: On Caring. New York, Harper & Row, 1972

Mill JS: On Liberty (1859). New York, Liberal Arts Press, 1956

Mill JS: Utilitarianism (1861). Priest O (ed): Indianapolis, Bobbs-Merrill, 1957

Morris C: Varieties of Human Value. Chicago, University of Chicago Press, 1956

Moscovice L, Nestegard M: The influence of values and background on the locus of decision of nurse practitioners. J Community Health 5:244–253, 1980

Muff J (ed): Socialization, Sexism, and Stereotyping. St Louis, CV Mosby, 1982

Murchison I, Nichols TS, Hanson R: Legal Accountability in the Nursing Process. St Louis, CV Mosby, 1978

Murphy CP: The moral situation in nursing. In Bandman EL, Bandman B (eds): Bioethics and Human Rights: A Reader for Health Professionals, pp 313–320. Boston, Little, Brown & Co, 1978

Murphy CP: Models of the nurse-patient relationship. In Murphy CP, Hunter H (eds): Ethical Problems in the Nurse-Patient Relationship, pp 9–24. Boston, Allyn & Bacon, 1983

Muyskens JL: Moral Problems in Nursing: A Philosophical Investigation. Totowa, NJ, Rowman & Littlefield, 1982

Namerow MJ: Integrating advocacy into the gerontological nursing major. Journal of Gerontological Nursing 8:149–151, 1982

National Institutes of Health Consensus Development Conference. JAMA 250:798, 1983

Natural Death Act: Section 7185-7195 of Chapter 3.9 California Health and Safety Code

Nesbitt J: Megatrends: Ten New Directions Transforming Our Lives. New York, Warner Books, 1982

Nightingale F: Notes on Nursing: What It Is and What It Is Not (1860). Philadelphia, JB Lippincott, 1946

Parsons T: Illness and the role of the physician: A sociological perspective. Am J Orthopsychiatry 21:454–460, 1951

Parsons T, Shils E: Toward a General Theory of Action. Cambridge, Harvard University Press, 1951

Pellegrino ED: Educating the humanist physician. JAMA 227:1293, 1974

Pence T: Ethics in Nursing—an Annotated Bibliography, 2nd ed (NLN 20-9189). New York, National League for Nursing, 1986

Piaget J: The Moral Judgment of the Child (1932). New York, Free Press, 1965

Pierce v Ortho Pharmaceutical Corporation, 84 NJ 58, 417 A 2d 505 (NJ 1980)

Plato: Euthyphro, Apology, Crito, and Symposium, Hadas M (trans). South Bend, IN, Gateway Editions, Ltd, 1953

President's Commission for the Study of Ethical Problems in Medicine and Biomedical and Behavioral Research: Summing Up. Washington, DC, Government Printing Office, March 1983

President's Commission for the Study of Ethical Problems in Medicine and Biomedical Behavioral Research. JAMA 246:2184–2186, 1984

President's Commission: Deciding to Forego Life-Sustaining Treatment. Washington, DC, Government Printing Office, 1983

Price R: A review of the principal questions in morals (1758, cited from 1787 ed). In Raphael DD (ed): British Moralists 1650–1800, vol 2. Oxford, Oxford University Press, 1969

Purtillo R, Cassell CK: Ethical Dimensions in the Health Professions. Philadelphia, WB Saunders, 1981

Rachels J: Active and passive euthanasia. New Engl J Med 292:1, 1975

Ramsey P: Patient As Person: Explorations in Medical Ethics. New Haven, Yale University Press, 1970

Ramsey P, McCormick R (eds): Doing Evil to Achieve Good: Moral Choice in Conflict Situations. Chicago, Loyola University Press, 1978

Raths L, Harmin M, Simon S: Values and Teaching, 2nd ed. Columbus, Charles E Merrill, 1978

Rest J: The research base of the cognitive developmental approach to moral education. In Hennessy T (ed): Values and Moral Development. New York, Paulist Press, 1976

Richards G: Critical care under PPS. Hospitals 59:66, 1985

Robb IH: Nursing Ethics: For Hospital and Private Use. Cleveland, C Koeckert, 1900

Rokeach M: Beliefs, Attitudes, and Values. San Francisco, Jossey-Bass, 1968

Rokeach M: The Nature of Human Values. New York, Free Press, 1973

Rosenberg MJ: An analysis of affective-cognitive consistency. In Rosenberg MJ, Hovland C, McGuire W, Abelson R, Brehm J (eds): Attitude, Organization and Change. New Haven, Yale University Press, 1960

Rosoff AJ: Informed Consent: A Guide for Health Care Providers. Rockville, MD, Aspen Systems, 1981

Safer P, Grenvik A: Organization and physician education in critical care medicine. Anesthesiology 47:82, 1977

Schlotfeldt RM: Accountability: A critical dimension in health care. Health Care Dimensions 3:137–148, 1976

Scott WA: Values and Organizations. Chicago, Rand-McNally, 1965

Shannon TA: Twelve Problems in Health Care Ethics. Lewiston, NY, E Mellen Press, 1984

Sherman EL, Skinner ER: Medical intensive care: Indications, interventions, and outcomes. N Engl Med J 302:938, 1980

Shields EA (ed): Highlights in the History of the Army Nurse Corps. Washington, DC, US Army Center of Military History, 1981

Shmavonian N: Human Values in Medicine and Health Care. Valley Forge, PA, Audiovisual Resources, United Ministries in Education, 1983

Silver M: Values Education. Washington, DC, National Education Association, 1976

Simon S, Howe L, Kirschenbaum H: Values Clarification: A Handbook of Practical Strategies for Teachers and Students. New York, Hart, 1972

Simpson MA: Dying, Death and Grief: A Critically Annotated Bibliography and Source Book of Thanatology and Terminal Care. New York, Plenum Press, 1979

Singer M: On duties to oneself. Ethics 69:202–205, 1959

Singer MG: Duties and duties to oneself. Ethics 73:133–142, 1963

Smith CS: Outrageous or outraged: A nurse advocate story. Nurs Outlook 28:624–625, 1980

Smith MB: Social Psychology and Human Values. Chicago, Aldine, 1969

Sollito S, Veatch R: Bibliography of Society, Ethics and the Life Sciences. Hastings-on-Hudson, NY, Institute of Society, Ethics and the Life Sciences, 1974 (rev by Fenner D, 1975; by Taylor NK, 1976–77)

Steinbock B (ed): Killing and Letting Die. Englewood Cliffs, Prentice-Hall, 1980

Tate BL: Nurse's Dilemma—Ethical Considerations in Nursing Practice. Geneva, International Council of Nurses, 1977

Taylor NK: Bibliography of Society, Ethics and the Life Sciences. Hastings-on-Hudson, NY, Institute of Society, Ethics and the Life Sciences, 1977

Taylor P: Principles of Ethics: An Introduction. Belmont, CA, Dickinson, 1975

Thibault GE, Mulley AG, Barnett GO, Goldstein RL, Rider VA, Sherman EL, Skinner ER: Medical intensive care: Indications, interventions, and outcomes. N Engl J Med 302:938, 1980

Thompson IE, Melia KM, Boyd KM: Nursing Ethics. New York, Churchill Livingstone, 1983

Thompson JB, Thompson HO: Ethics in Nursing. New York, Macmillan, 1981

Tuma J: Professional conduct (letter). Nurs Outlook 25: 546, 1977

Uustal D: Searching for values. Image 9:15–17, 1977

Uustal D: The use of values clarification in nursing practice. Journal of Continuing Education in Nursing 8:8–13, 1977

Uustal D: Values clarification in nursing: Application to practice. Am J Nurs 78:2058–2063, 1978

Uustal D: Values and Ethics: Considerations in Nursing Practice. Amherst, MA, S V Inc, 1978

Uustal D: Experiences in valuing. AORN Journal 31:188–193, 1980

Uustal D: Exploring values in nursing. AORN Journal 31:183–187, 1980

Uustal D: Values Education in Nursing Curricula throughout the United States. PhD diss, Amherst, University of Massachusetts, 1983

Uustal D: Values education: Opportunities and imperatives. Nurse Educator 9:9–13, 1984

Uustal D: Values and Ethics in Nursing: From Theory to Practice. East Greenwich, RI, Educational Resources, 1985

Veatch RM: A Theory of Medical Ethics. New York, Basic Books, 1981

Veatch RM, Fry ST: Case Studies of Nursing Ethics. Philadelphia, JB Lippincott, 1987

Walters L: Bibliography of Bioethics, vols 1–6; Detroit, Gale, 1975–80; vols 7-9, New York, Free Press, 1981–83; vols 10–11, Washington, DC, Georgetown University, Kennedy Institute of Ethics, 1984–85

Warthen v Toms River Hospital. 488, A 2d 229, 118 BNALRRMK 3179 (NJ Sup Ct 1985)

Weber M: The Protestant Ethic and the Spirit of Capitalism, Parsons T (trans). New York, Charles Scribner's Sons, 1958

Whitworth H: The World of Childrens Hospital. Los Angeles, Childrens Hospital, 1985

Winslade WJ, Ross JW: Choosing Life or Death: A Guide for Patients, Families, and Professionals. New York, Free Press, 1986

Winslow GR: From loyalty to advocacy: A new metaphor for nursing. Hastings Cent Rep :32–40, 1984

Woodruff AD: Personal values and the direction of behavior. School Review 50:32–42, 1942

Wright D: The Psychology of Moral Behavior. Baltimore, Penguin Books, 1971

Index